Noncardiac Surgery in the Cardiac Patient
Assessment and Management

Edited by

Stephen P. Glasser, M.D., F.A.C.P., F.A.C.C.

Fellow of the Council of Clinical Cardiology
of the American Heart Association

Professor of Medicine and Director,
Division of Cardiovascular Medicine
Department of Internal Medicine
University of South Florida College of Medicine

Chief of Cardiology,
James A. Haley Veterans Administration Hospital
Tampa, Florida

FUTURA PUBLISHING COMPANY
Mount Kisco, New York
1983

Dedication

To my children, Laurie Jeanne and Julie Anne.
To their maturity, wisdom, intellect, understanding, and wit

Contributors

Patricia P. Barry, M.D.

Assistant Professor of Medicine; Director, Division of Geriatric Medicine; Clinical Services Coordinator, Suncoast Gerontology Center, University of South Florida College of Medicine; Geriatric Medicine Academic Award, The National Institute on Aging

William M. Blackshear, Jr., M.D.

Assistant Professor of Surgery; Chief, Vascular Surgery, University of South Florida College of Medicine, James A. Haley Veterans Administration Hospital

Keith W. Chandler, M.D.

Assistant Professor of Medicine, Division of Pulmonary Disease, University of South Florida College of Medicine, James A. Haley Veterans Administration Hospital

Pamela I. Clark, R.N.

Assistant Professor of Medicine; Research Coordinator; University of South Florida College of Medicine, James A. Haley Veterans Administration Hospital

H. David Friedberg, M.D., F.R.C.P., F.A.C.C.

Professor of Medicine; Chief of Clinical Electrophysiology, University of South Florida College of Medicine

Stephen P. Glasser, M.D., F.A.C.P., F.A.C.C.

Professor of Medicine; Director, Division of Cardiovascular Medicine, University of South Florida College of Medicine; Chief of Cardiology, James A. Haley Veterans Administration Hospital

Willard S. Harris, M.D., F.A.C.P., F.A.C.C.

Professor of Medicine and Associate Chairman, Department of Medicine, University of South Florida College of Medicine; Chief, Medical Service, James A. Haley Veterans Administration Hospital

Eric E. Harrison, M.D., F.A.C.C., F.A.C.P.

Clinical Assistant Professor of Medicine; University of South Florida College of Medicine; Associate Director, The Cardiology Center, Tampa General Hospital

Randy B. Hartman, M.D.

Assistant Professor of Medicine, University of South Florida College of Medicine; Director, Coronary Care Unit, James A. Haley Veterans Administration Hospital

Leah E. Katz, C.R.N.A.

Adjunct Associate Professor of Anesthesiology; Director, Nurse Anesthesia Program, Department of Anesthesiology, University of California, Los Angeles; School of Medicine, Los Angeles, California iv

Ronald L. Katz, M.D., F.F.A.R.C.S. (Hon.)

Professor and Chairman, Department of Anesthesiology, University of California, Los Angeles; School of Medicine, Los Angeles, California

Thomas J. Linnemeier, M.D.

Fellow in Cardiology, St. Vincent Hospital, Indianapolis, Indiana

Jorge I. Martinez-Lopez, M.D., F.A.C.P., F.C.C.P., F.A.C.C.

Professor of Medicine (Cardiology), Department of Medicine, Louisiana State University Medical Center; Director, Cardiology Department, Charity Hospital of Louisiana, New Orleans, Louisiana

Patricia Miscioscia, R.N.

Peripheral Vascular Laboratory Nurse Technician, James A. Haley Veterans Administration Hospital

R. Joe Noble, M.D., F.A.C.C.

Cardiologist, St. Vincent Hospital, Indianapolis, Indiana; Clinical Professor of Medicine, Indiana University School of Medicine, Indianapolis, Indiana

Fred I. Rabow, M.D., F.A.C.C., F.R.C.P.

Clinical Assistant Professor of Medicine, University of South Florida College of Medicine

Sheldon S. Sbar, M.D.

Clinical Associate Professor of Medicine, University of South Florida College of Medicine; Director, The Cardiology Center, Tampa General Hospital

Peter Schulman, M.D., F.A.C.C.

Assistant Professor of Medicine, University of South Florida College of Medicine; Head, Cardiac Non-Invasive Laboratory, James A. Haley Veterans Administration Hospital

David A. Solomon, M.D., F.C.C.P., F.A.C.P.

Associate Professor of Medicine, Division of Pulmonary Disease, University of South Florida College of Medicine; Chief, Pulmonary Disease Section, James A. Haley Veterans Administration Hospital

Edward F. Steinmetz, M.D., F.A.C.C.

Chief of Cardiology, St. Vincent Hospital, Indianapolis, Indiana; Clinical Professor of Medicine, Indiana University School of Medicine, Indianapolis, Indiana

Drew H. Sterling, D.O., D.A.B.A., F.A.C.A.

Assistant Professor of Surgery, University of South Florida College of Medicine, Section of Anesthesia, James A. Haley Veterans Administration Hospital

James W. Williams, M.D.

Associate Professor of Surgery, Department of Surgery, The University of Tennessee College of Medicine, Memphis, Tennessee

Foreword

Meticulous preoperative evaluation of patients with heart disease is essential if they are to realize the proceeds of modern medicine and surgery. While such evaluation is important in all patients, the cardiac patient often has very special problems. Not the least of these is the increasing length of survival of patients with a wide variety of cardiac diseases. A very complex interface exists between the referring physician, be he/she a family physician, internist or cardiologist, and the surgeon. It is the purpose of this text to foster and maintain effective communication across this interface to assure that it does not become a gap into which the patient's care falls eventuating in an unsatisfactory operative outcome.

One of the principal problems which is necessary for good preoperative evaluation is often not generally clear, particularly when there is evidence of multi-system derangement. It also must be conceded that what is often done or is not done is a simple expression of the experience and background of the involved physician and not necessarily always appropriate to the problem at hand. The authors have effectively presented material, including indicated tests and procedures, which will derive, as accurately as possible, the operative risks which the patient will encounter. They have also clearly stated what the derived data mean, making it possible to avoid the high costs of indiscriminate testing for everything.

Those using the text as a reference will find an initial section devoted to physiologic stress of surgery and anesthesia. In this section particular emphasis is given to the vast array of drugs which are increasingly used in the management of their basic heart disease. The second section outlines in detail the variety of tests available to the physician for assessment. These are very adequately described, including stress testing and evaluation of ventilatory function.

Specific clinical entities that are apt to influence management are dealt with in the third section of this text. Here the problems peculiar to the aged are set forth along with those who are thought to have excess risk due to pulmonary disease, dental disease, or pregnancy. Specific cardiac problems of coronary disease, hypertension, congestive failure, and valvular heart disease, among others, are examined.

The authors have successfully presented a great deal of information which can be used by the referring physician and the surgeon alike in the intelligent management of patients with heart disease who face the necessity of either elective or emergency surgery. The text provides a common ground upon which these problems may be assessed and met, decreasing both morbidity and mortality in this group of patients whose numbers are ever increasing.

Roy H. Behnke, M.D.
Professor and Chairman
Department of Internal Medicine
University of South Florida
College of Medicine

Foreword

Continuing efforts are being made to further lower the morbidity and mortality of major surgical procedures, including those that must be performed in patients with cardiovascular disease of varying severity. The ever-increasing age of the population with the expected cardiopulmonary, renal, and vascular changes makes a thorough preoperative evaluation more important each year. The author of this text has brought together authorities in various fields of cardiorespiratory disease to present the indications for and the methods available for the competent preoperative evaluation of patients at increased operative risk because of concomitant cardiac or circulatory disease.

The surgeon as well as the internist–cardiologist must be aware of the modern-day methods of evaluating these patients preoperatively. The authors' goal is to provide better communication between the internist, cardiologist, and the surgeon, which in turn will undoubtedly improve patient care.

Some patients are all too ready to "get it over with" at the time of their first visit to a surgeon. It would be less difficult for the surgeon and safer for the patient if most cardiovascular and pulmonary evaluations were carried out before the initial surgical consultation. The prescheduling of operations may result in the use of shortcuts in preoperative evaluation. Some tests may indicate the need for more detailed investigation, and this may conflict with demands on the surgeon to adhere to an assigned day for operation. The steady growth of outpatient surgery and "same day admission" surgery mandate that all special medical testing must be preplanned before admission, except in cases of emergency.

It is important for both physicians and surgeons to suspect possible increased cardiovascular risk in some patients, even those with minimal complaints referable to this system. Biliary tract disease often produces symptoms mimicking heart disease, and the two may coexist. On the other hand, perhaps there is a danger of underestimating the significance of minor cardiovascular complaints when patients are to undergo abdominal surgery.

The physician should calculate the added stress of the surgical procedures, including the possible excess loss of blood and the effects of various medications used by the anesthesiologist. Medical responsibility must be sustained throughout the surgical procedure in the high-risk patient as well as in the management of immediate postoperative problems. The current trend toward fragmentation of care may make this difficult, but the interests of the patient must remain paramount. Communication between internist–cardiologist, anesthesiologist, and surgeon should be more commonplace. The expertise of the internist–cardiologist should not be excluded from either the recovery room or the intensive care facility.

This volume provides the internist–cardiologist as well as the surgeon with the current practical methods of evaluating the patient with cardiovascular disease for a noncardiac surgical procedure. The dramatic results in thoracic and cardiovascular surgery should not lull the physician into a false sense of security that everything will go well for other surgical procedures without expert preoperative evaluation and proper therapy.

Many complications will be avoided and lives will be saved if the practical principles presented in this book are carefully followed. It deserves the serious attention of both physician and surgeon, regardless of their fields of interest.

Robert M. Zollinger, M.D.
Professor and Chairman Emeritus
The Department of Surgery
Ohio State University College of Medicine

Preface

Currently, more than twenty-eight million persons in the United States have cardiovascular disease, and almost 700,000 acute coronary occlusions occur each year. The problems of the perioperative management of this group of patients are, therefore, an important part of medical practice and these problems are found to overlap many subspecialty areas. However, this topic has not received the attention it deserves in the literature, at conferences, or in texts, probably because the subject is so broad, because each case has unique features and circumstances which may not fit comfortably into any set of rules, and because this type of assessment is an art acquired primarily through experience.

This book is divided into three parts. The first section deals with the physiologic responses to surgery, the effects of anesthetics primarily as they relate to cardiac function, and a discussion of the cardiac medications patients with heart disease are most likely to be taking. The second section discusses the preoperative laboratory evaluation of the cardiac patient. This is not meant to obviate the importance of the history and physical examination, but represents the need to limit the discussion of so broad a subject. In the third section, specific problems of the cardiac patient are dealt with, and their preoperative, operative, and postoperative management are discussed.

The topics selected are not meant to be all-inclusive but, rather, represent those problems I deem either most frequent (arrhythmias, coronary artery disease, hypertension, congestive heart failure, etc.) or about which internists, in my experience (and I include myself here) know the least (the pregnant cardiac patient, pulmonary disease, and the elderly patient).

I have attempted, in this monograph, to bring together a group of specialists who have had considerable experience with the problems patients with cardiovascular disease experience when they are being considered for or are undergoing noncardiac surgery. Although some specific guidelines are set forth, the contributors have reviewed what is and is not known about the topic and have avoided a "cookbook" approach, since this is too complex a subject with too much controversy to allow for a simplistic approach.

Although I believe it is now timely to bring together the knowledge of this area, it is recognized that with the rapidly advancing information in the field of cardiovascular disease, continual updating will be required and, undoubtedly, new and critical information will already be available by the time this monograph is published. Nonetheless, it is hoped that this work will help to bring together the sometimes fragmented information into a more cohesive approach to the anachronism, "clear for surgery."

I cannot finish without a special acknowledgment to all the contributors, whose timeliness and cooperativeness must be recognized. And, a special acknowledgment to Pamela I. Clark, whose critical review of the entire manuscript was invaluable. It was also through her insistence that a noun and verb were placed in each sentence (hopefully?)—and that syntax was considered, to allow for easy reading. And finally, I would like to thank Betty Pac, who was responsible for typing and retyping and collating and recollating this manuscript.

STEPHEN P. GLASSER

Contents

Introduction

Stephen P. Glasser, M.D.

Almost 700,000 acute coronary occlusions occur each year among the more than twenty-eight million persons in the United States who have cardiovascular disease. Whether the physician is referring a patient for surgery or is called in by the surgeon as a consultant, the patient must be evaluated with great care. In this situation, one cannot base any meaningful assessment on the history or physical examination performed by another physician. Also, the consulting physician should keep in mind the possibility that a problem thought to be surgical might be a manifestation of a more basic medical problem. For example, in the patient with epigastric pain, considered to have gallbladder or peptic ulcer disease, the electrocardiogram may reveal an inferior wall myocardial infarction (Figure 1).

In the 1920s, it was generally believed that for the purposes of anesthesia and operations, a heart that was damaged but was carrying on an adequate circulation under normal conditions of life was the equivalent of a normal heart. This concept was supported even more recently by Ponka,[1] who found that in those subjects who had survived a previous myocardial infarction, had recovered, and were compensated without angina, anesthesia and operation were well tolerated with a postoperative complication rate of 6% and a mortality of 2.8%. Sprague,[2] in 1929, also made several observations that still apply. He noted that effort tolerance was a better guide to surgical risk than was the physical examination, that no type of heart disease, per se, excluded surgery entirely, that congestive heart failure increased surgical risk, while preoperative medical therapy reduced that increased risk, that the vital signs were the best guide to the patient's well-being during surgery, that age was an important prognostic factor in postoperative morbidity and mortality, and that when all was said and done, the skill of the anesthesiologist and surgeon overrode all the other factors.

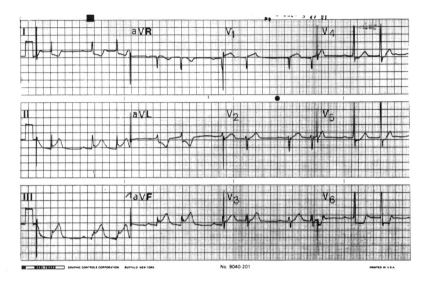

Figure 1. An electrocardiogram was obtained when a 62-year-old woman was admitted to the hospital with epigastric and right upper quadrant pain. Acute cholecystitis was suspected, but the ECG demonstrates an acute inferior myocardial infarction (the S-T segment elevation in V_1-V_3 was the result of right ventricular involvement).

Preoperative Evaluation

The preoperative evaluation, regardless of the etiology of the heart disease, should include a carefully obtained history and physical examination, chest x-ray, electrocardiogram, and selected noninvasive studies. A past history of anesthesia experience, drug reactions, and any familial problems related to these two factors should be included in the history. Preoperative evaluation should also include an assessment of drugs the patient might be taking with a consideration as to how they might interact with anesthetic agents. (It should be noted that almost all anesthetic agents decrease the force of myocardial contractility and/or increase the frequency of arrhythmias.[3]) The patient's effort tolerance should, at minimum, be directly observed by walking with the patient down the hall or up a flight of stairs.

Preoperative Risk Classification

A number of classifications have been utilized in an attempt to categorize patients as to their potential surgical risk. The American Society of Anesthesiology (ASA) physical status scale[4] consists of five classes, as listed in Table 1. Although descriptive, this classification has not proved to be very useful in predicting operative outcome, since it seems to demonstrate only that sicker patients are more likely to die. A similar classification that has also fallen short of providing reliable prognostic information in this setting is the Dripps–American Surgical Association classification[5] (Table 2). Several studies have attempted to use the New York Association classification for predicting operative outcome, as well. Prior to 1973, the New York Heart Association[6] recognized four classes (Table 3). However, it was realized that there were many limita-

Table 1

ASA Physical Status Scale

Class 1—Normal healthy individual
Class 2—Mild systemic disease
Class 3—Severe, but not incapacitating systemic disease
Class 4—Incapacitating illness that is a threat to life
Class 5—Moribund patient

Table 2

Dripps Classification

Class 1—Healthy patient having a limited operation
Class 2—Patients with a mild to moderate systemic disturbance
Class 3—Patients with a severe systemic disturbance
Class 4—A patient with a life threatening disturbance

Table 3

Pre 1973 New York Heart Association Classification

Class 1—No symptoms despite vigorous activity
Class 2—Symptoms with moderate activity
Class 3—Symptoms with minimal activity
Class 4—Symptoms at rest

tions of this classification, in general, and as it applied to the patient about to undergo surgery, specifically. Thus, a new classification was proposed by the New York Heart Association[7] in 1973 (Table 4). It is fair to say that, although simplistic, this newer classification has not as yet gained widespread popularity.

Continuing efforts to arrive at some prognostic classification have continued. Most recently, a risk index was developed at the Massachusetts General Hospital and a point score established, relating the incidence of complications to the operative mortality.[8] Their data are summarized in Table 5. Limitations of this study include the fact that it takes 25 points to predict a significantly high operative mortality, but to obtain this many points one would

Table 4
Post 1973 New York Heart Association Classification

Cardiac Status	Prognosis
1) Uncompromised	1) Good
2) Slightly compromised	2) Good with therapy
3) Moderately compromised	3) Fair with therapy
4) Severely compromised	4) Guarded despite therapy

Table 5
Correlation of Point Score and Operative Complications

Points	N	Life Threatening Complications	Mortality
0–5	537	4 (0.7%)	1 (0.2%)
6–12	316	16 (5%)	5 (2%)
13–25	130	15 (11%)	3 (2%)
25	18	4 (22%)	10 (56%)

Points are obtained in the following manner:

S_3 gallop or jugular venous distension	11 points
Myocardial infarction (within 6 months)	10 points
Rhythm other than sinus or PACs	7 points
>5 PVCs/minute	7 points
Age > 70 years	5 points
Emergency operation	4 points

Three points were allotted for deranged blood gases and electrolytes ($PO_2 < 60$, $PCO_2 > 50$, $K^+ < 3.0$, $BUN > 50$, etc.) and for intraperitoneal, intrathoracic and aortic operations.

almost certainly have to deal with an elderly patient who has had a recent myocardial infarction and is in flagrant heart failure, a situation which any physician intuitively would know carried a high surgical risk. Nonetheless, in this study the Dripps–ASA criteria could not match the multifactorial indexes' ability to isolate eighteen especially high risk patients (although there was a general correlation between the two classifications). Also, the risk index was used to identify potentially controllable (S_3, jugular venous distention, etc.) factors as well as serve as a guideline for indicating which patients might require additional medical consultation prior to surgery. Of interest, a number of factors that did *not* predict operative outcome included serum lipids, cigarette smoking, peripheral vascular disease, stable angina pectoris, hypertension (diastolic blood pressure < 120 mmHg), bundle branch block, and nonspecific ST-T wave changes on electrocardiogram.[9] It is, thus, obvious that there remains no ideal preoperative classification that readily and reliably predicts operative outcome. This should not be surprising, considering the complexity of the situation.

Preoperative Electrocardiogram (ECG)

It seems appropriate to obtain an ECG in patients with heart disease prior to surgery. But, it is the requirement in most hospitals that a preoperative ECG should be performed before surgery in *all* persons over the age of 35–40. Yet, the paucity of studies available supporting the value of mandatory preoperative ECGs is surprising. Howland et al.[10] suggested that a preoperative ECG was indicated for every patient scheduled for surgery, but this recommendation was formed on the basis of routine *post*operative electrocardiographic ECG evaluation. In 1978, Ferrer[11] assessed the prevalence of abnormal ECGs obtained routinely *pre*operatively (Table 6). As expected, the percent of abnormal ECGs was greater in older patients. Overall, 19% (198 subjects) of the total study population were found to have ECG abnormalities. Table 7 lists the type of abnormalities she found. As noted from this table, almost half were changes in the ST segment and T waves (48%), of which 27% were changes in the T wave only. Left anterior fascicular block, PR prolongation, right and left bundle branch

Table 6
Percent of Abnormal ECGs Obtained Routinely Preoperatively in 1,068 Patients*

Age	Male	Female
29	0	0
30–40	17	7
41–50	10	11
51–60	17	18
61–70	32	19
71–30	48	48

*adapted from Ferrer[11]

Table 7
Types of Abnormalities Found on Routine Preoperative ECGs in 198 Subjects*

ST-T wave changes	48
Arrhythmias (atrial and ventricular)	14
Left anterior fascicular block	8
Prolonged PR interval	6
Myocardial infarction	6
Right bundle branch block	4
Left bundle branch block	3
Left ventricular hypertrophy	3

*adapted from Ferrer[11]

block, old myocardial infarction, left ventricular hypertrophy, and left atrial abnormality were present in 3–8%. The second most common ECG abnormality was arrhythmias (14%), of which 6% were ventricular premature beats. Atrial fibrillation (3%), atrial flutter (1.4%), and other less significant atrial arrhythmias made up the difference. Although in Ferrer's concluding remarks she suggested that an ECG be made an obligatory laboratory test for all preoperative patients, regardless of age, she also noted that the meaning of an abnormal ECG taken preoperatively cannot be determined solely from the interpretation of the tracing. With these general comments in mind, the ensuing chapters will discuss specific areas of the perioperative assessment and management of patients with cardiac disease.

References

1. Ponka JA: Arteriosclerotic heart disease and surgical risk. *Am Heart J* 93:1, 1977.
2. Sprague HB: The heart in surgery. *Surg Gynecol Obstet* 49:54, 1929.
3. Price HL: *Circulation During Anesthesia and Operation.* Springfield, Charles C. Thomas Publisher, p. 27, 1967.
4. Owens WS, Felts JA, Spitnagel EL: ASA physical status classification: A study of consistency of ratings. *Anesthesiology* 49:239, 1978.
5. Dripps RD, Lamod A, Eckenhoff JE: The role of anesthesia in surgical mortality. *JAMA* 1978:261, 1961.
6. Criteria Committee of the New York Heart Association: *Disease of the Heart and Blood Vessels: Nomenclature and Criteria for Diagnosis.* Sixth Edition. Little Brown Company, p. 112, 1953.
7. Ibid: Seventh Edition. Little Brown Company, p. 286, 1973.
8. Goldman L, Caldera DL, Nussbaum SR, et al.: Multifactorial index of cardiac risk in non cardiac surgical procedures. *N Engl J Med* 297:845, 1977.
9. Goldman L, Caldera DL, Southwick FS, et al.: Cardiac risk factors and complications of non cardiac surgery. *Medicine* 57:357, 1978.
10. Howland WS, Schweizer O, and LaDue JS: Evaluation of routine postoperative electrocardiography. *NY State J Med* 62:1941, 1962.
11. Ferrer IM: The value of obligatory preoperative electrocardiograms. *JAMWA* 33:459, 1978.

Overview

In this Section, a general overview of the subject is presented with comments relating to the attempts to render a preoperative risk classification and the value and indications of routine preoperative electrocardiography. The first chapter discusses the physiologic responses to surgery in general, and Chapter II includes an overview of the types of anesthetics available today and their effects on myocardial function and cardiac conduction. Finally, a discussion of the drugs many cardiac patients will be taking at the time of their noncardiac surgery with specific reference as to their continuation or discontinuation in the perioperative period is presented.

Chapter i

Physiologic Response to Surgery

James W. Williams, M.D.

There are a number of physiologic adaptations that occur in subjects suffering trauma. Patients with cardiac disease may have limited ability to respond to stress. Surgery represents one such stress.

The physiologic changes in healthy man following trauma have been studied and well documented. These changes are designed to: maintain maximal intravascular volume in the stressed or injured subject by augmenting water and sodium economy; augment perfusion of skeletal and cardiac muscle by raising cardiac output and increasing resistance in other arterial beds (sympathetic activity); and maximally utilize stored sources of energy and protein. The first two of these will be discussed in this chapter. Energy and protein utilization are important but, as far as is known, are not of major importance in determining risk of surgery in patients with cardiac disease. These physiologic responses will be discussed as they are affected by the pituitary-hypothalamic axis, by the cardiac compensatory mechanisms, and by the acid-base and electrolyte changes seen in the perioperative period (Table 1).

Physiologic responses to stress and bodily injury, which affect every surgical patient, evolved millions of years ago. These phenomena were presumably selected and preserved because they gave the injured animal a better chance of surviving that injury, its associated hemorrhage and tissue destruction, and limited starvation. These adaptive responses were not designed to preserve the animal with a failing or diseased heart since, in many instances, the physiologic response itself may place considerable stress on the cardiovascular system. These responses also did not evolve in the

1

Table 1
Physiologic Responses to Surgery and Their Potential Adverse Effects

Physiologic Responses	Potential Adverse Effect
Pituitary-Hypothalamic	Na^+ and H_2O retention $\rightarrow$ Pulmonary
↑ ACTH	and venous congestion
↑ Cortisol	
↑ ADH	
↑ Epi and Norepinephrine	↑ MVO_2 $\rightarrow$ Ischemia and arrhythmia
Cardiac	
Peripheral Vascular	↑ MVO_2 ⎫
Resistance	⎬ Ischemia and arrhythmia
2–3 DPG	↓ Tissue O_2 ⎭
Acid-base and Electrolyte	
Alkalosis	Cerebral vasoconstriction
Hypokalemia	Arrhythmia

↑ = increase
↓ = decrease
MVO_2 = maximal oxygen consumption

environment of sophisticated general anesthesia, nasogastric suction, venous cannulation, Ringer's lactate infusion, blood replacement, and hyperalimentation. Therefore, once man attempts to restore homeostasis via external sources, the naturally evolved response may be no longer appropriate and may, in fact, be harmful. Surgical advances which may be lifesaving for the young, healthy patient may be received by the patient with heart disease in a drastically different manner. One example of this phenomenon is the usually beneficial brisk catecholamine and steroid release following injury, which may be harmful to the patient with marginal cardiac reserve.

Pituitary and Hypothalamic Responses

Stress results in an increase in antidiuretic hormone (ADH) and ACTH, epinephrine, and norepinephrine secretion. The pituitary gland, as directed by strategically located volume receptors and by the central nervous system, releases ADH in response to decreased blood volume, tissue injury, and trauma itself. Because of increased blood levels of ADH, the postoperative patient has decreased water clearance which may last for days. The result is increased water retention through decreased urine output.

ACTH secretion by the pituitary gland is regularly increased by the stress of surgery. The adrenal glands respond with increased cortisol production and, to a lesser extent, aldosterone production. The normal kidneys will not excrete appropriate sodium or water, in the presence of high levels of ADH and cortisol, despite a significant intravascular volume excess. If the surgery is free of complications, levels of these hormones quickly return to normal. Of particular significance to the cardiac patient, however, are the water and sodium retaining properties of these steroids.

Secretion of epinephrine and norepinephrine from the adrenal medulla is under the control of the sympathetic nervous system. Increased levels of circulating epinephrine may be secondary to apprehension as well as the stress of surgery, fever, sepsis, and hypoglycemia. The hypothalamus initiates these changes in response to decreased blood volume, decreased blood pressure, or afferent nerve impulses from higher levels in the central nervous system. Increased circulating levels of catecholamines increase the heart rate, increase peripheral resistance, and increase the strength of contraction of the heart, all of which may favorably influence recovery from trauma, but which also increases the work of the heart and its oxygen requirements. In addition, these catecholamines lower the excitability threshold and are, thereby, arrhythmogenic.

Cardiac Responses to Surgery

Elevated cardiac output and increased peripheral resistance to cardiac ejection are seen in association with catecholamine release, fever, local inflammatory processes, sepsis, shivering, increased work of breathing, etc. The catabolic state of the injured patient is also associated with heightened cardiac output.

The rise in cardiac output may also result from changes in hemoglobin affinity for oxygen (the left-shifted oxyhemoglobin phenomenon), which decreases oxygen delivery to the tissues. Alkalosis and decreased levels of red blood cell 2–3 diphosphoglycerate (2–3 DPG) are causes of this situation. Although there are conflicting opinions regarding the magnitude of harm imposed by the shifted oxyhemoglobin curve, under experimental conditions, particularly in association with alkalosis or anemia, significant changes in cardiac output have been observed. Prudence would, therefore, dictate that one minimize the clinical situations which are known to impair oxyhemoglobin dissociation. Once again, these changes may be beneficial, but the patient with heart disease (who may not be able to sustain a rise in cardiac output in the face of increased peripheral resistance, a common situation in the postoperative state), may develop several problems, such as: decreased renal perfusion, resulting in fluid retention with congestion of the lungs and/or acute pulmonary edema; cardiac arrhythmias, which may be related to increased demands on marginally perfused myocardium in the presence of an increased circulating level of catecholamines; and progressive peripheral ischemia which may result in inadequate perfusion causing acidosis, and progressively deteriorating cardiac function, finally ending in primary heart failure and cardiogenic shock. An accurate assessment of cardiac reserve is, therefore, of extreme importance in considering a patient for elective surgery.

Electrolyte and Acid-Base Changes

Part of the physiologic response to surgery is a change in the acid-base and electrolyte composition of extracellular fluid; a strong trend toward alkalosis is usually seen. This is related to increased levels of aldosterone, which increases reabsorption of sodium and encourages, in its place, excretion of hydrogen and potassium ions, thereby diminishing the kidneys' ability to excrete an alkaline urine. The oxidation of infused materials, such as citrate from blood and lactate from intravenous fluids, adds to the alkalotic load with which a patient must deal. Removal of gastric juice by nasogastric suction and the tendency toward hyperventilation seen in anxiety and in painful situations, further adds to the alkalosis. This state may be exaggerated in patients receiving corticosteroids, those with severe liver disease, and those on long-term diuretic drugs.

If this early trend toward alkalosis reaches a more serious state with pH levels in excess of 7.5, several consequences may be seen. Among these are a left-shifted oxyhemoglobin dissociation curve which can cause decreased peripheral oxygenation. Additionally, hypokalemic cardiac arrhythmias or digitalis toxicity may develop. Cerebral vasoconstriction results from severe alkalosis and produces central nervous system hypoxia. In the patient with cerebrovascular insufficiency, further hyperventilation, further alkalosis, and coma may ensue. Since metabolic alkalosis can be difficult to correct, prevention is of obvious importance. Prevention includes adequate replacement of potassium and chloride to permit adequate exchange for hydrogen ion in the kidney, and provision for adequate fluid volume.

Regulation of potassium levels in the extracellular fluid is also affected by many of the physiologic and metabolic changes seen following trauma or surgery. The increased aldosterone effect causes loss of potassium in the urine. Alkalosis tends to cause an exchange of sodium or potassium for hydrogen at the cellular level which further depresses extracellular fluid concentrations of potassium. Nasogastric removal of hydrogen and chloride ions and potassium ion from the stomach may also add to this deficit. Aggravating this is the fact that many patients with cardiac disease are treated with diuretics which cause further renal loss of potassium. The added importance of maintaining normal potassium balance in patients with heart disease is obvious.

The above responses to trauma may be viewed collectively as a challenge to the cardiovascular system. The success with which the cardiovascular system can deal with these challenges is dependent upon the functional reserve of the heart and cardiovascular system, the physician's understanding of the forces at work, and the skill both in minimizing the surgical challenge and optimally managing fluid, electrolyte, and acid-base balance in the postoperative period.

Suggested Reading

Clowes GK, George HA, Del Guercio L: Circulatory response to trauma of surgical operations. *Metabolism* 9:67, 1950.

CHAPTER II

Effects of Anesthetics on Myocardial Function

Fred I. Rabow, M.D.
and Drew H. Sterling, D.O.

General Anesthetics

Every anesthetic agent in current use is capable of causing an alteration of cardiovascular function to some degree. Anesthetic agents may change autonomic tone and circulating catecholamine levels, affecting changes in preload and afterload and, thus, cardiac output. Likewise, the direct actions of anesthetics on myocardial contractility and on the conduction system may have dramatic effects. As the pharmacology and actions of the following agents and techniques are reviewed, it is well to remember that the way in which technique is utilized and the care with which it is employed is often more important than the actual anesthetic chosen.

Halogenated Inhalation Agents

Inhalation agents are generally used for the maintenance of general anesthesia. Prior to the 1960s, diethyl ether, cyclopropane, and nitrous oxide were the most commonly used agents. In the late 1950s, a series of volatile, halogenated anesthetics were synthesized and their use has become widespread. These agents have the advantages of high potency, of being noninflammable, and of having a low incidence of nausea and vomiting.

7

Halothane

In the past twenty years, halothane (Fluothane) has emerged as the most commonly used primary general anesthetic in the United States. It is a clear, colorless liquid that is administered to the patient via a calibrated vaporizer. Due to the rather high potency of halothane, (less than 1% inspired concentration for maintenance of anesthesia), it can be used effectively with a high inspired oxygen tension.

Other than the central nervous system alterations, the most pronounced effects of halothane are on the cardiovascular system. Following induction, a lowering of the blood pressure is the rule, and is progressive, varying directly with the depth of anesthesia. The effects are due to halothane mediated alterations in both determinants of blood pressure, namely, peripheral vascular resistance and cardiac output.

Peripheral vascular resistance tends to decrease progressively with increasing blood levels of halothane.[1,2] Peripheral vasodilatation, primarily at the arteriolar level, is clinically observed with skin and muscle blood flow tending to increase at the expense of the splanchnic circulation. Cardiac output also decreases directly with the blood levels of halothane and is due to both a decrease in stroke volume and heart rate. Alterations in both contractility and preload are responsible for the decrease in stroke volume. Contractility varies inversely with the blood halothane level due to a direct action on the myocardium.[3] Preload tends to decrease because of dilatation of the venous capacitance vessels with a resultant relative hypovolemia. The decreased heart rate is due to slowing of sinoatrial node discharge secondary to a decrease in the slope of phase 4 depolarization.[4]

The previously mentioned fall in peripheral vascular resistance tends to moderate the fall in cardiac output, but the net effect is still a reduction in output that varies directly with the blood halothane level. This fall in cardiac output is in the range of 25% at a steady rate and 2% inspired concentration in healthy patients. It is interesting to note that even with a fall in cardiac output of that magnitude, neither metabolic acidoses nor a fall in mixed venous oxygen tension develops. This is probably due to both an approximate 20% reduction in metabolic rate and an elevation of the arterial oxygen concentration due to an increased inspired oxygen tension. Thus, using the Fick formula:

$$\text{cardiac output} = \frac{\text{metabolic O}_2 \text{ consumption}}{\text{arterio-venous O}_2 \text{ difference}}$$

some authors postulate that the decrease in cardiac output noted is at least partially due to homeostatic mechanisms. Despite the effects on cardiac output, anesthesiologists routinely administer halothane to patients with cardiovascular disease with good results. This may be in part due to the ease of administration of halothane and its rapid titratability of dose to effect, so that rapid changes in concentration can be effected according to the status of the patient.

Dysrhythmias are rather frequently noted in patients undergoing halothane anesthesia. Accelerated junctional rhythm in the range of 80–100 beats per minute is most common. These are usually well tolerated except in the patient with a compromised myocardial reserve who needs the "atrial kick" to maintain adequate ventricular filling. A significant fall in blood pressure may occur in this group, occasionally necessitating pharmacologic intervention. Ventricular dysrhythmias are also frequently noted during halothane anesthesia. They have been attributed to both re-entry and increased automaticity.[5,6] Ventricular arrhythmias are usually associated with elevated blood catecholamine levels from either endogenous sources ("light anesthesia," hypoxia, hypercarbia, acidosis) or exogenous sources (surgically injected for hemostasis). Treatment usually involves correction of the metabolic problem, limiting the amount of epinephrine injected, and the use of intravenous lidocaine, if needed. Rarely, propranolol may be used either therapeutically or prophylactically.

Enflurane

Although less potent than halothane, enflurane (Ethrane) has a qualitatively similar effect on the cardiovascular system. While it shares with halothane the depressant effect on the A-V node and conduction system, it tends to have a slightly positive chronotropic effect on the S-A node.[7] The net effect is maintenance of a relatively stable heart rate with increasing anesthetic depth, as opposed to the slowing seen with halothane. Recent studies have shown enflurane to have less of a sensitizing effect on the myocardium to catecholamines.[8]

Methoxyfluorane

While still occasionally used at low concentrations for analgesia, notably in obstetrics, methoxyfluorane (Penthrane) use has been declining over the past several years due to its proven nephrotoxic effect.[9] Again, the alterations to the cardiovascular system are similar to those of halothane, with a few exceptions. Methoxyfluorane has a biphasic effect on the S-A node with a mild decrease in heart rate at low concentrations which is then followed by an increase in rate.[4] At high blood levels, junctional and ventricular dysrhythmias can be seen, similar to halothane. Methoxyfluorane also sensitizes the heart to catecholamines.

Nonhalogenated Inhalation Agents

Nitrous Oxide

Nitrous oxide is a biologically inert gas that is administered almost universally during general anesthesia. The inspired concentration normally used is 40–60%. Because nitrous oxide is a weak anesthetic, it is almost always administered in conjunction with another inhalation or intravenous agent.

For years it was thought that nitrous oxide did not depress the cardiovascular system, but recent studies have demonstrated that this is not the case. Inhalation of 40% nitrous oxide has been shown to depress myocardial function in patients with coronary artery disease.[10] The changes noted in these patients include decreased blood pressure, decreased myocardial contractility, and elevated left ventricular end-diastolic pressure. The same inspired concentration in patients without coronary artery disease does not change these parameters.[10] The effects of nitrous oxide are even more pronounced when this agent is added to other anesthetics such as narcotics or halothane.[11,12] The mechanism for these changes seems to be a direct effect on the myocardium.[12,13] Even though the above effects are statistically significant, nitrous oxide has only about one-fourth the cardiac depressant effect as an equi-anesthetic concentration of halothane.

Cyclopropane

The use of cyclopropane has been declining in recent years as flammable agents are phased out of practice. The cardiovascular effects of cyclopropane are varied and pronounced. There is a significant release of catecholamines during the administration of cyclopropane which tends to support blood pressure even though the net effect in the isolated heart–lung preparation is that of myocardial depression. Blood pressure is maintained due to the effects of the circulating catecholamines increasing peripheral vascular resistance. Even with the high catecholamine level, heart rate generally does not rise due to reflex bradycardia and parasympathetic stimulation. Ventricular arrhythmias are commonly seen with hypoxia, hypercarbia, acidosis, and with the administration of atropine and catecholamines.

Diethyl Ether

Although also declining in popularity in the United States due to the phasing out of flammable agents, diethyl ether is still the most widely used general anesthetic in the world. In the isolated heart–lung preparation, heart rate and blood pressure are well maintained in spite of the direct depressant effect. It has been determined that the positive chronotropic effect of ether is neither catechol-mediated nor due to a direct beta adrenergic effect but, rather, is a result of a direct action on the sinoatrial node.[14] Peripheral vascular resistance is maintained by a direct vasoconstrictive effect on vascular smooth muscle. The incidence of ventricular arrhythmias is very low with this agent.

Intravenous Barbiturates

Intravenous agents are used in the majority of general anesthetics in this country. Because of a rapid, smooth, pleasant loss of consciousness, barbiturates are the most commonly used agents for induction of anesthesia. The most frequently used barbiturates are methohexitol (Brevital), thiamylol (Suritol) and sodium thiopental (Pentothal). Because the cardiovascular responses of this entire group of drugs are similar, they will be discussed together using sodium thiopental as the prototype.

Following a test dose of thiopental, incremental doses are administered until consciousness is lost. At that point, anesthesia can be maintained with the same drug or another agent may be added. Most of the cardiovascular effects observed are due to a direct depressant effect on the vasomotor center.[15] This causes peripheral arteriolar vasodilatation with increasing limb and skin blood flow at the expense of splanchnic and renal perfusion. When given gradually in small doses, this effect is minimized, but when given as a rapid bolus to a patient who has a compromised cardiovascular system, profound hypotension may result. Vasodilatation of the capacitance vessels leading to decreased venous return also contributes to the fall in blood pressure. The result is a fall in cardiac output of 25% or more, a fall not generally well tolerated in the compromised patient. Other cardiovascular effects include a decrease of baroreflex sensitivity, leading to diminished heart rate response and hypotension.[16]

Intravenous Nonbarbiturate Tranquilizers

Diazepam

The benzodiazepines are another group of intravenous medicants that are finding greater use, both for induction and maintenance of anesthesia. Diazepam (Valium) is a sedative-amnesic drug that, when given in the dose range of 0.1 to 0.2 mg/kg, causes loss of consciousness with a minimum of cardiovascular effects. Blood pressure, heart rate, and cardiac output are all fairly well maintained with the lower clinical doses. Larger doses, however, cause a significant decrease in cardiac output even in the healthy patient.[17,18] Electrophysiologically, there appears to be a mild antidysrhythmic effect due to an elevation of the ventricular diastolic threshold.[19]

Droperidol

The major tranquilizers also have a place in anesthesia. Droperidol (Inapsine) is a butyrophenone derivative that is used as a sedative–hypnotic by itself and in combination with the narcotic fentanyl. The combination is known as Innovar. In either form, this agent is used for preoperative sedation, induction, and maintenance of anesthesia with good hemodynamic stability. Large intravenous doses occasionally lead to profound hypotension secondary to the alpha-blocking properties of droperidol. It also has been shown to have a mild quinidine-like effect in inhibiting ventricular dysrhythmias.[20]

Narcotics

Narcotics are widely used as premedicants as well as primary and adjunctive anesthetic agents. When used as the analgesic component of a "balanced anesthetic," it is usually combined with nitrous oxide and often a hypnotic, such as a barbiturate. Morphine may be given this way in doses from a few milligrams as an analgesic to 3 mg/kg as the sole anesthetic for major surgery.

Morphine

The effects of morphine on the cardiovascular system are dose related. At low doses, cardiovascular effects are minimal and, thus, morphine is very safe for use in the high risk patient. At doses approaching 0.5 to 1.0 mg/kg, one starts to see a slowing of the heart rate due to depression of the S-A node. Venodilatation and some arteriolar vasodilatation can occur, caused by both histamine release and central vasomotor depression. This preload and mild afterload reduction causes a mild decrease in mean arterial pressure, but is accompanied by improved ventricular performance as evidenced by elevations of stroke volume index and cardiac index. When nitrous oxide is added to morphine anesthesia, a further decrease in mean arterial pressure occurs due to a decrease in cardiac index and stroke volume.[21,22]

Meperidine

When given in large intravenous doses, as might occur during maintenance of anesthesia, meperidine (Demerol) may reduce stroke volume, cardiac output, systemic vascular resistance, and mean arterial pressure.[23] Due to a very mild atropine-like effect, heart rate usually remains fairly constant. When nitrous oxide is added to the technique, a further decrease in stroke volume and cardiac output are noted again with little change in heart rate. Blood pressure remains stable due to a rise of peripheral vascular resistance with the addition of nitrous oxide.[23] At equi-analgesic doses, meperidine causes less histamine release than morphine.

Fentanyl

Fentanyl (Sublimaze) may be administered parenterally, either alone or as Innovar, which is a fixed combination with droperidol. Uses of fentanyl range from premedication to primary anesthetic agent. On a milligram to milligram basis, fentanyl is 80 to 100 times more potent than morphine. The rapid onset and short duration of action of fentanyl makes it uniquely suited to anesthesia. Following normal intravenous doses, fentanyl has an onset of action in about one minute, peaks at about four minutes, and has a duration of action of about 45 minutes. These short time intervals allow for easy titration of dose to effect. Like other narcotic analgesics, fentanyl may cause a decrease in blood pressure by a minor histamine release, and perhaps a central vasomotor depression. Heart rate generally decreases with therapeutic levels. The combination of fentanyl with droperidol tends to provide a smooth, stable anesthetic with a minimum of cardiodepressant effects. The addition of nitrous oxide to this combination does not appear to cause myocardial depression, as it does with morphine.

Dissociative Agents

Ketamine

Ketamine (Ketalar) is a unique anesthetic of the so-called dissociative class of agents. Following parenteral administration of clinical doses, the patient appears to be awake with open, moving eyes, spontaneous respiration, and even spontaneous movements and vocalizations. This activity is inappropriate and not in response to surgical stimulae. Ketamine has a cardiovascular stimulant effect. Following intravenous administration, increases in heart rate, blood pressure, cardiac index, and pulmonary artery pressure are recorded. Stroke volume index remains unchanged. Elevation of myocardial oxygen consumption is a consistent finding.[24] The above cardiovascular effects are explained by ketamine's central sympathetic stimulating and parasympathetic inhibiting effects. Serum catecholamine levels are consistently elevated following ketamine administration.

General Anesthetic Adjunctive Agents

Depolarizing Muscle Relaxants

Succinylcholine

The prototype of the depolarizing type of relaxants is succinylcholine. Chemically, it is composed of two acetylcholine molecules. Succinylcholine acts at acetylcholine receptors with a similar but more prolonged action due to its slower breakdown by hydrolysis. Following an intravenous dose of succinylcholine, there is frequently a slowing of the heart rate. This is seen more commonly with children, but may be noted in adults with second and subsequent doses. This effect is probably due to a direct action on myocardial cholinergic receptors, but a secondary vagal effect from stimulation of great vessel pressor receptors may also play a role.[25]

Potassium is released from skeletal muscle fibers during depolarization, and the resultant rise in serum levels may lead to dysrhythmias. The elevation in potassium is normally in the range of 0.2 mEq/liter, but in persons with recent burns, muscle trauma, neuromuscular disease, or immobilization with casts, the rise could be much greater. Transient values as high as 12 to 14 mEq/liter have been recorded.[26]

Nondepolarizing Muscle Relaxants

D-tubocurarine

Competitive or nondepolarizing muscle relaxants are represented by D-tubocurarine. The cardiovascular effect of a large intravenous dose of curare is a lowering of blood pressure. This is primarily due to histamine release, but ganglionic blockade leading to vasodilatation with a decrease in both preload and afterload plays some role.

Dimethyl-tubocurarine

A semisynthetic derivative of D-tubocurarine is dimethyl-tubocurarine (Metubine). On a milligram to milligram basis, it is about three times as potent as the parent drug. At clinical doses, there appears to be fewer cardiovascular effects because of a higher ratio of affinity to motor end-plates versus ganglionic receptors. Histamine release is also relatively less at clinical doses.

Gallamine

A synthetic, nondepolarizing relaxant that has only limited popularity is gallamine (Flaxedil). Following normal clinical doses, a rather marked positive chronotropic and perhaps a positive inotropic effect are noted. These actions are due primarily to vagolytic action, although some evidence of a direct beta effect is present.[27]

Pancuronium

This is another fairly new, synthetic nondepolarizing relaxant that has been enjoying increasing use in all phases of general anesthesia, especially with the high risk patient. At clinical doses, pancuronium (Pavulon) causes neither significant histamine release nor ganglionic blockade. An increase in heart rate is normally seen, but this effect is less marked than with gallamine. The positive chronotropic effect is due to a vagolytic, atropine-like action; an increase in heart rate is not seen in a patient who has been pretreated with atropine.[28] Tachydysrhythmias are occasionally noted following large doses administered through a central venous catheter. Because these adverse actions are minimal, pancuronium is considered by most anesthesiologists as the relaxant of choice for the high risk cardiac patient in whom mild elevations in heart rates would not be detrimental.

Muscle Relaxant Reversal Agents

Anticholinesterases are agents used to reverse the effects of non-depolarizing muscle relaxants. Since the actions of the major anticholinesterases in clinical use (neostigmine, pyridostigmine, and edrophonium) are qualitatively similar, they will be discussed together using neostigmine as the example. These drugs combine reversibly with true cholinesterase, temporarily inactivating this enzyme. This effect allows the concentration of acetylcholine to increase at the myoneural junction. The increased acetylcholine concentration at the endplates displaces the competitive relaxant molecules from their receptor and allows for normal muscle contraction. Because anticholinesterases are not specific for their sites of action, acetylcholine levels are increased in all areas of the body.

The cardiovascular actions of increased acetylcholine levels are complex because of several excitatory and inhibitory phenomena acting at once. The most prominent effect noted is a vagal-like response with bradycardia. This slowing of conduction, particularly through the A-V node, can result in various degrees of A-V block. At the same time, the increased acetylcholine levels cause epinephrine to be released from adrenal medullary cells. It has also been demonstrated that neostigmine, per se, interferes with the re-uptake of norepinephrine after it has been released from adrenergic nerve endings. When the high level of circulating catecholamines is superimposed on varying degrees of conduction disturbance in the presence of an ischemic myocardium, dysrhythmias should not be unexpected. Because of the varying factors at work, these dysrhythmias may range from sinus arrest to ventricular fibrillation. It should be noted that the maintenance of adequate oxygenation and the avoidance of hypercarbia and acidosis, along with the usual concomitant use of a vagolytic agent, prevents most arrhythmias.

Anti-sialogues

Atropine is the prototype of a group of drugs widely used for their vagolytic effect. These drugs have been classified as anticholinergic, but are more accurately antimuscarinic since only the muscarinic effects of acetylcholine are antagonized. In addition to drying secretions as premedicants, antimuscarines are used to abolish vagal reflexes at any time during anesthesia. They are routinely administered with anticholinesterases so that the nicotinic effects of acetylcholine predominate.

The major action of atropine on the cardiovascular system is an increase in heart rate. Dysrhythmias are occasionally noted following the administration of atropine. These include premature junctional beats, junctional rhythms, and premature ventricular contractions. Ventricular tachycardia and ventricular fibrillation have also been reported following intravenous atropine, more commonly with cyclopropane or halothane than with other agents.

The other commonly used antimuscarinic drugs, scopolamine and glycopyrrolate (Robinul), differ mainly in their potency, onset and duration of action, and central nervous system effects.

Regional Anesthesia

Regional anesthesia refers to the installation of local anesthetics either centrally (spinal cord) or peripherally (directly around the peripheral nerves), in order to produce anesthesia in particular areas of the body. The most common forms are spinal anesthesia, epidural anesthesia, and regional nerve blocks.

Local Anesthetic Agents—the Amides

The main drugs in this group are lidocaine hydrochloride (Xylocaine), mepivacaine hydrochloride (Carbocaine), bupivacaine hydrochloride (Marcaine), and etidocaine hydrochloride (Duronest). They are all structurally and functionally similar, differing mainly in their duration of action, potency, and toxicity. Lidocaine has the shortest duration of action of the three, bupivacaine and etidocaine the longest, and mepivacaine intermediate. This group represents the most commonly used local anesthetic agents.

All local anesthetics have direct negative inotropic properties, but at serum levels achieved with regional anesthesia, significant myocardial depression is rarely observed. A lidocaine level of over fifteen μg/cc is necessary for significant myocardial depression, which is high enough to afford a considerable margin of safety. However, in the setting of pre-existing myocardial dysfunction, or advanced liver disease, the hepatic clearance of lidocaine is slower, possibly allowing a higher than expected serum level of local anesthetic to be reached.[29] In general, the local anesthetic agents of the amide group, when used for regional anesthesia, are hemodynamically safe, even in the face of significant cardiac disease.

The amide local anesthetics also have electrophysiologic properties which are important in the treatment of arrhythmias. Lidocaine decreases automaticity by decreasing the slope of phase 4 depolarization in pacemaker fibers. By altering the rate of rise of the action potential, re-entrant ventricular arrhythmias are also suppressed. Atrioventricular conduction is insignificantly affected by lidocaine, as evidenced by very little alteration of His bundle electrographic intervals.[30]

Local Anesthetic Agents—the Esters

Procaine

One of the first local anesthetics developed, procaine (Novacaine) has been generally replaced by the more popular amide agents and is, thus, rarely used.

Tetracaine

This is the most potent local anesthetic available and has the longest duration of action. Tetracaine (Pontocaine, Methocaine) is presently used mainly for spinal anesthesia, although it is also used topically in the eye and mucous membranes. When used for spinal anesthesia, it is employed in very small doses, and cardiovascular effects arise not from the drug itself but from the sympathetic blockade, which will be discussed below.

Cocaine

Cocaine is used solely as a topical anesthetic for the nose and pharynx. It is particularly useful because of its local sympathomimetic property, resulting in vasoconstriction. This action decreases bleeding and shrinks congested membranes. However, in addition to vasoconstriction, tachycardia and hypertension can occur. The sympathomimetic effects are due to the blocking of norepinephrine uptake at the presynaptic level. Although it is used topically, care should still be exercised when used on patients with cardiac disease.

Although toxicity of local anesthetic agents can be manifest as circulatory collapse, it should be emphasized that by far the most common toxic effects are neurologically related. Central nervous system depression and, less commonly, generalized seizures can occur, usually at lidocaine levels greater than 10 μg/ml.

Allergic responses to the amide group of local anesthetics are rare, at most. The notoriety of allergy to procaine and other ester-linked anesthetics has carried over to the more commonly used amide preparations. However, proper evidence of allergy to any of the amides is, indeed, lacking. In fact, many of the "side effects" of local anesthesia such as palpitations, dizziness, sweating, and tremulousness are due to the added epinephrine.

Local Anesthetic Agents—Epinephrine

Discussion of local anesthetic agents is not complete without mention of epinephrine. This drug is frequently added to local anesthetic solutions because of its vasoconstrictive properties, which retard absorption of the local anesthetic. The benefits thus derived are decreased circulating levels of the local anesthetic, prolongation of the anesthesia, and less local bleeding. However, this potent catecholamine has adverse effects of its own. It has both alpha and beta-adrenergic properties, which will increase contractility and heart rate, thus increasing the work of the heart. Also, arrhythmogenicity may be facilitated. Peripherally, the alpha affect of epinephrine can produce significant hypertension, but at low serum levels epinephrine will have a predominant beta effect on the peripheral circulation, thus lowering systemic vascular resistance and possibly inducing hypotension. Although only small amounts are used and even smaller concentrations reach the systemic circulation, epinephrine should be cautiously used in patients with coronary artery disease or congestive heart failure.

Mepivocaine has been described to have some degree of inherent vasoconstrictive properties, thus precluding the necessary addition of epinephrine. However, this effect is presently controversial.

Local Anesthetics—Technique

More important than the direct effects of local anesthesia on cardiovascular function is the indirect effect produced by the particular technique used.

Spinal Anesthesia

This involves the injection of local anesthetic into the subarachnoid space. The technique provides excellent abdominal, pelvic, and perineal anesthesia, including muscle relaxation. The dermatome level of the ensuing block can be adjusted by altering both the position of the patient and the dosage, volume, or specific gravity of the local anesthetic solution used. In addition to the desired block of motor sensory fibers, sympathetic nerve impulses are also interrupted, producing peripheral vasodilatation. This can result in significant hypotension. The level of blood pressure drop is related directly to the following:

—The higher the level of the block, the more extensive the autonomic blockade. In addition, if the block extends above the fourth thoracic level, the effect of cardiac sympathetic denervation may lead to decreased myocardial contractility and heart rate.[31,32]

—The higher the pre-existing systolic blood pressure, the greater the potential fall in blood pressure.

—Hypovolemia will also contribute to a drop in blood pressure.

Because of the frequent hypotension, it is often necessary to administer a pure alpha-adrenergic agonist such as methoxamine, neosynephrine, or a mixed alpha and beta agent such as ephedrine.

Most of the hypotension is produced by a decrease in peripheral vascular resistance. However, cardiac output can also fall, probably due to a decrease in venous return secondary to decreased venomotor tone.[31,32] Decreased endogenous catecholamines (secondary to the block) producing a decrease in heart rate and contractility may also contribute to a fall in cardiac output.

Epidural Anesthesia

This entails delivery of the local anesthetic into the space surrounding the dura mater. The regional anesthesia produced is similar to that of spinal anesthesia; however, there are differences in dose, duration, and sequela. It has become especially popular for obstetrical use because of the ease of continuous anesthesia by means of indwelling catheters.

The hemodynamic effects, particularly hypotension, of epidural anesthesia can occur similarly to that described for spinal anesthesia[33,34] except that for a given level of block, the fall in blood pressure is usually less marked with epidural anesthesia. However, because of the increased vascularity of the epidural space, and the fact that approximately five times more local anesthetic is needed for epidural anesthesia to achieve the same level block as with spinal anesthesia, increased absorption of the local anesthetic may be significant enough to produce systemic cardiovascular effects.

Regional Nerve Blocks

These involve the installation of local anesthetic into the tissue surrounding the peripheral nerve(s) to be blocked. The possible sites are numerous, varying from a brachial plexus block for upper extremity anesthesia to individual nerve blocks (e.g., perineal nerve). Potential hemodynamic problems can arise from absorption of the local anesthetic producing systemic effects.

A particular type of regional nerve block that should be mentioned is intravenous regional anesthesia. This is used frequently for relatively brief surgical procedures on the hand, wrist, or forearm. The technique involves the intravenous injection of a local anesthetic at a distal site in the extremity with a tourniquet inflated proximally to contain the local anesthetic within the extremity. Potential adverse effects can occur when the tourniquet is deflated at the termination of surgery and a bolus of local anesthetic is released into the circulation. However, at the dosages routinely used, the maximum serum levels of local anesthetic is less than that with other regional techniques (e.g., brachial blocks or epidural), provided the procedure has lasted long enough to allow the drug to become fixed to tissues (usually thirty minutes).

General Anesthesia and Cardiac Disease

Ventricular dysfunction

It should be remembered that all anesthetic agents have the ability to decrease contractility. With maintenance of general anesthesia, the halogenated inhalation agents are more cardiodepressant than the intravenous agents (e.g., narcotics). Patients with significant ventricular dysfunction and valvular disease are particularly sensitive to the vasodilatation produced by the anesthetic agents. Since a majority of such problems will occur during induction of anesthesia, induction should be carried out slowly and carefully in the high risk patient. It may be wise to monitor arterial and/or pulmonary artery pressures during induction, administering fluids or vasopressors as necessary.

Coronary Artery Disease

Anesthesia may negatively alter myocardial oxygen balance predominantly by increasing myocardial oxygen consumption, but also by decreasing myocardial oxygen delivery. The increase in myocardial oxygen consumption is usually produced by an increase in heart rate and systolic blood pressure associated with induction and/or light anesthesia. Therefore, induction should be carried out slowly and carefully to keep the blood pressure and heart rate response somewhat moderated. Measures to achieve this would include deeper anesthesia before intubation, more extensive topical anesthesia, or even administering intravenous nitroglycerin or nitroprusside. Decreased myocardial oxygen delivery can occur if the anesthetic causes significant hypotension, thereby compromising coronary blood flow.

Arrhythmias

The development or exacerbation of supraventricular or ventricular arrhythmias may be seen with light anesthesia, with intubation, or with the administration of endogenous catecholamines. Halothane and cyclopropane, in particular, sensitize the myocardium to the effects of catecholamines in producing ventricular arrhythmias.

Significant bradyarrhythmias may occur with vagal reactions during intubation or with intraoperative traction of the peritoneal or extraocular muscles. The anticholinesterases, used in reversing some muscle relaxants, and hypoxia may also lead to slowing of the heart rate. Treatment is directed towards eliminating the primary cause and administering atropine, if necessary.

Regional Versus General Anesthesia in the Cardiac Patient

The question often arises as to the preference of regional versus general anesthesia in a patient with cardiac disease. In the few studies comparing the two, no significant difference in morbidity and mortality has been demonstrated.[35,36] Advantages of regional anesthesia in the cardiac patient include less myocardial and respiratory depression and the avoidance of sympathetic or parasympathetic stimulation associated with intubation. A well executed regional block in the appropriate patient probably causes the minimum of hemodynamic disturbances. Because of the preload and afterload effects, regional anesthesia would probably be most applicable to the congestive heart failure patient, providing significant hypotension is avoided. However, it should be remembered that hypovolemic and fixed cardiac output states are contraindications to spinal and epidural anesthesia because of the potential percipitous fall in blood pressure secondary to peripheral vasodilatation.

A factor to be considered in choosing an anesthetic technique is the psychologic status of the patient. If the patient is very apprehensive about the prospect of surgery and/or regional anesthesia, his endogenous catecholamine release may do more harm than a carefully administered general anesthetic. Certain other physical problems may be present that mitigate a specific technique. For example, spinal and epidurals are contraindicated in patients with either a superficial infection on the lower back or with a bleeding diathesis (risk of an epidural hematoma). Also, the surgical site often determines the type of anesthesia that must be used. Although a few anesthesiologists are skilled enough to anesthetize almost any area of the body by nerve block, most clinicians confine their regional techniques to lower abdominal and extremity work.

It should be emphasized that the care which an anesthetic is administered is often more important than the type of technique chosen. This, together with an appropriate matching of pathophysiology to expected hemodynamic alteration, would seem to give the patient the best chance for a good outcome.

References

1. Black GW, McArdle L: The effects of halothane on the peripheral circulation in man. *British Journal of Anesthesiology* 34:2, 1962.
2. Price HC, Price MC: Relative ganglionic blocking potencies of cyclopropane, halothane, nitrous oxide and the interaction of nitrous oxide with halothane. *Anesthesiology* 28:349, 1967.
3. Price HC: Circulatory actions of general anesthetic agents. *Clin Pharmacol Ther* 2:163, 1961.
4. Reynolds AK, Chez JF, Pasquet AF: Halothane and methoxyflurane. A comparison of their effects on cardiac pacemaker fibers. *Anesthesiology* 33:602, 1970.
5. Zink J, Sasyniuk RI, Dresel PE: Halothane-epinephrine induced cardiac arrhythmias and the role of heart rate. *Anesthesiology* 43:548, 1975.
6. Myerberg RJ, Steward JW, Hoffman BF: Electrophysiological effects of canine A-V conduction system. *Circ Res* 26:361, 1970.
7. Krishna G, Paradise RR: Mechanisms of inotropic effects of volatile inhalation anesthetics. *Anesth Analg* 56:173, 1977.
8. Johnson RR, Eger EI II, Wilson C: A comparative interaction of epinephrine with enflurane, isoflurane, and halothane in man. *Anesth Analg* 55:709, 1976.
9. Mazze RI, Cousins MJ: Renal toxicity of anesthetics with specific reference to the nephrotoxicity of methoxyflurane. *Canadian Anesthesia Society Journal* 20:64, 1973.
10. Eisele JH, Smith NT: Cardiovascular effects of 40% nitrous oxide in man. *Anesth Analg* 51:956, 1972.
11. Smith NT, Eger EI II, Gregory GA, et al.: The cardiovascular and sympathetic responses to the addition of nitrous oxide to halothane in man. *Anesthesiology* 32:410, 1970.
12. Toppos DG, Buckley MJ, Taver MB, et al.: Left ventricular performance and pulmonary circulation following addition of nitrous oxide to morphine during coronary artery surgery. *Anesthesiology* 43:61, 1975.
13. Bennett MD, Loerer EA, et al.: Cardiovascular responses to nitrous oxide during enflurane and oxygen anesthesia. *Anesthesiology* 46:227, 1977.

14. Krishna G, Trueblood MS, Paradise RR: The mechanism of positive chronotropic action of diethyl ether on rat atria. *Anesthesiology* 34:312, 1975.
15. Peiss PN, Manning JW: Effects of sodium pentobarbitol on electrical and reflex activation of the cardiovascular system. *Circ Res* 14:228, 1964.
16. Bristav SD, Prys-Roberts C, Fisher A, et al.: Effects of anesthesia on baroreflex control of heart rate in man. *Anesthesiology* 31:42, 1969.
17. Rao S, Sherbanink RW, Rasod K, et al.: Cardiopulmonary effects of diazepam. *Clin Pharmacol Ther* 14:182, 1973.
18. Cote P, Gueret P, Bourassa M: Systemic and coronary hemodynamic effects of Diazepam in patients with normal and diseased coronary arteries. *Circulation* 50:1210, 1974.
19. Dunbar RW, Boettner RB, Haley JV, et al.: The effects of diazepam on the antiarrhythmic response to lidocaine. *Anesth Analg* 50:685, 1971.
20. Kern R, Einwachter HM, Haas HO, et al.: Cardiac membrane currents as affected by neuroleptic agent: Droperidol. *Pfleugers Archives* 35:262, 1971.
21. Stoelting RK, Gibbs PS: Hemodynamic effects of morphine and morphine-nitrous oxide in valvular heart disease and coronary artery disease. *Anesthesiology* 38:45, 1973.
22. Wang KC, Martin WE, Hornbein TF, et al.: Cardiovascular effects of morphine sulfate with oxygen and nitrous oxide in man. *Anesthesiology* 38:542, 1973.
23. Stanley TH, Bidwai AV, et al.: Cardiovascular effects of nitrous oxide during meperidine infusion in the dog. *Anesth Analg* 56:836, 1977.
24. Tweed WA, Munich M, Wymis D: Circulatory responses to ketamine anesthesia. *Anesthesiology*, 1971.
25. Galindo A, Wyte SR, Witherhold JW: Junctional rhythm induced by halothane anesthesia. *Anesthesiology* 37:261, 1972.
26. Tobey RE: Paraplegia, Succinylcholine, and cardiac arrest. *Anesthesiology* 32:359, 1970.
27. Brown BR, Crout JR: The sympathomimetic effects of gallamine on the heart. *Journal of Pharmacology and Experimental Therapeutics* 172:266, 1970.
28. Miller RD, Eger EI II, Stevens WC, et al.: Pancuronium-induced tachycardia in relation to alveolar halothane, dose of pancuronium, and prior atropine. *Anesthesiology* 42:352, 1975.
29. Collinsworth KA, Kalman SM, Harrison DC: The clinical pharmacology of Lidocaine as an antiarrhythmic drug. *Circulation* 50:1217, 1974.
30. Rosen MR, Hoffman BF, Wit AL: Electrophysiology and pharmacology of cardiac arrhythmias V. cardiac antiarrhythmic effects of lidocaine. *Am Heart J* 88:380, 1974.
31. Shimosato S, Etsten BE: The role of the venous system in cardiocirculatory dynamics during spinal and epidural anesthesia in man. *Anesthesiology* 30:619, 1969.

32. Ward RI, Bonica JJ, Freund FG, et al.: Epidural and subarachnoid anesthesia. Cardiovascular and respiratory effects. *JAMA* 19:275, 1965.
33. Bonica JJ, Berges PU, Morikawa KI: Circulatory effects of peridural block = 1. Effects of level of analgesia and dose of lidocaine. *Anesthesiology* 33:619, 1970.
34. McLean APH, Mulligan GW, Otton P, et al.: Hemodynamic alterations associated with epidural anesthesia. *Surgery* 62:79, 1967.
35. Arkins R, Smessaert AA, Hicks RG: Mortality and morbidity in surgical patients with coronary artery disease. *JAMA* 190:485, 1964.
36. Sapala JA, Ponka JL, Duvernoy WF: Operative and intraoperative risks in the cardiac patient. *J Am Geriatr Soc* 23:529, 1975.

CHAPTER III

Cardiac Medications

Peter Schulman, M.D.

Management of perioperative medications for the cardiac patient presents a number of difficulties. Medications adequate to control the manifestations of heart disease under the usual conditions of daily living may be inadequate under the added burdens imposed by anesthesia and surgery. Additionally, oral outpatient regimens may be unsuitable for perioperative use. Information from published literature reviews, large clinical trials, or controlled studies is sparse. Furthermore, disagreement exists concerning the perioperative use of some agents, like the beta blockers, while consensus has changed dramatically regarding the use of others, like the long-acting nitrates. With these points in mind, available data concerning the perioperative use of five major classes of cardiac medications will be reviewed. Based on available data, clinical logic, and favorable experience, recommendations are presented for prescribing these drugs to the cardiac patient undergoing noncardiac surgery.

Digitalis Preparations

Digitalis preparations are probably the drugs most commonly used by cardiac patients facing noncardiac surgery. The fundamental actions of these agents on the intact heart can be divided into two areas, mechanical and electrophysiological. Mechanically, digitalis increases the strength of myocardial contraction, improving cardiovascular performance in the patient with heart failure. In persons with normal cardiac function, however, peripheral ad-

29

justments prevent an increase in cardiac output. The electrophysiological effects of digitalis are both indirect, mediated through vagal augmentation, and direct. In therapeutic doses, digitalis slows conduction through the atrioventricular node and, thus, controls the ventricular rate in atrial flutter or fibrillation. In patients with sinus rhythm, a slight slowing of the sinus rate usually occurs.

Manifestations of digitalis toxicity fall into two major categories: depressed conduction, leading to bradyarrhythmias, and increased automaticity, giving rise to tachyarrhythmias. A characteristic digitalis-toxic rhythm is supraventricular tachycardia with block, combining elements both of increased automaticity and of depressed conduction (Figure 1). Noncardiac toxic effects include disturbances of gastrointestinal, central nervous, or visual systems. These noncardiac toxic symptoms follow the onset of cardiac rhythm disturbances in more than 50% of digitalis-intoxicated patients, and one cannot rely on their presence or absence to diagnose or exclude toxicity.

Digoxin is the most commonly used digitalis preparation and will be primarily considered in the following discussion. Digitoxin, by virtue of its four- to six-day half-life, is less suitable for perioperative use because adjustments in total glycoside effect are too slowly accomplished with this long-acting agent. We suggest that patients taking digitoxin be switched over to digoxin, first by withholding all glycoside for several days and then, starting digoxin at the usual therapeutic dose. A recent review[1] details the methods used to convert a patient from one digitalis preparation to another.

Digoxin is available in both oral and intravenous form. In normal subjects, its half-life is 36 hours and 85% is excreted unchanged by the kidneys.[2] Several conditions potentiate the effect of digitalis on the heart and thus, predispose to digitalis toxicity (Table 1). Quinidine has recently been shown to alter digitalis effect; by mechanisms incompletely understood, serum digoxin levels will rise when quinidine is introduced to a patient on a stable digoxin dose.[3] A number of other drugs also adversely interact with digitalis preparations (Table 2). Because of digoxin's low therapeutic index and high potential for drug interactions and because several of these agents are commonly used in the perioperative setting, special attention must be given to the patient on digoxin.

The patient should be questioned and examined for signs and symptoms of underdigitalization (e.g., *un*compensated heart fail-

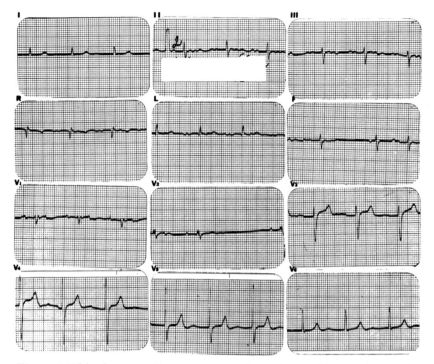

Figure 1. This electrocardiogram was performed on a 68-year-old female with hypertension and mild renal dysfunction. She was taking 0.25 mgm of digoxin P.O. every day, and complained of nausea. An atrial rate of 140 bpm with a ventricular rate of 70 bpm is present, consistent with the diagnosis of atrial tachycardia with 2:1 block. Note in Lead V_2 that a long pause occurs at an almost exact multiple of the inherent atrial rate. This suggests sinus node exit block. Her serum digoxin level was 3.2 ng%. Digoxin was discontinued and when her symptoms and arrhythmia abated, the medication was reinstituted at 0.125 mgm P.O. each day.

ure, arrhythmia) as well as overdosage (arrhythmia, gastrointestinal, central nervous system, visual disturbances) which might need correction. Hypokalemia is common since many patients taking digoxin also take a potassium-depleting diuretic. Routine measurements of magnesium, calcium, and thyroxin levels are not necessary unless the suspicion of an abnormality exists. Likewise, a routine serum digoxin level is generally not required if renal function is normal. However, if renal function is impaired, serum di-

Table 1
Conditions which Potentiate Cardiac Glycoside Effect

Acid-Base Disturbance	Hypomagnesemia
Drugs	Hypothyroidism
Hypercalcemia	Hypoxia
Hypokalemia	Myocardial Disease

Table 2
Drug Interactions with Digitalis*

Drug	Digitalis Effect	Mechanism
Antacids	Decreased	Decreased absorption
Barbiturates	Decreased	Increased degradation
Cholestyramine	Decreased	Intestinal binding
Diuretics (not K+ sparing)	Increased	Hypokalemia
Kaolin Pectin	Decreased	Decreased absorption
Neomycin	Decreased	Unknown
Quinidine	Increased	Altered binding and excretion
Rifampin	Decreased	Increased degradation

*Adapted from Adverse Interactions of Drugs. *The Medical Letter* 23:17–28, 1981.

goxin levels may be high without appropriate dose reduction. Guidelines for the use of digoxin in renal failure are available.[2,4]

In preparation for surgery, the stable cardiac patient should continue his usual oral digoxin dose right up to the day of surgery. In the early postoperative period, if the patient is NPO, the daily digoxin dose can temporarily be given intravenously. However, since bioavailability is 20 to 50% greater by the intravenous route, prolonged I.V. use necessitates appropriate dose reduction. Should renal function deteriorate postoperatively, the dose must also be reduced. In this setting, serum digoxin levels are useful.

Patients in chronic atrial fibrillation who have well-controlled ventricular rates in the basal state may develop acceleration of the ventricular rate during the perioperative period due to increases in sympathetic tone from the stresses of surgery. When this occurs, small additional intravenous doses of digoxin (e.g., .125 to .25 mg) may be given to slow the ventricular response. Alternately, 0.5 to

1.0 mg increments of intravenous propranolol can be used. When using propranolol for tachyarrhythmias, extreme caution must be exercised in the patient with a history of heart failure.

One occasionally encounters patients taking digitalis for unknown or unclear reasons. In such patients, one may be tempted to discontinue the drug entirely. Interestingly, one study has shown that 86% of 56 patients in sinus rhythm on chronic digitalis therapy, instituted mainly for "reasonable" indications, suffered no clinical hemodynamic or dysrhythmic deterioration when digitalis was withdrawn under careful surveillance.[5] However, these results are preliminary, and one cannot recommend discontinuation of digitalis in any chronically digitalized patient prior to elective surgery unless this drug is clearly contraindicated.

Data pertaining to digitalis pharmacology has special relevance to certain subsets of surgical patients. Since digitalis can elevate splanchnic resistance, there is a danger of precipitating mesenteric insufficiency in patients with marginally adequate perfusion when the drug is given.[2] In malabsorption syndromes, oral digoxin is erratically absorbed,[11] and the drug is best given intravenously. Bile salts and pancreatic enzymes, however, are not required for digitalis absorption, so that pancreatic insufficiency does not necessarily preclude the use of oral digoxin.

The prophylactic use of digoxin for the surgical patient is controversial. Two retrospective studies, one by Wheat and Burford,[6] the other by Shields and Ujiki,[7] reported lower incidences of perioperative tachyarrhythmias in patients given prophylactic digoxin prior to surgery. On the other hand, two other retrospective studies by Juler et al.[8] and Selzer and Walter[9] showed no advantage to predigitalization. In certain animal models, digoxin affords protection fron anesthetic-induced decline in myocardial function.[10] However, the extent to which this animal data applies in vivo is speculative. Additionally, metabolic rates and PaO_2 and serum potassium levels fluctuate in the perioperative setting, and an unpredictable glycoside effect can result in any given patient. Thus, we feel that prophylactic digitalization adds a potential source of complication and should be avoided when no clear therapeutic indication exists. Should digoxin be clearly indicated following surgery, there would then be no uncertainty about how much digoxin is already "on board."

Propranolol

A potent therapeutic tool in the management of angina pectoris, hypertension, tachyarrhythmias, IHSS, thyrotoxicosis, and other conditions, propranolol was until a few years ago the only beta-adrenergic blocking agent commercially available in the United States. Other agents offering certain potential advantages over propranolol are now available. Because of limited experience with these agents in the perioperative setting, this section will deal primarily with propranolol.

Propranolol is available for oral and intravenous use. Oral propranolol is nearly completely absorbed, but is only 20 to 50% bioavailable because of extensive "first pass" hepatic uptake. The total daily dose required for control of angina can vary from as low as 40 mg to over 480 mg, largely because of differences in hepatic extraction. In patients with diminished hepatic blood flow (e.g., CHF), first pass uptake declines and serum levels will rise. In persons with normal hepatic blood flow, the serum half-life of propranolol is about 4 to 6 hours, yet the effect of beta-blockade persists much longer; residual effects can be demonstrated for as long as 24 to 36 hours in some subjects. Therefore, although the regimen is not yet FDA-approved at this writing, propranolol has been prescribed for angina on a twice-a-day basis.

Intravenous propranolol avoids the problem of hepatic extraction, and bioavailability is more complete. As a result, 1 mg I.V. is roughly equivalent to 15 to 20 mg of oral propranolol.

Whether to continue the patient's propranolol in the perioperative period has been extensively debated. Prospective controlled studies on the benefits and hazards of propranolol in the setting of noncardiac surgery have not been reported, but analogous studies during coronary bypass surgery have been carried out. Results of these studies suggest that propranolol can be safely maintained by the oral route right up to the time of coronary bypass surgery, and can even be given intravenously in the hours following surgery.[12] Data relating to bypass surgery, however, may not directly apply to noncardiac surgery because, in bypass surgery, postoperative coronary blood flow has been greatly augmented. Additionally, the patient undergoing coronary bypass is generally more closely monitored in the perioperative period than the patient undergoing noncardiac surgery.

The principal argument against continuing propranolol throughout the operative period relates to the known myocardial depressant effect of virtually all anesthetic agents, which the concomitant use of propranolol could potentiate. Given the added demands on the heart in the perioperative period, the argument goes, heart failure could ensue. Viljoen[13] has reported five cases of intraoperative heart failure, thought to be related to the use of propranolol. Other potential hazards of propranolol in the surgical patient are: blunting of the appropriate tachycardic response to hypovolemia, thereby masking the presence of volume depletion; impairing pulmonary function due to the unopposed (bronchoconstrictive) alpha stimulation; and potentiating sinus bradycardia or A-V block in association with intense vagal stimuli.

On the other hand, a study from the Texas Heart Institute[14] has failed to demonstrate potentiation of propranolol's beta-blocking activity by morphine or halothane, two agents commonly used on cardiac patients. Furthermore, three subsequent clinical studies[12, 15, 16] demonstrated improved outcome when propranolol was maintained. The improved results in these later clinical studies may be due to unrelated surgical advances occurring in the six years elapsed since Viljoen's study. More likely, however, the improved outcome is due to the ability of propranolol to prevent myocardial ischemia by blunting excessive heart rate and blood pressure rises resulting from the stresses of anesthesia and surgery. The protective effect of propranolol in preventing ischemia and arrhythmias remains the principal rationale for continuing the drug.

Citing the risk of myocardial depression, Hillis and Cohn[17] advocate gradual withdrawal of propranolol over two to four preoperative days, while the patient's activities are limited. In addition to the *potential* benefits of having the propranolol largely removed from the system prior to surgery, they point out that gradual tapering avoids the problem of sudden propranolol withdrawal syndrome.[18] This phenomenon is characterized by a rebound increase in episodes of angina, myocardial infarction, hypertension, and arrhythmias two to six days following abrupt discontinuation of propranolol. Although the pathophysiology is not completely understood, it is thought to be related to an increase in the sensitivity to catecholamines following abrupt withdrawal of propranolol (but not necessarily other beta-blockers). It is avoided by gradual tapering of the drug prior to discontinuation.

In contrast to the recommendations of Hillis and Cohn,[17] Goldman,[19] writing from the same institution, contends that the safest strategy is to continue the usual propranolol dose until the morning of surgery, and to restart the drug orally as soon as possible postoperatively. Should signs of adrenergic excess appear, such as tachycardia, hypertension, angina, or arrhythmias, and other potential causes (e.g., fluid overload hypoxia) are excluded, oral or intravenous propranolol is advocated.

We concur with the recommendations of Goldman.[19] Our stable angina patients continue taking propranolol up to the morning of noncardiac surgery. Generally, the drug is restarted at the full dose as soon as possible following surgery. If oral intake is proscribed for prolonged periods, or if signs of withdrawal syndrome appear shortly after surgery, propranolol is given intravenously, 0.5 to 1 mg as a test dose followed by 1 to 5 mg every two to four hours. In our experience, clinically important myocardial depression, bradyarrhythmias, or bronchoconstriction have not occurred with this regimen. If congestive heart failure supervenes, and propranolol is deemed at fault, we discontinue propranolol and administer isoprotenenol, titrated carefully to override the beta-blockade.

When postoperative hypotension and tachycardia occurs, it can be difficult to distinguish between hypovolemia and myocardial depression as the cause. If results of a careful examination and chest x-ray are equivocal, a Swan-Ganz catheter can be inserted to determine the pulmonary capillary wedge pressure and to guide further therapy.

Nitroglycerin and Organic Nitrates

These agents are potent vasodilators used in the treatment of classic angina, variant angina due to coronary artery spasm, and congestive heart failure. Nitrates relieve angina by improving the myocardial oxygen supply–demand ratio. The principal action of nitrates in classic angina is due to a lowering of intraventricular pressure and a diminution of chamber sizes, both of which reduce myocardial oxygen consumption. In vasospastic angina, nitrates directly dilate the coronary artery segment in spasm. The beneficial effects in congestive heart failure result from peripheral pooling of blood, the so-called "internal phlebotomy." This action lowers cardiac preload and relieves pulmonary congestion.

Table 3
Nitroglycerin and Nitrate Preparations

Agent	Route	Usual Dose	Duration of Action
Nitroglycerin	Sublingual	.3–.6 mg q 5 min	2–30 min
Nitroglycerin	Oral	6.5–19.5 mg q 4–6 hr	4–6 hr
Nitroglycerin	Topical	½–2 inches (7.5–30 mg)	3–6 hr
Nitroglycerin	Intravenous	10–50 mcg/min or more	4–9 min
Isosorbide dinitrate	Sublingual	2.5–10 mg q 2–4 hr	1.5–3 hr
Isosorbide dinitrate	Oral	10–60 mg q 4–6 hr	4–6 hr
Isosorbide dinitrate	Chewable	5–10 mg q 2–4 hr	2–3 hr
Pentaerythritol tetranitrate	Oral	40–80 mg q 4–6 hr	3–5 hr

A large number of short and long-acting nitrate preparations are available (Table 3). Despite prior published reports to the contrary, it has now been conclusively shown that "long-acting" nitrate effects persist for several hours.[20] Thus, durations of actions range from minutes for intravenous nitroglycerin to over six hours for topical nitroglycerin and oral isosorbide dinitrate.

Organic nitrates, along with beta-blockers, are the first line drugs in the management of patients with coronary artery disease. It follows that the medical consultant must manage nitrate therapy in the vast majority of coronary patients undergoing noncardiac surgery.

Prior reviews[17,21–24] do not directly address the management of nitrate therapy in the perioperative period. We are unaware of controlled studies to determine optimal perioperative nitrate regimens. Our recommendation must ultimately be based on our favorable experience and upon therapeutic logic.

In general, nitrates are recommended for patients with known or suspected coronary disease who undergo surgery. Patients with severe or unstable angina should be considered for myocardial revascularization prior to any elective, noncardiac operation. For emergency noncardiac surgery in patients with severe angina, intravenous nitroglycerin should be considered in addition to invasive hemodynamic monitoring.

For the patient with stable angina, long-acting nitrates are recommended. If the patient is to be NPO for more than a few hours, on the day of surgery or 24 hours earlier, nitroglycerin ointment, one to two inches, applied topically, every four hours is begun. This regimen can temporarily substitute for prior outpatient regimens, allowing for uninterrupted nitrate therapy throughout the perioperative period and avoiding oral or sublingual agents. When the patient is no longer NPO following surgery, the preoperative nitrate regimen can be restored.

Glasser et al.[25] provide further helpful general guidelines for nitrate therapy in the surgical setting. These include: checking for postural changes prior to surgery on the same nitrate regimen intended for surgery; avoiding nitrates when hypovolemia is present; avoiding abrupt discontinuation of any long-acting nitrate regimen; and avoiding the placement of nitroglycerin ointment over the surgical site where it will surely be wiped off in the operating room. It is also wise to avoid placing nitroglycerin over the patient's precordium in order to avoid transmitting unwanted vasodilator from patient to patient via the physician's stethescope.

Anticoagulants

Virtually all patients with mechanical valve prostheses and many patients with artificial tissue valves require lifelong anticoagulation to prevent thromboembolism. The perioperative management of these patients and other cardiac patients taking oral anticoagulants for conditions such as ventricular aneurysm, rheumatic heart disease or venous thromboembolism requires planning that must begin before the patient arrives in the hospital.

In formulating guidelines for the use of warfarin in the cardiac patient undergoing surgery, the risk of surgical hemorrhage must be weighed against the danger of serious embolization. Data from two studies support the largely-held assumption that the risk of hemorrhage is excessive when anticoagulation is continued during the perioperative period. In one retrospective series of Katholi et al.,[26] there was a 44% incidence of unanticipated hemorrhage resulting in one death among patients continued on anticoagulants. Not surprisingly, unanticipated hemorrhage did not occur in their series when anticoagulation was discontinued. In a subsequent prospective study of 45 operative procedures performed on patients with mechanical prosthetic valves by the same group,[27] unexpected (but controllable) bleeding occurred in three patients given heparin in the perioperative period. Dental extractions in their patients were performed with full anticoagulation, without adverse sequela.

Data on the risk of thromboembolism upon cessation of anticoagulation is also available. In Katholi's earlier study,[26] there were no thromboembolic events in 25 patients with aortic prostheses when anticoagulation was stopped three to five days preoperatively. On the other hand, there were two perioperative thromboembolic episodes, resulting in death, in ten operations performed on patients with mitral or multiple valve prostheses when anticoagulation had been discontinued.

Tinker and Tarhan[28] reviewed the records of 159 patients with mechanical heart valves who underwent 180 noncardiac operations at the Mayo Clinic between 1962 and 1975. In 113 operations where anticoagulation was discontinued one or more days before surgery, no thromboembolic episodes occurred in the perioperative period. Virtually all of the bleeding complications occurred in patients who had continued anticoagulants or had a prolonged elevation of prothrombin time following cessation of the medication.

Because patients with prosthetic valves are especially prone to thromboembolism, these data on the risk of emboli can logically extend to most anticoagulated patients. For most orally anticoagulated patients facing major elective surgery, warfarin can be discontinued with reasonable safety approximately three days prior to operation. It can be restarted at former doses within one to three days postoperatively when hemostasis is assured. If the prothrombin time is near normal just prior to surgery, the risk of excessive surgical bleeding is small. Furthermore, with this regimen the risk of thromboembolism during the perioperative period is low. For patients deemed at *excessively* high risk for embolic phenomena during cessation of anticoagulation (e.g., patients with a history of previous emboli or selected patients with mitral prostheses), the period of time the patient is left "unprotected" can be shortened by instituting full dose heparin at the time warfarin is discontinued. In that case, heparin is administered by constant intravenous infusion, titrating the dose to maintain the partial thromboplastin time 1½ to 2½ times control values. Immediately prior to surgery, heparin effect is reversed by intravenous administration of protamine sulfate. Shortly after surgery, when bleeding

Table 4
Anticoagulant Management in Patients Deemed at High Risk for
Thromboembolism

- Discontinue warfarin three days before surgery
- Simultaneously begin heparin by constant infusion, maintaining PTT 1½ to 2½ times normal
- Immediately prior to surgery, administer protamine to reverse heparin effect
- Shortly after surgery, restart I.V. heparin and p.o. warfarin
- Discontinue heparin infusion when the prothrombin time is therapeutic

is controlled, both intravenous heparin and oral warfarin are restarted until the prothrombin time and partial thromboplastin time is again in the therapeutic range (Table 4). It is judged that the number of patients deemed at the high risk for emboli to require such tight control of anticoagulation is quite small.

Patients undergoing minor surgery, dental extractions, and certain other procedures such as herniorrhaphy, where excessive bleeding is readily visualized and controlled, may safely continue anticoagulation therapy throughout their surgery and hospitalization.

When emergency surgery is required, the anticoagulant effect of warfarin can be rapidly reversed with 25 to 50 mg of intravenous vitamin K, injected slowly. In most patients, the prothrombin time begins to normalize in one to two hours, and returns to normal in 8 to 12 hours after this dose. If more rapid restoration of clotting function is needed, fresh frozen plasma, 500 ml given intravenously, will immediately normalize clotting function, but there is an increased risk of hepatitis.

Heparin Prophylaxis

Based upon the results of several large scale clinical trials in the 1970s (Table 5), the Council on Thrombosis of the American Heart Association has concluded that mini-dose heparin administered to hemostatically competent patients over the age of 40 undergoing elective major abdominal or thoracic surgical procedures, will reduce the incidence of postoperative pulmonary emboli by 80%.[29]

Table 5
Indications for Heparin Prophylaxis

Definite benefit
    Elective major abdominal surgery
    Elective thoracic surgery
Limited value
    Open prostatectomy
    Repair of femoral fracture
    Hip and knee reconstruction
Not recommended
    Eye or brain surgery
    Spinal anesthesia

It is reasonable to extend these recommendations to virtually all hemostatically competent cardiac patients, who would tolerate poorly any thromboembolic complications. The following guidelines are suggested. Cardiac patients not taking oral anticoagulants are candidates for low dose heparin prophylaxis. Hematocrit, prothrombin time, partial thromboplastin time, and platelet count should be normal prior to surgery. Aspirin and platelet-active agents are withheld for five days before surgery, and warfarin is avoided in the perioperative period. Heparin, 5,000 USP units, is administered subcutaneously two hours preoperatively and is repeated every 8 to 12 hours postoperatively until hospital discharge. No laboratory tests are required to monitor therapy. Trials have shown that low dose heparin prophylaxis is of limited value in open prostatectomy, repair of femoral fracture, and hip and knee reconstruction. Because of the slightly increased risk of minor wound hematoma, this regimen is not recommended for eye or brain surgery or with spinal anesthesia. This regimen is also not intended for the prosthetic valve patient requiring full anticoagulation pre- and post-operatively.

Management of Antiarrhythmic Medication

Perioperative management of antiarrhythmic medication must take into consideration both the initial indications for treatment and the current antiarrhythmic regimen. Because of still unresolved issues, indications for antiarrhythmic therapy, especially with respect to ventricular ectopy, vary widely among practitioners. For example, virtually all physicians would aggressively treat premature ventricular beats in a patient with episodic syncope caused by ventricular tachycardia. On the other hand, the indications for treating an asymptomatic middle-aged male with thirty unifocal ventricular premature beats per hour are less clear-cut. Clearly, a more cautious approach must be taken when a patient with symptomatic ventricular arrhythmia faces major surgery. However, when we find patients taking antiarrhythmic medications for questionable or improper indications, we have found it is safe to carefully discontinue antiarrhythmic medications preoperatively under electrocardiographic monitoring.

Four antiarrhythmic agents are available in both oral and intravenous forms: digoxin, propranolol, procainamide, and phenytoin. The perioperative management of digoxin and propranolol therapy has been previously discussed. The intravenous forms of procainamide and phenytoin have a bioavailability equivalent to their oral counterparts so that the respective oral and intravenous dosage can be readily substituted. A patient taking one of these agents orally can simply be given the same dose in intravenous form in the perioperative period. Quinidine can also be given orally or parenterally, but serious hypotension can result when given intravenously, and it is probably best avoided. Intravenous lidocaine remains the most effective intravenous agent for suppression of ventricular ectopy.

When perioperative antiarrhythmic therapy is required, the patient's usual regimen is continued throughout the perioperative period, using parenteral substitutions as needed. Where parenteral substitutions are unavailable or unsuitable, as in the case of a patient taking disopyramide or quinidine, intravenous lidocaine is given in bolus injections of 100 mg to 200 mg over a 20 minute period followed by a constant infusion of 2 to 4 mg/min.

Because of quinidine's curare-like effect on skeletal muscle, this drug can impair postoperative pulmonary mechanics and delay the return of spontaneous respiration. Consequently, the anesthesiologist should be made aware of any patient's preoperative use of quinidine.

Medical consultants are frequently called to the recovery room or to the operating suite to assist in the management of arrhythmias developing during surgery or in the immediate postoperative period. Katz and Bigger[30] have pointed out that arrhythmias occur in the vast majority of patients undergoing surgery, even in the absence of underlying heart disease. In the majority of cases, the arrhythmia is due to transient and readily reversible factors such as surgical manipulations, inadequate or excessive anesthesia, hypoxia or electrolyte disturbance, and it is abolished when the cause is eliminated. Specific antiarrhythmic medication is rarely needed. When it is not possible to cease surgical manipulation or otherwise eliminate the cause of the arrhythmia, and it is felt that deleterious cardiovascular consequences could result from the arrhythmia, specific antiarrhythmic therapy is indicated. The selection of agents is based on the usual criteria that prevail in the nonsurgical setting. Intravenous lidocaine is usually the drug of first choice.

References

1. Marcus FI: Digitalis pharmacokinetics and metabolism. *Amer J Med* 58:452, 1976.
2. Smith TW: Digitalis glycosides. *New Engl J Med* 288:719, 942, 1973.
3. Leahey EB, Reiffel JA, Drusin RE, et al.: Interaction between quinidine and digoxin. *JAMA* 240:533, 1978.
4. Jelliffee RW, Brooker RW: A nomogram for digoxin therapy. *Amer J Med* 57:63, 1974.
5. Johnston GD, McDevitt DG: Is maintenance digoxin necessary in patients with sinus rhythm? *Lancet* 1:467, 1979.
6. Wheat MW, Burford TR: Digitalis in surgery: Extension of classical indications. *J Throacic Cardiovasc Surg* 41:162, 1961.
7. Shields T, Ujiki GT: Digitalization for prevention of arrhythmias following pulmonary surgery. *Surg Gynec Obstet* 126:743, 1968.
8. Juler GL, Stemmer EA, Connolly JE: Complications of prophylactic digitalization in thoracic surgical patients. *J Thoracic Cardiovasc Surg* 58:352, 1979.
9. Selzer A, Walter RM: Adequacy of preoperative digitalis therapy in controlling ventricular rates in postoperative atrial fibrillation. *Circulation* 34:119, 1966.
10. Goldberg AH, Maling HM, Gaffner TE: The value of prophylactic digitalization in halothane anesthesia. *Anesthesiology* 23:207, 1962.
11. Heizer WD, Smith TW, Goldfinger SE: Absorption of digoxin in patients with malabsorption syndromes. *New Engl J Med* 285:257, 1971.
12. Oka Y, Frishman W, Becker RM, et al.: Clinical pharmacology of the new beta-adrenergic blocking drugs. Part 10. Beta-adrenoreceptor blockade and coronary artery surgery. *Am Heart J* 99:255, 1980.
13. Viljoen JF, Estafanous FG, Kellner GA: Propranolol and cardiac surgery. *J Thorac Cardiovasc Surg* 64:826, 1972.

14. Slogoff S, Keats AS, Hibbs CW, et al.: Failure of general anesthesia to potentiate propranolol activity. *Anesthesiology* 47:504, 1977.
15. Slogoff S, Keats AS, Ott E: Preoperative propranolol therapy and aortocoronary bypass operation. *JAMA* 240:1487, 1978.
16. Boudoulas H, Snyder GL, Lewis RP, et al.: Safety and rationale for continuation of propranolol during coronary bypass operation. *Ann Thorac Surg* 26:222, 1978.
17. Hillis LD, Cohn PF: Noncardiac surgery in patients with coronary artery disease. Risks, precautions and perioperative management. *Arch Intern Med* 138:972, 1978.
18. Miller RR, Olson HG, Amsterdam EA, et al.: Propranolol withdrawal rebound phenomenon. Exacerbation of coronary events after abrupt cessation of antianginal therapy. *New Engl J Med* 292:416, 1975.
19. Goldman L: Noncardiac surgery in patients receiving propranolol. Case reports and recommended approach. *Arch Intern Med* 141:193, 1981.
20. Abrams J: Nitroglycerin and long-acting nitrates. *New Engl J Med* 302:1234, 1980.
21. Perlroth MG, Hultgren HN: The cardiac patient and general surgery. *JAMA* 232:1279, 1975.
22. Rose SD, Corman LC, Mason DT: Cardiac risk factors in patients undergoing noncardiac surgery. *Med Clin North America* 63:1271, 1979.
23. Wolf MA, Braunwald E: General anesthesia and noncardiac surgery in patients with heart disease. In Braunwald E, Ed, *Heart Disease*. Philadelphia: W. B. Saunders, pp. 1911–1922, 1980.
24. Logue RB, Kaplan JA: Surgery in patients with heart disease. Part A. Medical management in noncardiac surgery. In Hurst JW, et al., Eds, *The Heart*. New York: McGraw-Hill, pp. 1762–1777, 1978.
25. Glasser SP, Spoto E Jr, Solomon DA, et al.: When cardiac patients become surgical patients. *Hospital Practice* 165, March, 1979.
26. Katholi RE, Nolan SP, McGuire LP: Living with prosthetic heart valves. Subsequent noncardiac operations and the risk of thromboembolism or hemorrhage. *Am Heart J* 92:162, 1976.
27. Katholi RE, Nolan SP, McGuire LP: The management of anticoagulation during noncardiac operations in patients with prosthetic heart valves. *Am Heart J* 96:163, 1978.
28. Tinker JH, Tarhan S: Discontinuing anticoagulation therapy in surgical patients with cardiac valve prosthesis. Observations in 180 operations. *JAMA* 239:738, 1978.
29. Council on Thrombosis of the American Heart Association: Prevention of venous thromboembolism in surgical patients by low-dose heparin. *Circulation* 55:423A, 1977.
30. Katz RL, Bigger JT: Cardiac arrhythmias during anesthesia and surgery. *Anesthesiology* 33:193, 1970.

The Preoperative Assessment

In this Section, an attempt is made to discuss the laboratory evaluation of cardiac patients as it relates to their preoperative risk. The electrocardiogram is one of the most common tools utilized in this regard, and the significance of different electrocardiographic patterns as it relates to the presence and/or significance of cardiac disease is discussed. Some comments regarding postoperative electrocardiographic changes are also included here. The exercise test and echocardiography have also achieved an important place in the evaluation of suspected or proven heart disease. These two sections approach the subject from the standpoint of symptom presentation. Thus, it attempts to answer the question, for instance, "What is the value of an exercise test in the preoperative assessment of the chronic stable angina patient?" or, "What is the value of preoperative echocardiography in a patient about to undergo a cholecystectomy who is found to have a systolic murmur?"

Since many patients with coronary artery disease will have concomitant peripheral vascular disease (and vice versa), the evaluation of the presence and severity of the peripheral vascular disease is important. Therefore, a discussion of the noninvasive work-up of such patients is included here. Also, it is common for patients with heart disease to have associated pulmonary disease. Thus, a discussion of the preoperative pulmonary risk factors and the evaluation of pulmonary function is next presented. Finally is the question, "Which patients with suspected or proven cardiac disease need cardiac catheterization?" This question defies simplistic answers, but an attempt is made to provide some insight into this difficult problem and to suggest a schema of how to evaluate cardiac patients for noncardiac surgery.

CHAPTER IV

The Electrocardiogram

H. David Friedberg, M.D.

The Electrocardiogram

The electrocardiograph is an instrument invented by Einthoven at the beginning of this century. It soon achieved great significance in Medicine because it supplied the first physical sign of coronary artery disease. Its use is now almost universal. This chapter is not meant either to teach or to delve deeply into electrocardiographic diagnosis, but is meant, rather, to emphasize the value and limitations of the electrocardiogram, both in regard to preoperative evaluation and postoperative care, with emphasis upon the contour of the QRS complex, S-T segment, and T and U waves. In the perioperative situation, two great errors abound: over-reading—the preoperative electrocardiogram does not substitute for a careful history and physical examination; and a failure to take sufficient repeated serial tracings after surgery.

Technical Errors

Errors in the technique of recording the tracing may give rise to spurious findings and may easily mislead the unwary. Such errors, which include faults in standardization, calibration, filtering, damping, and centering of the tracing, are more common in single channel electrocardiographs used at night than in the more modern three channel machines used during the day. There are many ways of misconnecting the electrodes and of mislabeling the trac-

47

ing. In practice, before one considers that any electrocardiogram shows a definite change, one must be careful to consider the technical quality of the tracing.

Acute Myocardial Infarction

Classically, acute myocardial infarction is diagnosed by the combination of clinical, electrocardiographic, and laboratory changes. In the acute postoperative state, the clinical features and most of the laboratory findings may be misleading. Electrocardiographic changes and, in particular, *serial* electrocardiographic changes may be the best diagnostic clue available. Furthermore, electrocardiographic changes may be the only sign of an acute postoperative infarction.

Serial Electrocardiographic Changes

In order to make a confident diagnosis of acute myocardial infarction, serial electrocardiographic changes must be found. A common cause of missing this important diagnosis is failure to take repeated tracings in people who are likely to have this complication after surgery. Daily electrocardiograms must be taken until the condition is either diagnosed or excluded.

The QRST complex may be divided into three parts. A *pathological Q wave* (or its equivalent) is an indicator of myocardial cell death or necrosis. The *elevated S-T* segment is held to indicate injured myocardium, which may either recover or die. As the condition progresses, the S-T segment returns to the base line and the *T wave inverts*. The T wave is said to reflect ischemic myocardium. The reasons given are somewhat simplistic, but the facts are nevertheless there. These changes will accurately diagnose most transmural myocardial infarctions.

Infarctions without Q Waves

A subendocardial infarction produces changes in the T wave, but does not alter the QRS complex or S-T segment (Figure 1).

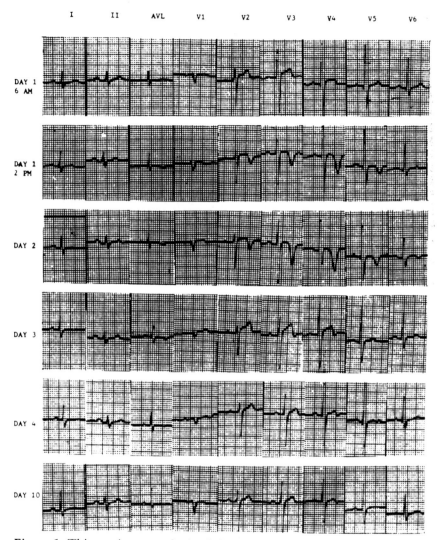

Figure 1. This tracing was obtained from a 54-year-old strawberry farmer admitted to the hospital with lower sternal heaviness. It demonstrates marked diffuse T-wave inversion, which evolved over a four-day period and was associated with elevation in total CPK and CPK-MB consistent with a subendocardial myocardial infarction. Six weeks later, coronary angiography revealed double vessel coronary disease. (Reprinted with permission of John Wright, PSG Inc., from Martinez-Lopez JI, Glasser SP, Clarke PI: *A Casebook of Electrocardiographic Tracings*, p. 133, 1982)

The T waves are deeply inverted, pointed, and symmetrical. They progress slowly. As many other conditions (for example: subarachnoid hemorrhage) may produce similar changes, the diagnosis cannot depend on the electrocardiogram alone.

If there is pre-existing complete or incomplete *left bundle branch block,* the acute infarction pattern may be masked and Q waves may not appear. Usually, some very suggestive change in the S-T segment and T wave will be found.

The appearance of axis shift, bundle branch block, or arrhythmia is *not* prima facie evidence of myocardial infarction. If the QRS complex is highly abnormal in the preoperative electrocardiogram, subtle changes may not be apparent after a postoperative myocardial infarction, and the diagnosis may, therefore, be missed.

Old or Stable Infarction Patterns

With the passage of time, the S-T segment returns to the baseline, the T wave reverts to normal, and only the Q wave remains as evidence of the prior heart attack (Figures 2A and 2B). Further, in 8–10% of cases, even the Q wave disappears so that the electrocardiogram is entirely normal.

The P Wave

In the preoperative electrocardiogram, abnormalities of the P wave may be reported as left (or right) atrial hypertrophy, enlargement, strain, or some similar expression. These terms all have an unwarranted precision. The lateralization is *not* reliable. Often, all that can be said is that there is most likely something wrong with an atrium, and the term "atrial abnormality" is, therefore, preferred.

In the postoperative electrocardiogram, however, a change in the P wave is of great diagnostic value: the development of tall and pointed P waves in the inferior leads may indicate an increase in pressure in the right atrium, such as may occur with an acute pulmonary embolism; the development in the postoperative electrocardiogram of a large negative component of the P wave in lead VI or V2 represents acute left atrial strain. This strongly suggests

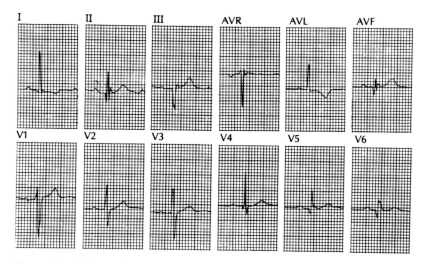

Figure 2A. This tracing was obtained from an asymptomatic 60-year-old man who stated that he had a "heart attack" six years ago. Inferior wall (Leads II, III, and aVF) Q waves are evident.

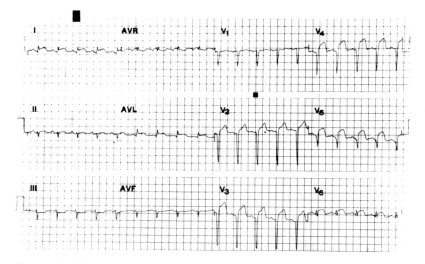

Figure 2B. This tracing was recorded from a 49-year-old man with substernal chest pain, diaphoresis, and nausea. Anterolateral Q waves ($V_1 - V_6$ + I and aVL) associated with marked S-T segment elevation in those same leads suggests an acute myocardial infarction.

left ventricular failure. Resolution of the P wave changes reflects a drop in the end-diastolic pressure in the left ventricle. These changes are due to increase in tension in the wall of the atrium. This predisposes the chamber to the development of premature beats, tachycardias, flutter, and/or fibrillation.

The S-T Segment

S-T Segment Elevation

Elevation of the S-T segment is a classic finding in acute myocardial infarction. However, it occurs in other conditions. An elevated S-T segment is often a *normal variant*, especially in young men (Figure 3), but it usually will not change markedly in successive tracings. It may, however, cause much iatrogenic unhappiness because of an erroneous diagnosis. This error may be prevented by a high index of suspicion.

Elevation of the S-T segment is also often seen in *pericarditis*. This is related to the diffuse epicardial injury caused by the inflammation and is, therefore, seen in most electrocardiographic

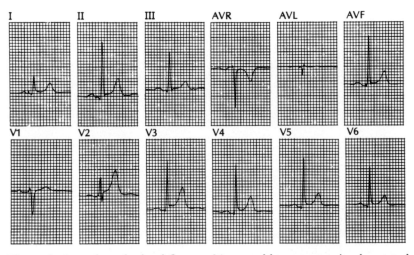

Figure 3. A tracing obtained from a 21-year-old army recruit who stated that he had a prior abnormal ECG. Comparison with that tracing revealed no change. Exercise "normalized" the S-T segment changes.

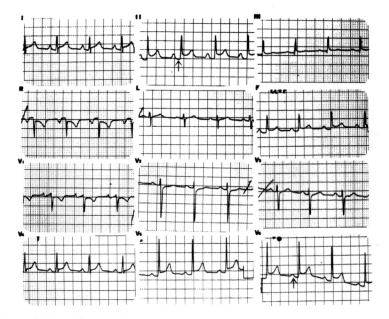

Figure 4. This 27-year-old woman was admitted to the hospital with chest pain and a pericardial friction rub. S-T segment elevation is noted in most leads. In addition, The P-R segment (arrows) is depressed in most leads, but elevated in aVR.

leads. An atrial injury current may also aid in diagnosis (Figure 4). The S-T segment (in contrast to the normal variant S-T elevation) evolves and returns to the base line very slowly. The T waves then invert, but changes in the QRS complex are not seen.

Persistent elevation of the S-T segment after an acute myocardial infarction is an indication of a *ventricular aneurysm*. In this situation, it may be very difficult to diagnose fresh injury or extension of the infarction (Figure 5).

S-T Segment Depression

Depression of the junction point between the QRS complex and the S-T segment is a physiological condition associated with an increased cardiac output, such as occurs normally with exercise (Figure 6).

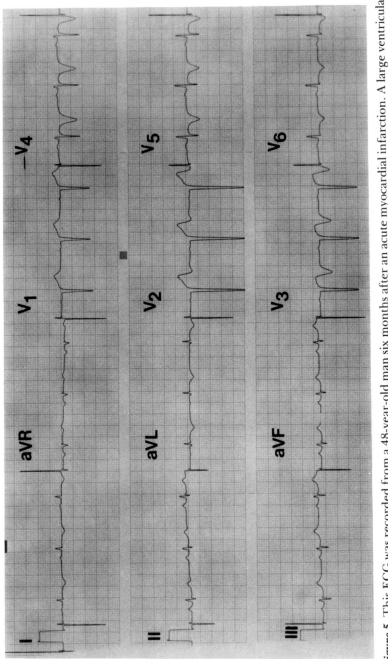

Figure 5. This ECG was recorded from a 48-year-old man six months after an acute myocardial infarction. A large ventricular aneurysm was evident on chest x-ray and echocardiography.

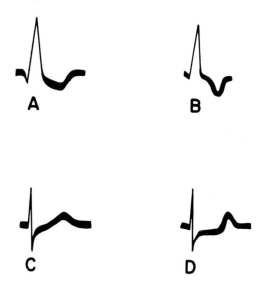

Figure 6. Figure showing diagrams of various S-T segment abnormalities. 'A' represents digitalis effect. 'B' represents the "left ventricular strain" pattern. 'C' represents physiologic junctional S-T segment depression. 'D': this S-T segment is straight and depressed—plane depression of the S-T segment.

An S-T segment that is *plane* or horizontal and straight for at least 0.10 seconds is abnormal and reflects some disease of the left ventricle, usually ischemia. This is more ominous if associated with S-T segment depression (Figure 6), as it may indicate a compromised left ventricular blood supply.

A downward sloping S-T segment is abnormal. This also suggests left ventricular disease, but not necessarily ischemic. For example, digitalis produces a downward sloping but straight S-T segment (Figure 6), although it does not influence the T wave. In a left ventricular *strain pattern*, the S-T is convex and the T is inverted. This is abnormal but nonspecific.

It is perfectly possible for junctional S-T segment depression to coexist with other abnormalities of the S-T segment. Comparison with the preoperative tracing and with serial tracings is helpful in differential diagnosis.

Other Changes

Alterations in the serum concentration of calcium and potassium may produce characteristic changes in the S-T segment (See below).

Elevation of the J point (junction of QRS complex and S-T segment) is a sign of *hypothermia.*

Summary

In general, it is possible to separate normal and abnormal S-T segment variations. Horizontal depression of the S-T segment is characteristically ischemic. Other forms of S-T segment depression are not specific, but are clearly abnormal. This is in marked contrast to the situation with regard to the T wave where it is often very difficult to distinguish the normal from the abnormal, and pathognomic changes are rare.

The T Wave

No part of the electrocardiogram is as fraught with traps for the unwary and tricks for both physician and patient as the T wave. Many physicians avoid problems with interpretations of changes in the T wave by using the expression "nonspecific ST-T changes." As explained above, a great deal of diagnostic information can be extracted from S-T segment changes. They may not be specific, but they may be serious. T wave changes are another matter. Certainly, an effort should be made to decide whether T wave variations are, perhaps, normal; perhaps, of great significance; but, seldom will an ironclad diagnosis result.

The Normal T Wave

Variations in Shape of T Wave

Normally, the T wave is in the same direction as the QRS complex: it has smooth onset, apex, and offset, but it is not symmetrical.

In *hyperkalemia,* the T wave may be tall and symmetrical, or tented, somewhat like an equilateral triangle. In the early phase of *acute myocardial infarction,* tall upright T waves may be seen. Symmetrical T waves may also be seen with head injuries, or other intracranial lesions. The discovery of such changes in the postoperative electrocardiogram should arouse suspicion. No other change in shape of an upright T wave is of diagnostic importance.

T Wave Inversion

T wave inversion is often regarded as suspicious of coronary artery disease and many a patient has had this label applied because of an electrocardiographic overdiagnosis.

Inverted T waves may be *normal* if the QRS complex in that lead is predominantly negative. In *youth,* T wave inversion in the anterior chest leads is normal. When there is bundle branch block, or other intraventricular conduction defect, the T wave is usually opposite in direction to the end of the QRS complex in that lead. This is a *secondary* change and has no intrinsic significance.

Changing T Waves

T waves can change with physiological stimuli that produce tachycardia in a manner very similar to that of ischemic disease. Postoperative pain, fever, and anxiety are amongst such stimuli. Even the taking of the tracing may cause the T wave to vary. Certain pharmacological stimuli can similarly produce T wave inversion. Anesthetic drugs may do this as well as isoprenaline and epinephrine.

Noncoronary Causes

Inverted T waves may indicate cardiac disease, but the disease may not necessarily be coronary in origin. Any disease affecting the left ventricle, such as aortic incompetence, may do this.

Another cause is simply the fact of pacing. When a patient has had a permanent pacemaker for some time, he may have deep T wave inversion in the normally conducted beats.

Noncardiac Causes

The T wave inversion may indicate a disease that is not even in the heart. Stimulation of the sympathetic trunks and ganglia can alter the T waves. So can lesions producing an increased intracranial pressure, or involving the floor of the fourth ventricle. Other causes include anemia and hypovolemia, which are common postoperatively.

Inverted T Waves with Normal Heart

The following conditions may produce T wave inversion or other changes in the T wave, even though the heart is normal: tachycardia, hyperventilation, anxiety and fear, exercise, a large meal, posture, cooling, anesthesia, and incorrect placing of the chest leads.

Isolated T Wave Changes on the Preoperative Electrocardiogram

A *T wave is known by the company it keeps.* If the S-T segment or QRS complex is definitely abnormal, the T wave must be regarded as abnormal. Problems arise in the preoperative consultations when the T wave is an isolated abnormality.

Many maneuvers have been recommended to help elucidate this problem:

Ensure that the patient is not hyperventilating and is relaxed.

Take additional exploratory leads.

Take a fasting electrocardiogram.

Mild exercise may normalize T waves and, indeed, a graded exercise stress test may be needed.

The use of a large dose of potassium chloride (10 grams) by mouth may also normalize the T wave.

A quite simple maneuver is to give the patient 40 mgm of propranolol by mouth and repeat the electrocardiogram an hour later. If the changes are due to anxiety or tachycardia, they should normalize. If both anxiety and disease are present, the T wave may return partly, not completely, to normal.

There are certain T wave changes that are frequently suggestive of *coronary insufficiency:* the T wave of coronary insufficiency has symmetrical limbs and a sharp, pointed vertex: this is called the "coronary" T wave. T wave configurations from other causes usually show asymmetrical limbs without a peaked vertex.

The U Wave

Prominent Upright U Waves

Prominent upright U waves (that is, in the same direction as the normal T wave in that lead) are found after exercise. These are usually normal findings unless associated with a low serum potassium.

Inverted U Waves

Inverted U waves, by contrast, are nearly always abnormal. If the T wave and the U wave are inverted *(concordant T-U inversion)* this may be regarded as confirmatory evidence that the T wave inversion is abnormal. This often happens with left ventricular strain or ischemia.

If the U wave is inverted and the T wave is not *(discordant U wave inversion)* this is a subtle sign of ischemia, or perhaps some left ventricular strain. It should always arouse suspicion, as it is rarely normal (Figure 7).

The Value of Stress Tests

A graded exercise stress test should be considered before elective surgery in any patient who presents with a history suggestive of ischemic heart disease, or who has suggestive electrocardiographic

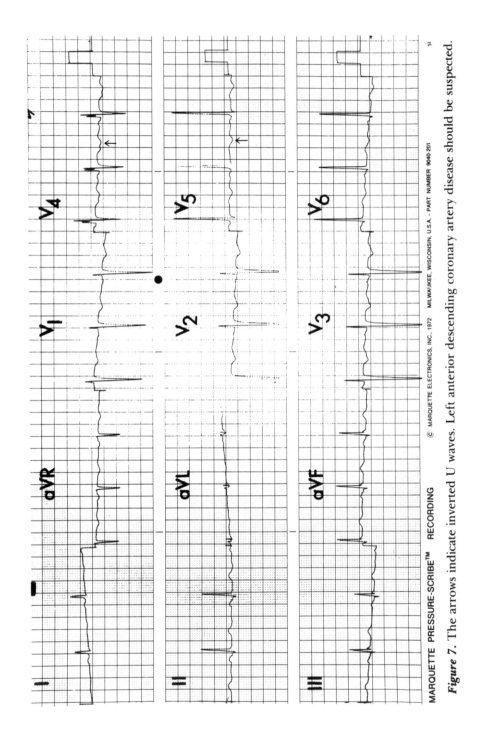

MARQUETTE PRESSURE-SCRIBE™ RECORDING   © MARQUETTE ELECTRONICS, INC. 1972   MILWAUKEE, WISCONSIN, U.S.A. - PART NUMBER 9040-201

Figure 7. The arrows indicate inverted U waves. Left anterior descending coronary artery disease should be suspected.

abnormalities of the QRS complex, S-T segment, or T wave. Any protocol may be followed using either a bicycle ergometer or a treadmill. A symptom-limited test also permits the assessment of the functional cardiac reserve. Furthermore, one may be fore-warned by the appearance of arrhythmias. An abnormal stress test is not necessarily a contraindication to surgery. However, if the patients cannot perform work at the level of 5 mets, the risk of surgery may be increased, and coronary arteriography may be in-dicated in some situations (See Chapter 9).

Acute Cor Pulmonale

The electrocardiographic findings associated with a pulmonary embolism and resulting acute cor pulmonale are:

Nothing: Very often no electrocardiographic changes are found: a normal electrocardiogram does *not* rule out this diagnosis.

Sinus Tachycardia is common.

Right Atrial Abnormality: tall pointed P waves in leads II, III, and aVF.

Q3-S1 Pattern: The association of a Q wave in lead III without a Q wave in lead aVF, but with an S wave in lead I, and usually an inverted T wave in lead III, is a classical finding in pulmonary embolism. This is a variant of posterior hemiblock and may be misdiagnosed as an acute inferior infarction. A good rule is that if the inferior leads suggest an inferior infarction and the chest leads suggest an anterior infarction, consider acute cor pulmonale.

Marked left axis deviation: The development of marked left axis deviation (anterior hemiblock) occurs not uncommonly.

Lead V1 may show a tall R wave or the pattern or *incomplete right bundle branch block* (rsR). Complete right bundle branch block is not common.

T wave inversion may be seen in the anterior leads.

Atrial premature beats are a prelude to atrial tachycardia, atrial flutter, and fibrillation, which are uncommon.

Changes in Electrolyte Concentrations

Hypokalemia

Lowered concentrations of serum and cellular potassium results in a prominence of the U wave. The T wave is somewhat diminished in amplitude and often the two waves are of equal size. Slight depression of the S-T segment may also be seen. These changes are usually first recognized in a transitional lead, such as lead V3. It is not correct that the Q-T interval is prolonged in this condition.

Hyperkalemia

Increased serum potassium concentrations produce tall upright pointed *symmetrical* T waves. The QRS is distorted and broadened. The P wave may disappear and a slow succession of highly abnormal QRS complexes and T waves may result. Emergency treatment is indicated.

Hypocalcemia

Low serum calcium produces a prolongation of the Q-T interval entirely due to prolongation of the S-T segment. The appearance is characteristic (Figure 8).

Hypercalcemia

An increase in the serum calcium produces a shortening of the Q-T interval entirely due to a shortening of the S-T segment, to the point that the T wave may begin at the end of the QRS complex. This is also a characteristic finding.

Alkalosis

Postoperative alkalosis is often associated with sinus tachycardia and some prolongation of the Q-T interval. The P wave then seems

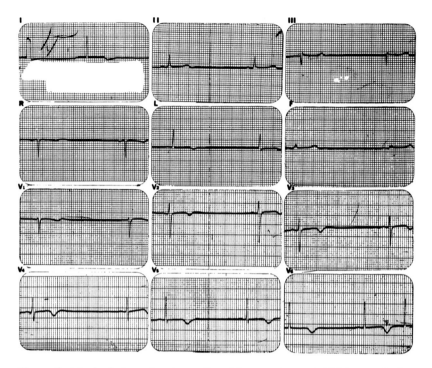

Figure 8. Marked sinus bradycardia with a prolonged QT interval (QT = .60 sec QT$_c$ = 0.48 second) is present. This tracing was obtained from a 60-year-old man with chronic renal insufficiency. His serum calcium was low.

to sit upon the end of the preceding T wave. If the U wave is prominent, the P wave may be superimposed. This is the P on U (or P on T) phenomenon and suggests a disturbance in acid-base metabolism.

Combined Electrolyte Abnormalities

Often, multiple abnormalities of electrolyte concentrations are present at the same time. The electrocardiogram may indicate only one change. The major value of the electrocardiogram in this situation is to direct the physician's thinking towards an abnormality of body chemistry.

Digitalis

The effects of digitalis on the electrocardiogram are: prolongation of the P-R interval; a downward sloping deformity of the S-T segment without significant change in the T wave; the QRS complex is not affected. (For digitalis toxic arrhythmias, see Chapter 3.)

Other Drugs

Certain other drugs, such as Quinidine and Procainamide, may prolong the QRS complex in toxic doses.

Left Bundle Branch Block

Left bundle branch block may be due to interruption of the fibers of the main left bundle, or to interruption of both the fascicular branches, or to damage to the peripheral Purkinje cells and network. Therefore, left bundle branch block may be the result of any condition that affects the left ventricle, such as hypertension, aortic valve disease, or coronary artery disease. It may occasionally be due to conduction system disease in which the myocardium is relatively intact. The presence of left bundle branch block in the preoperative electrocardiogram, therefore, should be regarded as evidence of serious disease of the left ventricle. Furthermore, since left bundle branch block will mask earlier changes in the electrocardiogram, most of the diagnostic value of the tracing is lost.

The appearance of left bundle branch block in the postoperative period should be regarded as evidence of severe left ventricular stress or myocardial ischemia or infarction. It usually indicates severe muscle damage and carries a poor prognosis.

Left bundle branch block may on occasion be found in apparently healthy people. It may represent a normal variance, or may be the first sign of a degenerative condition of the cardiac conducting tissue—Lenegre's Disease—a global electrical heart disease.

Right Bundle Branch Block

Right bundle branch block may be found in conditions that impose a load upon the right ventricle such as atrial septal defect, or cor pulmonale. It may be due to coronary artery disease: in this case, it nearly always indicates significant disease of the left anterior descending artery. It may also be due to disease of the conducting system with a relatively intact myocardium. It may also be a normal variant. Hiss and Lamb reported this finding in 2% of young, asymptomatic air force recruits.

Generally, right bundle branch block has a much better prognosis than its left-sided sister, as it does not imply significant damage to the left ventricle. The major concern is the possibility of further disease of the AV conducting system and the development of Stokes-Adams attacks.

The presence of right bundle branch block in the preoperative electrocardiogram warrants a search for possible causative factors. The development of true right bundle branch block in the postoperative electrocardiogram is not common.

Aberration

This is a physiologic variation of intraventricular conduction. The usual manifestation is a temporary right bundle branch block with the development of a higher heart rate (rate-related bundle branch block). This is a common cause of the presence of transient right bundle branch block in the postoperative period. Note that other forms of aberrations exist; these include left bundle branch and either hemiblock. Occasionally, aberration occurs with slowing of the heart (bradycardia dependent bundle branch block).

Axis Deviation

Marked Left Axis Deviation

Marked left axis deviation produces dominantly negative complexes in leads II, III, and aVF, and is due to interruption of the anterior fascicle of the left bundle branch (anterior hemiblock). This finding may reflect any disease that affects the left ventricle or the intrinsic conduction system. It is a common isolated abnormality in older people. The fresh appearance of left axis deviation in the postoperative electrocardiogram is abnormal, but not diagnostic. It may even be the result of acute cor pulmonale. Left axis deviation may also result from inferior myocardial infarction.

Right Axis Deviation

Right axis deviation produces dominantly positive deflections in leads II, III, and aVf, with lead I showing a negative or zero net QRS deflection. Right axis deviation is normal in young people and may result from right ventricular hypertrophy or anterolateral myocardial infarction. If these conditions are ruled out, then posterior hemiblock (due to interruption of the posterior fascicle of the left bundle branch) is probably present. This has a more serious significance than does anterior hemiblock because the posterior fascicle is a much wider structure. Posterior hemiblock rarely develops after surgery but, if it does, should be regarded as evidence of significant disease of the AV conduction system.

The Wolff-Parkinson-White Syndrome

The Wolff-Parkinson-White Syndrome (WPW) is an interesting electrocardiographic variant that has the following features: a shortened P-R interval; an abnormally widened QRS complex with a slurred beginning—the delta wave; the distance from the beginning of the P wave to the end of the QRS complex (the P-S interval) is normal; there are secondary ST-T changes; and there is a tendency to paroxysmal tachycardias and atrial fibrillation.

This syndrome has importance because the delta wave may lead to an incorrect diagnosis of myocardial infarction, bundle branch block, or left or right ventricular hypertrophy. The ST-T wave changes may lead to an incorrect diagnosis of myocardial ischemia or strain. Most of the signs of myocardial infarction are obscured by the abnormalities of the WPW syndrome. The diagnosis of infarction in the presence of WPW syndrome is, therefore, difficult.

The WPW syndrome may intermit. This means that, at various times, sinus beats may be conducted normally through the ventricle. The resulting QRS-T complex is normal in shape and contains all the diagnostic information.

Attacks of paroxysmal tachycardia may occur. The rate is characteristically very rapid, in excess of 190 beats per minute. Attacks can be terminated by vagotonic maneuvers or by propranolol. Electrocardioversion is nearly always successful. Propranolol is a useful drug for the prevention of tachycardia.

Suggested Reading

1. Chung EK: *Electrocardiography*. Hagerstown, Harper & Row, 1974.
2. Marriott HJL: *Workshop In Electrocardiography*. Oldsmar, Tampa Tracings, 1972.
3. Schamroth L: *The Electrocardiology of Coronary Artery Disease*. Oxford, Blackwell Scientific Publications, 1975.
4. Marriott HJL: *Practical Electrocardiography, Ed. 6*. Baltimore, Williams & Wilkins, 1977.
5. Schamroth L: *An Introduction to Electrocardiography, Ed. 5*. Oxford, Blackwell Scientific Publications, 1976.
6. Hiss RG, Lamb LE: Electrocardiographic findings in 122,043 individuals. *Circulation* XXV:947, 1962.

CHAPTER V

Exercise Testing

Pamela I. Clark, R.N.
and Stephen P. Glasser, M.D.

Graded exercise stress testing can play a significant role in the selection of cardiac patients for elective noncardiac surgery, and can influence the perioperative management of the surgical patient. It allows the physician to observe the patient's physiological adaptation to stress and, as such, is a valuable extension of the standard history and physical examination. Generally, exercise testing can be of some benefit in any patient who does not have limiting noncardiac problems (such as orthopedic limitations) and in whom a 12-lead electrocardiogram is considered in the preoperative assessment. The diagnostic yield of the routine 12-lead electrocardiogram is very small compared to the exercise ECG (which includes a resting tracing), and extensive physiologic information can be gained by observation during exercise. The recommendation of exercise testing, prior to elective surgery, should therefore be limited primarily by cost and logistics. The impact of information gained by that testing on future medical or surgical management depends primarily upon the clinical presentation of the patient being tested.[1]

The Patient with Chronic, Stable Angina

Over 90% of patients presenting with typical angina pectoris will have significant coronary artery disease, so exercise testing can be expected to have little *diagnostic* impact in this group. However,

69

when an individual is to undergo noncardiac surgery, and has a well-documented history of chronic, stable angina, exercise testing may be of help in selecting a subgroup with "critical" coronary narrowing. Patients with left main, left main "equivalent" (proximal left anterior descending and circumflex), triple vessel, or proximal left anterior descending coronary obstructive disease will often produce "markedly positive" exercise tests. A "markedly positive" test is defined as S-T segment depression of greater than 2 mm at a low work load or a low heart rate (Figure 1). Table 1 summarizes several studies[2–6] of the "markedly positive" test and shows that such a test is capable of predicting "critical" lesions in 23% to 82% of patients, the greater sensitivity being found in studies using the less rigid definition of S-T depression. The greater the degree of S-T depression seen and the earlier it appears during exercise, the more certain one can be that critical disease is present. In addition, Margolis[7] demonstrated that in a population with known coronary disease, the two-year survival was related to the stage of exercise at which ischemic S-T segment depression appeared (Table 2).

Table 3 looks at the incidence of "markedly positive" exercise ECG responses in patients with known left main coronary artery disease, and emphasizes the importance of the test in defining this particularly high risk group.[2–4,8,9] It is important to note also that therapy with propranolol does not seem to mask an ischemic response to exercise in patients with left main disease.

The Patient with Atypical Angina

Of greater *diagnostic* impact is the exercise test on the patient who presents with a chest pain syndrome that is not wholly typical for angina. Table 4 shows the potential impact of a normal or abnormal exercise test on the probability of disease in individuals with atypical angina, raising the probability of disease from approximately 50% (pretest) to 88% (post-test) with an abnormal test and lowering disease probability to around 25% with a normal test.[1]

Emphasis on the electrocardiographic response to exercise has been the rule throughout the history of exercise testing, and this myopic view has resulted in periodic disillusionment with the test.

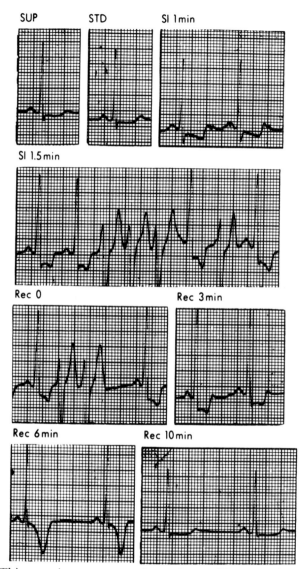

Figure 1. This exercise test was performed on a 67-year-old male school teacher who complained of classic angina pectoris. He was taking only sublingual nitroglycerin as needed. As shown in the figure, during exercise he developed ventricular tachycardia associated with 4 mm downsloping S-T depression, occurring at a low heart rate and workload. Subsequent coronary angiography demonstrated triple vessel disease with 100% obstruction of the left anterior descending, 90% obstruction of the left circumflex, and 95% obstruction of the right coronary artery.

Table 1

Relationship of a Marked Depth of S-T Segment Depression to the Extent of Coronary Artery Disease

Study	Kleiner et al.[2]	Cheitlin et al.[3]	Levites et al.[4]	Williams et al.[5]	Goldman et al.[6]
Number Patients with S-T Depression	35　2 mm	45　2 mm	26　2 mm	32　3 mm	26　3 mm
Percentage with LM Disease	23 LM	24 LM	15 LM	100% LM or LAD	0 LM
Percentage with LME Disease		29 LME	35 LME		
Percentage with LAD Disease		22 LAD		100% LM or LAD	92 LAD
Percentage with Multivessel Disease		82 Double or Triple vessel	50 ("Other lesions")	100 Double or Triple vessel	69 Triple vessel

LM = left main, LME = left main equivalent, LAD = left anterior descending
(Reprinted with permission of Harper & Row from: Glasser SP, Clark PI: *The Clinical Approach to Exercise Testing*, p. 34, 1980.)

Table 2
Comparison of Bruce Stage in which S-T Depression Occurs and the
Two-Year Medical and Surgical Survival

Stage	Medical (%)	Surgical (%)
I	54	82
II	67	86
III	84	92
IV	99	98

(Reproduced with permission of Harper & Row from: Glasser SP, Clark PI: *The Clinical Approach to Exercise Testing*, p. 29, 1980.)

Table 3
Incidence (%) of 2-mm or Greater S-T Depression in Subjects with Left
Main or Left Main Equivalent Disease from Five Studies

Kleiner et al.[2]	100
Cheitlin et al.[3]	100
Levites et al.[4]	100
Ellestad et al.[8]	67*
Salem et al.[9]	70†

*20% had negative S-T response
†4% had negative S-T response
(Reprinted with permission of Harper & Row from: Glasser SP, Clark PI: *The Clinical Approach to Exercise Testing*, p. 34, 1980.)

Table 4
Post-test Odds and Probabilities of Disease Related to Pretest Odds and
Probabilities

Clinical Presentation	Pretest Odds/Prob	Positive Test Post-test Odds/Prob	Negative Test Post-test Odds/Prob
Typical Angina	9:1/90%	63:1/98%	9:3/75%
Atypical Angina	1:1/50%	7:1/88%	1:3/25%
Asymptomatic	1:9/10%	7:9/44%	1:27/4%

(Reprinted with permission of Harper & Row from: Glasser SP, Clark PI: *The Clinical Approach to Exercise Testing*, p. 16, 1980.)

It is important to remember that the graded exercise test is an ideal extension of the patient's history and physical examination, and can provide valuable information about reproduction of symptoms and signs. Chest pain production during exercise has equal diagnostic impact to that of S-T segment depression (Table 5).[10] Failure of blood pressure or heart rate to rise with exercise is an ominously abnormal sign. The development of rales, S_3 or S_4 gallops, or new murmurs, excessive dyspnea, or excessive heart rate at low workloads may signal exercise-induced left ventricular dysfunction. Attention to all exercise parameters dramatically increases the ability of exercise testing to establish a functional assessment of the preoperative patient with suspected coronary obstructive disease.

The Asymptomatic Patient

When an adequate stress test fails to reveal ischemic S-T segment shifts, chest pain, or other abnormal signs and symptoms, it is unlikely that a clinical coronary event will be manifest over the ensuing few years. On the other hand, when an asymptomatic person develops S-T depression during exercise testing, he or she has a significantly increased risk (10 to 15 times) of a coronary

Table 5

Comparison of Exercise S-T Depression and Exercise Angina in the Diagnosis of Coronary Artery Disease (CAD) and Multivessel Disease (MVD)

	Number	Angiographic CAD (%)	MVD (%)
+ECG +EA	76	91	93
+ECG −EA	85	65	76
−ECG +EA	40	72	72
−ECG −EA	80	35	50

+ECG = ischemic S-T changes   −ECG = no S-T changes
+EA = exercise-induced angina   −EA = no angina with exercise
(Reprinted with permission of Harper & Row from: Glasser SP, Clark PI: *The Clinical Approach to Exercise Testing*, p. 49, 1980.)

event occurring within five to ten years. Bruce et al.[11] evaluated three test variables: exercise duration of less than six minutes, exercise-induced chest pain, and S-T segment depression. The combination of these variables appeared helpful in identifying apparently healthy men at risk of developing coronary disease. The risk of suffering a coronary morbid or mortal event is particularly striking when an asymptomatic individual has had a previously normal exercise test, followed by a "stress test conversion" to abnormal.[12] Abnormal exercise examination, therefore, represents a very powerful risk factor, and is even more significant than the standard risk factors.

The practice of treadmill testing for latent coronary artery disease in asymptomatic people has been criticized because of the high incidence of false–positive tests. Redwood et al.[13] argued that a positive test in an asymptomatic patient presents the physician (and patient) with a dilemma. On the one hand is the psychological impact that such a test result has on the patient, especially considering the high probability that no disease is present; on the other hand are the ethics involved in using the test result as a "threat" to induce the patient to practice better control of risk factors, when the odds may be against the patient having significant coronary disease. They concluded that the "physician who elects to conduct routine screening exercise tests should also be prepared to proceed with coronary arteriography despite its attendant inconvenience, cost, and risk."[13] We cannot agree with their conclusions. We feel that the discovery of an abnormal S-T response in an asymptomatic subject should be considered information that influences therapy. With a proper approach and sound advice, along with careful follow-up and serial testing, the abnormal test can be put in proper perspective to the patient's benefit.

We feel that exercise stress testing of the asymptomatic subject is indicated preoperatively in some patients, such as those known to be at high risk of latent coronary artery disease: hypertensives, smokers, those with known lipid abnormalities, those with strong family histories of premature coronary disease, and especially in those patients with other occlusive arterial disease. The finding of an abnormal stress test in such a patient should lead either to further diagnostic work-up or at least to more vigorous medical management and monitoring during surgery.

The Patient with Left Ventricular Dysfunction

Physical performance (functional) capacity is defined (for clinical purposes) as the maximal oxygen uptake an individual can achieve without experiencing limiting symptoms or signs.[14] The exercise test has been used to evaluate the functional capacity of patients with heart disease and is believed to be a more accurate measurement of the degree of cardiac impairment than the physician's assessment of functional classification by history. The relative lack of correlation between capacity for physical work and other objective measurements of the severity of cardiac lesion may at first seem to invalidate exercise testing as a clinical method. However, one should not lose sight of the fact that the patient's capacity for physical work provides a measure of the functional impact of a given lesion on the total oxygen transport system and, thus, does not necessarily correlate with the severity of the lesion in terms of anatomy or hemodynamic measurements.

When assessing the preoperative patient for functional capacity, there are several indices that we evaluate. Among them are the total exercise time, the functional aerobic impairment, and the percent of predicted oxygen consumption achieved. The total time a subject spends exercising in a given protocol can be used as an indicator of functional capacity by comparing his or her performance with that of age and sex matched individuals and, using standard nomograms, functional aerobic impairment can be estimated. Functional aerobic impairment is defined by Bruce as "the percentage deviation between the observed and predicted values for VO_2 max."[15] If the Bruce protocol is used for testing, and the patient is not allowed to bear any weight on the handrails, the treadmill duration time plotted against age on a standard nomogram[16] yields a functional aerobic impairment that is of adequate accuracy for clinical use.

Maximum oxygen consumption (VO_2 max) is the highest level of oxygen uptake that an exercising subject can achieve; that is, if physical work is further increased, oxygen consumption will fail to increase, having reached physiologic limits. Oxygen consumption is limited by cardiac output and by extraction of O_2 by the peripheral tissues (arteriovenous O_2 difference). Predicted VO_2 max for a healthy subject is influenced by age, sex, body weight, and level of habitual physical activity. The percent of predicted oxygen consumption that an individual achieves at peak exercise can also be estimated without complicated analysis of expired air. Since the functional aerobic impairment is the percent reduction in predicted oxygen uptake, the percent of normal predicted VO_2 max can be estimated by subtracting the functional aerobic impairment from 100%.[15] Thus, an individual with 30% impairment would have achieved approximately 70% of the VO_2 max predicted for his age, sex, and level of activity. A person with 0% impairment is estimated to have reached 100% of his predicted VO_2 max.

The exercise test can also be invaluable in assessing functional reserve by way of a thorough cardiovascular physical examination before and after exercise. New appearance of S_3 or S_4 gallops, murmurs of papillary muscle dysfunction, or rales are indicators of stress-induced left ventricular dysfunction. Significant shortness of breath and inappropriately high heart rate for a given exercise load are less specific, but may also indicate left ventricular failure. Failure of blood pressure or heart rate to rise with increasing work loads is a very ominous sign, placing the patient at very high risk for future cardiac morbid or mortal events.

The Patient with Valvular Heart Disease

Clinical quantification of decreased exercise tolerance is often difficult and unreliable in the presence of chronic valvular heart disease. The insidious onset of disease usually leads to gradual disability, which the patient may be unaware of or willing to disregard. Objective exercise testing can help to quantitate the degree of impairment of exercise capacity.

The degree of impairment of exercise capacity is a fairly good indicator of severity of mitral valve stenosis.[17] Exercise increases heart rate and decreases diastolic filling time; left atrial pressure rises, producing pulmonary capillary congestion and dyspnea. Limitation of exercise duration by fatigue is also a common finding, probably resulting from an inability to increase cardiac output to exercising muscles because of the fixed mitral obstruction.

The role of exercise testing in the functional evaluation of other forms of valvular heart disease is less well established. Aortic regurgitation, in particular, presents a therapeutic dilemma. Patients with aortic insufficiency may tolerate the lesion well, remaining asymptomatic for years, but once they become symptomatic, they may follow a rapid downhill course, when irreversible myocardial damage may be present. Unfortunately, dynamic exercise testing may prove of little value in detecting subclinical dysfunction. Exercise probably tends to normalize the hemodynamics of aortic regurgitation: higher heart rates reduce the regurgitant fraction, lower aortic diastolic pressure allows relatively early left ventricular decompression, and the lower peripheral resistance favors forward flow by reducing afterload.

Exertion can often uncover the symptoms of significant aortic stenosis (fatigue, dyspnea, dizziness, angina) but because significant aortic stenosis carries a risk of lethal ventricular arrhythmias and sudden death with exertion,[18] we are reluctant to routinely test these patients in the exercise laboratory and usually recommend early cardiac catheterization.

There are many situations in which the results of an exercise stress test would not significantly alter medical or surgical management, and the performance of the test itself might induce additional risk to the patient. The following case illustrates poor judgment in the application of exercise stress testing to preoperative assessment.

> A 55-year-old carpenter had a filling defect on barium enema that was thought to represent carcinoma of the colon. He had a history of chest pain thought by his physician to probably be angina, but with several atypical features. He had been taking a digitalis preparation for three years because of cardiomegaly and symptoms of congestive heart failure. Exercise testing was recommended by the Internal Medicine Consultant in order to evaluate his atypical chest pain. Because digitalis will cause exercise S-T segment depression in the absence of coronary artery disease, the test—and therefore the surgery—was postponed for two weeks for digitalis withdrawal. One week after discontinuing digitalis, the patient went into overt pulmonary edema and suffered an acute myocardial infarction.

In this case, the decision to perform exercise stress testing was, at best, ill-considered. The contemplated surgery was not elective in nature; no matter what the results of exercise testing, the surgery would have been necessary, and strict perioperative cardiac monitoring required. Preparation for stress testing off digitalis led to a situation of even higher risk for nonelective surgery.

On the other hand, exercise testing can provide information which leads to modification of management. An illustrative case is that of a 57-year-old high school physics teacher with known gallbladder disease. An episode of acute cholecystitis prompted scheduling for cholecystectomy. He had had chronic, stable angina for three years which was well controlled with propranolol and nitroglycerine. Exercise stress testing was performed without withdrawal of propranolol and yielded 3 mm S-T segment depression and chest pain at a low work load and heart rate. He underwent cardiac catheterization which revealed 90% obstruction of his left main coronary artery and 70% right coronary artery obstruction. He underwent aortocoronary bypass surgery and his gallbladder disease was treated conservatively.

As these cases illustrate, the safety and utility of exercise stress testing as a part of the preoperative management of the cardiac patient is individually related to the judgment with which the candidate for testing is selected. Of equal importance is the optimal choice of exercise end-points. It is good practice to consider all possible test results prior to testing and ask the question, "How will these results affect overall management?" Keeping these points in mind, the exercise stress test can become a powerful tool in preoperative assessment.

References

1. Glasser SP, Clark PI: *The Clinical Approach to Exercise Testing.* Hagerstown, Harper & Row, 1980.
2. Kleiner JP, Boland JM, Brundage BH: The markedly positive stress test. Is it an indicator of left main coronary disease (abstr). *Circulation* (Suppl) 53,54(II):206, 1976.
3. Cheitlin MD, Davia JE, DeCastro CM, et al.: Correlation of "critical" left coronary artery lesions with positive submaximal exercise tests in patients with chest pain. *Am Heart J* 89:305, 1975.
4. Levites R, Anderson GJ: Detection of critical coronary artery lesions by treadmill exercise testing (abstr). *Circulation* (Suppl) 53,54(II):11, 1976.
5. Williams DO, Capone RJ, Most AS: The "strongly positive exercise test": An indication for aggressive management of angina pectoris (abstr). *Circulation* (Suppl) 53,54(II):10, 1976.
6. Goldman S, Tselos S, Cohn K: Marked depth of ST-segment depression during treadmill exercise testing. Indicator of severe coronary artery disease. *Chest* 69:729, 1976.

 7. Margolis JR: Treadmill stage as a predictor of medical and surgical survival in coronary disease (abstr). *Circulation* (Suppl) 51,52(II):109, 1975.
 8. Ellestad MH: *Stress Testing.* Philadelphia, FA Davis, 1975.
 9. Salem BI, Terasawa M, Mathur VS, et al.: Exercise testing and left main coronary artery disease: Experience with 57 patients. *Cardiovascular Diseases,* Bulletin of the Texas Heart Institute 5:384, 1978.
10. Weiner DA, McCabe C, Hueter D, et al.: The predictive value of chest pain as an indicator of coronary disease during exercise testing (abstr). *Circulation* (Suppl) 54,55(II):10, 1976.
11. Bruce RA, DeRouen TA: Exercise testing as a predictor of heart disease and sudden death. *Hospital Practice* September 1978, p. 69.
12. Doyle JT, Kinch SH: The prognosis of an abnormal electrocardiographic stress test. *Circulation* 41:545, 1970.
13. Redwood DR, Borer JS, Epstein SE: Whither the S-T segment during exercise? Editorial. *Circulation* 54:703, 1976.
14. Blomqvist CG, Mitchell JH: Heart disease and dynamic exercise testing. In Willerson JT, Sanders CA (Eds.): *Clinical Cardiology.* New York, Grune & Stratton, p. 213, 1977.
15. Bruce RA: Progress in exercise cardiology. In Yu PN, Goodwin JF (Eds.): *Progress in Cardiology,* Vol. 3. Philadelphia, Lea & Febiger, 1974.
16. Bruce RA, Kusumi F, Hosmer D: Maximal oxygen intake and nomographic assessment of functional aerobic impairment in cardiovascular disease. *Am Heart J* 85:546, 1973.
17. Chapman CB, Mitchell JH, Sproule BJ, et al.: The maximal oxygen intake test in patients with predominant mitral stenosis. *Circulation* 22:4, 1960.
18. Jokl E, McClellan JT (Eds.): *Exercise and Cardiac Death.* Baltimore, University Park Press, p. 41, 1971.

CHAPTER VI

Echocardiography

Stephen P. Glasser, M.D.
and Pamela I. Clark, R.N.

Echocardiography has joined the other established noninvasive modalities (history, physical examination, electrocardiogram, and chest x-ray) as an important means of helping to assess many heart problems that arise in clinical practice. In some situations, an echocardiogram will support a suspected diagnosis or define a differential diagnosis, provide important information regarding severity and prognosis, and may be useful in follow-up to assess progression of disease, effect of therapy, or need for surgical intervention. An echocardiogram can often supply information not obtainable by any other diagnostic technique, or may yield information otherwise available only via cardiac catheterization. The use of echocardiography may, thus, avoid or delay the need for catheterization in some patients.

The echocardiogram may be useful in the perioperative evaluation of patients with heart disease in a number of ways. Table 1 lists some clinical subsets and the relative value of the technique in the diagnosis of heart disease or in assessing its severity. Echocardiography is not a substitute for a careful history and physical examination, but when the usual clinical assessment fails to satisfactorily explain a patient's presentation, or when further definition of the severity of heart disease is required, echocardiography may be extremely helpful.

The use of echocardiography as it relates to the perioperative period will be briefly discussed according to the outline presented in Table 1.

Table 1

Clinical Presentations in which Echocardiography May Be Helpful

---

HEART MURMUR
    Unexplained
        Valvular heart disease (D)
        Idiopathic hypertrophic subaortic stenosis (D)
        Mitral annular calcification (D)
        Myxoma (D)
        Congestive heart disease (S)
        Functional murmur versus bicuspid valve (S)
        Infective endocarditis (S)
    Valvular heart disease
        Aortic stenosis (S)
        Aortic insufficiency (S)
        Mitral stenosis (D)
        Myocardial infarction (S)
        Mitral valve prolapse (D)

ASSESSMENT OF LEFT VENTRICULAR FUNCTION (S)
    Cardiomegaly (D)

HYPERTENSION (S)

CHEST PAIN
    Coronary artery disease/ventricular aneurysm (S)
    Mitral valve prolapse (D)
    Idiopathic hypertrophic subaortic stenosis (D)
    Aortic stenosis (S)
    Dissection (S)
    Pericarditis with pericardial effusion (D)

POSTOPERATIVE FEVER (S)

(D) = Diagnostic
(S) = Suggestive

Assessment of Left Ventricular Function

Perhaps the most frequent and effective application of echocardiography to preoperative assessment is in the patient with suspected left ventricular dysfunction. Harlan et al.[1] have shown that some of the standard signs and symptoms of congestive heart failure may have poor sensitivity and/or specificity (see Chapter 16), resulting in a poor predictive accuracy for the diagnosis of heart disease. Table 2[1] demonstrates that dyspnea, for example, occurred in 66% of patients with congestive heart failure (sensitivity).

Table 2

Sensitivity, Specificity, and Predictive Value (n = 329) of Descriptors
Related to Congestive Heart Failure

Descriptor	Sensitivity %	Specificity %	Predictive Value* %
Dyspnea	66	52	23
Orthopnea	21	81	2
Paroxysmal nocturnal dyspnea	33	76	26
Edema by history	23	80	22
History of inotropic therapy	47	77	34
Heart rate 100/min at rest	7	99	6
Rales	13	91	27
Edema by examination	10	93	3
Ventricular gallop sound (S₃)	31	95	61
Neck vein distension	10	97	2
Hepatojugular reflux**	17	91	—
Cardiomegaly by radiography	62	67	32

*Predictive value[12] = $\dfrac{(P)\,(Se)}{(P)\,(Se) + (1 - P)\,(1 - Sp)}$, where *P* is prevalence, *Se* is sensitivity, and *Sp* is specificity. For each symptom or sign, this value indicates the likelihood that a positive test will identify an affected individual in a population where the prevalence of failure (as defined in this study) is approximately 20%.

**Available only on 121 patients. (Reprinted with permission of American College of Physicians and William R. Harlan, M.D.: Harlan WR, Oberman A, Grimm R, Rosati RA: *Annals of Internal Medicine* 86:133, 1977.)

However, dyspnea occurs in many situations where congestive failure is not the cause, and in Harlan's study the specificity of this symptom for heart failure was 52%. The resultant predictive value of dyspnea for congestive heart failure, therefore, was only 23%. In contrast, neck vein distention was noted in only 3% of subjects without congestive heart failure (specificity 97%); but, since it occurred in only 10% of patients with congestive heart failure (sensitivity 10%), the predictive value was again low (2%).

Echocardiography has been used to evaluate left ventricular function, but a number of constraints are present.[2] Years ago, it was suggested that the shape of the left ventricle approximates that of a prolate ellipse. A prolate ellipse is a geometric structure in which the short diameters are one-half the length and this allows one to calculate its volume, using the formula:

$$V = 4/3 \; II \cdot \frac{L}{2} \cdot \frac{D_1}{2} \cdot \frac{D_2}{2}$$

Since the left ventricle contracts primarily by shortening its minor diameter, it was felt that one could approximate end systolic and end diastolic volumes (and, thereby, stroke volume; ejection fraction and/or cardiac output) by measuring the left ventricular transverse diameter at end systole and end diastole. Because of the number of assumptions made but, more importantly, because these tenets hold only in normally shaped left ventricles (Figure 1) these measurements are gross, at best. Nonetheless, there are a number of other echographic parameters that do correlate with impairment of left ventricular function (LV dilatation, change in systolic to diastolic dimension less than 25%, poor aortic root motion, early aortic valve closure, inordinate mitral to septal separation, etc.). It is unlikely that an entirely normal echocardiogram will be recorded in the presence of significant left ventricular dysfunction.

Cardiomegaly

Cardiomegaly found on physical examination or chest x-ray is another common presentation of cardiac disease. The signs and symptoms of cardiac disease are relatively limited, but a common denominator of almost all lesions of hemodynamic significance is cardiac enlargement.

Although a clinical examination will suggest cardiomegaly and an x-ray of the chest will show an enlarged cardiac silhouette, they cannot differentiate the causes of cardiomegaly. Echocardiography is an excellent noninvasive tool for this purpose, since it can delineate specifically which chamber or chambers are enlarged (Figure 2), suggest possible etiologies, and assess hemodynamic severity. The echocardiogram might reveal that the enlarged cardiac silhouette is not heart at all but, rather, due to pericardial effusion.

Hypertension

Hypertensive heart disease remains the single most common cause of congestive heart failure. Because left ventricular hypertrophy usually precedes overt failure, its early and accurate diagnosis is important and may influence mortality, morbidity, and care

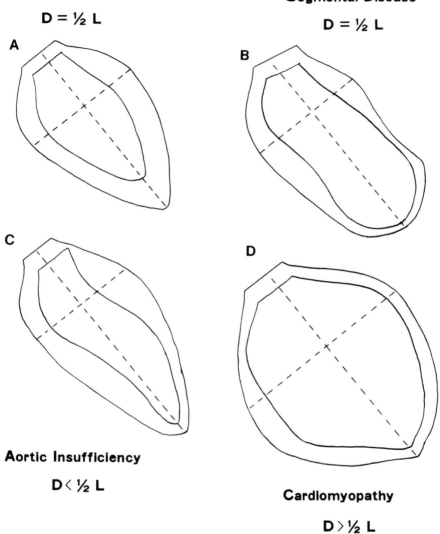

Figure 1. M-mode echocardiography to estimate left ventricular function must be utilized cautiously. The volume formula for a prolate ellipse applies only to the normal ventricle A. Note the possible errors by improper utilization of the formula in B. Segmental nature of coronary disease, C. Aortic insufficiency, and D. Cardiomyopathy. D = diameter, L = length.

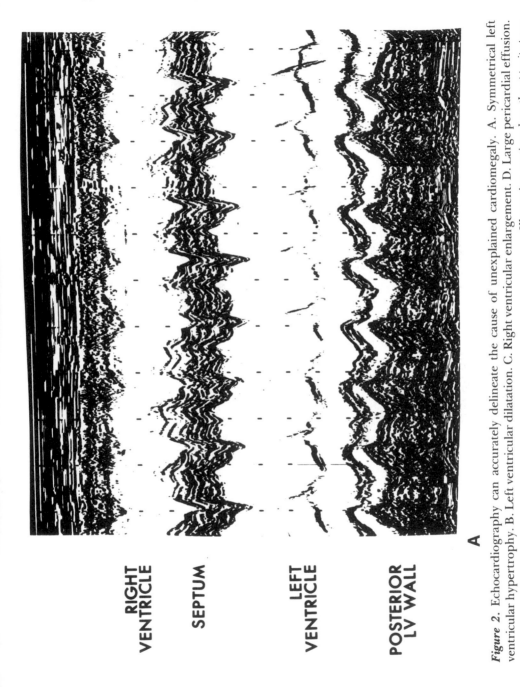

RIGHT VENTRICLE

SEPTUM

LEFT VENTRICLE

POSTERIOR LV WALL

A

Figure 2. Echocardiography can accurately delineate the cause of unexplained cardiomegaly. A. Symmetrical left ventricular hypertrophy. B. Left ventricular dilatation. C. Right ventricular enlargement. D. Large pericardial effusion.

Illustration continued on the opposite page

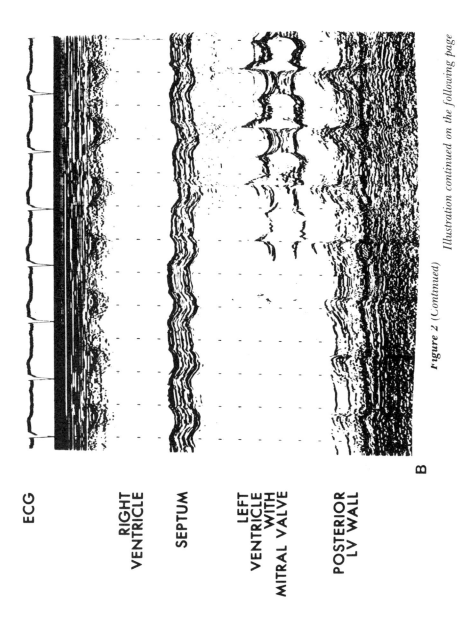

ECG

RIGHT VENTRICLE

SEPTUM

LEFT VENTRICLE WITH MITRAL VALVE

POSTERIOR LV WALL

B

Figure 2 (Continued)

Illustration continued on the following page

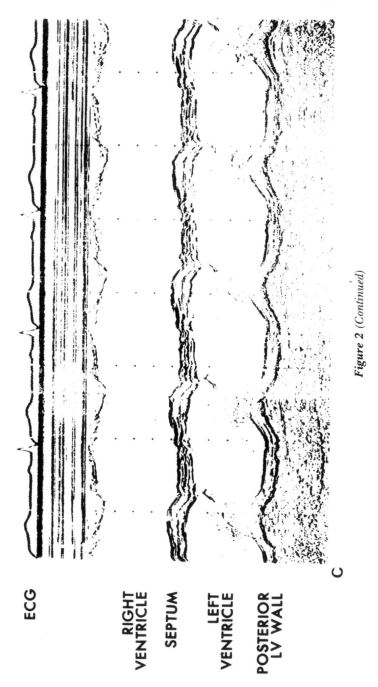

Figure 2 (*Continued*)

Illustration continued on the opposite page

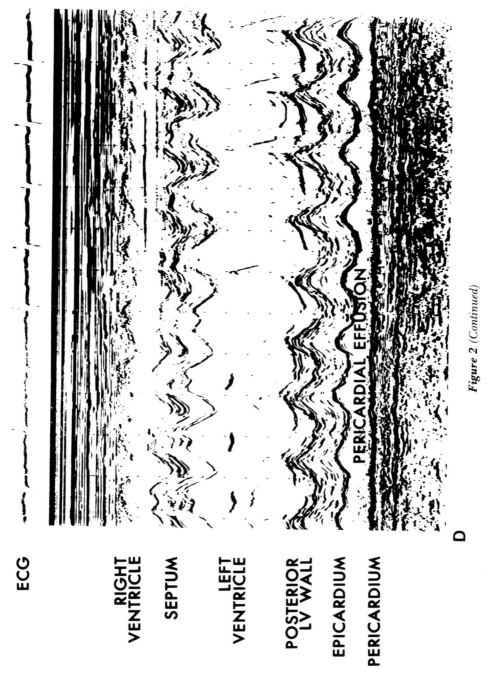

ECG

RIGHT
VENTRICLE

SEPTUM

LEFT
VENTRICLE

POSTERIOR
LV WALL

EPICARDIUM

PERICARDIUM

PERICARDIAL EFFUSION

D

Figure 2 *(Continued)*

Illustration continued on the following page

(see Chapter 15). Echocardiography provides a direct means of assessing both functional and anatomic abnormalities of the heart (Figure 2) and several studies have applied this knowledge to the evaluation of the hypertensive patient. Savage et al.[3] studied 234 asymptomatic subjects with mild to moderate systemic hypertension and found increased ventricular septal and/or left ventricular wall thickness in 61%. Other abnormalities included left atrial enlargement, left ventricular enlargement, and aortic root enlargement (5–7%), decreased mitral valve closing velocity (E-F slope) in 6%, and a decreased ejection fraction in 15%. In contrast, less than 10% of those same hypertensive subjects had abnormal 12-lead ECGs or abnormal chest x-rays. This demonstrated the high prevalence of cardiac abnormalities in a population of asymptomatic subjects. It is not yet known how this may affect a patient in the perioperative period.

Unexplained Murmur

When cardiac murmurs are heard, but the etiology remains unclear, the following causes should be considered:

Valvular heart disease   Mitral subannular calcification
Cardiomyopathy   Congenital heart disease
  Hypertrophic   Left atrial myxoma
  Congestive   Functional murmur

Valvular Heart Disease

The importance of echocardiography in the diagnosis of valvular heart disease is well established. Abnormalities of cusp motion or unusual thickening, narrowing of the valve orifice, and increased echo density (suggesting fibrosis or calcification) provide specific qualitative information. The common valvular lesions in adults are, of course, stenosis or incompetency of the aortic or mitral valves.

Valvular aortic stenosis presents echocardiographically as a dense band of echoes recorded from the aortic cusps (Figure 3). The degree of cusp separation roughly coincides with the severity of the stenosis, but many factors interfere with the accuracy of measurement of separation so that, in any individual case, quan-

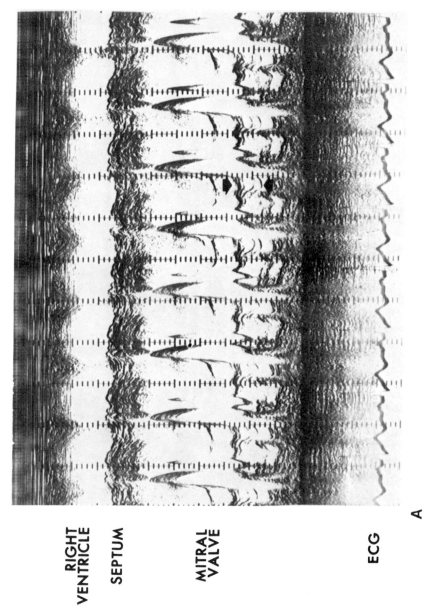

RIGHT
VENTRICLE

SEPTUM

MITRAL
VALVE

ECG

A

Figure 3. The unexplained systolic murmur may be evaluated by echocardiography. A. Mitral valve prolapse. B. Aortic stenosis with marked left ventricular dysfunction. C. Idiopathic hypertrophic subaortic stenosis. D. Flail mitral leaflet.

Illustration continued on the following page

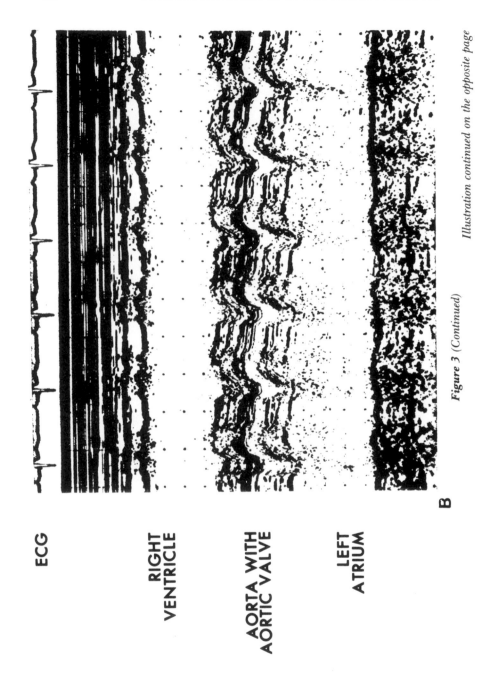

ECG

RIGHT
VENTRICLE

AORTA WITH
AORTIC VALVE

LEFT
ATRIUM

B

Illustration continued on the opposite page

Figure 3 (Continued)

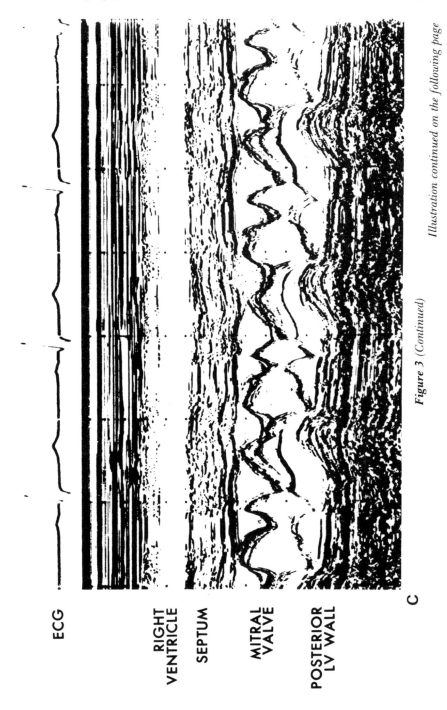

ECG

RIGHT VENTRICLE

SEPTUM

MITRAL VALVE

POSTERIOR LV WALL

C

Figure 3 (Continued)

Illustration continued on the following page

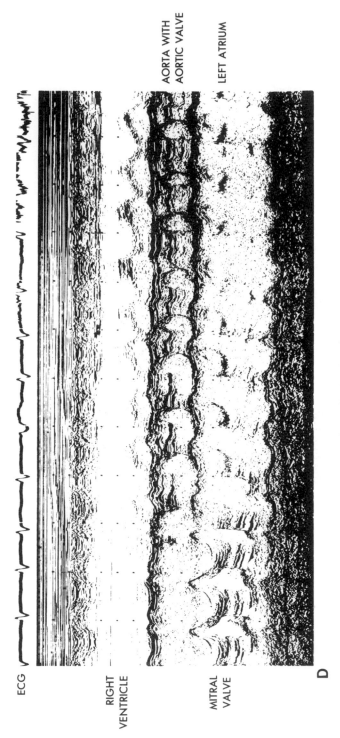

ECG

RIGHT
VENTRICLE

MITRAL
VALVE

AORTA WITH
AORTIC VALVE

LEFT ATRIUM

D

Figure 3 (Continued)

tification of cusp excursion has limited value. The severity of stenosis is better assessed by the associated degree of left ventricular hypertrophy and assessment of wall motion. Two dimensional echocardiography will probably prove to be a superior method for directly measuring the aortic valve orifice. Thus, the need for bacterial endocarditis prophylaxis would be indicated if abnormal valve echoes were visualized, and a reassessment of the severity of the aortic valve obstruction or need for preoperative cardiac catheterization may be necessary if left ventricular hypertrophy or poor aortic valve cusp separation is present.

Aortic regurgitation can also be suggested by echocardiography. Valvular abnormalities, as described above, may be present but the characteristic finding is a fine high frequency fluttering of the anterior mitral valve leaflet and/or septal wall during diastole, thought to result from the regurgitant jet striking these structures (Figure 4). The oscillations do not indicate severity, however; again, severity of the lesion is best judged by its consequences on left ventricular size and function. One sign of severe aortic insufficiency is premature closure of the mitral valve, a result of inordinately high left ventricular diastolic pressure, with a larg regurgitant volume filling a normal sized, relatively noncompliant left ventricle. As with aortic stenosis, antibiotic prophylaxis is indicated but, more importantly, left ventricular size and left ventricular wall contractility will reflect left ventricular function.

The echocardiogram may be helpful in suggesting the etiology of mitral regurgitation. In rheumatic mitral insufficiency, the valve leaflets are thickened and opening motion and diastolic motion is abnormal. Due to commissural fusion, abnormal posterior leaflet motion may also be evident. On the other hand, when mitral regurgitation is due to mitral valve prolapse (Figure 3), valve excursion is increased, and systolic posterior (rather than anterior) motion is present. Calcification of the mitral annulus and idiopathic hypertrophic subaortic stenosis also have characteristic echocardiographic features. All probably indicate the need for antibiotic prophylaxis (although there is some controversy with mitral prolapse and, perhaps, mitral annular calcification).

The echocardiographic features of mitral stenosis are characteristic and quite diagnostic (Figure 4). They consist of thickening of the leaflets with increased density (suggesting the accompanying fibrosis and/or calcification), decreased closing velocity of the anterior mitral leaflet (E–F slope) reduced excursion of the anterior leaflet (D–E) and abnormal motion of the posterior mitral leaflet

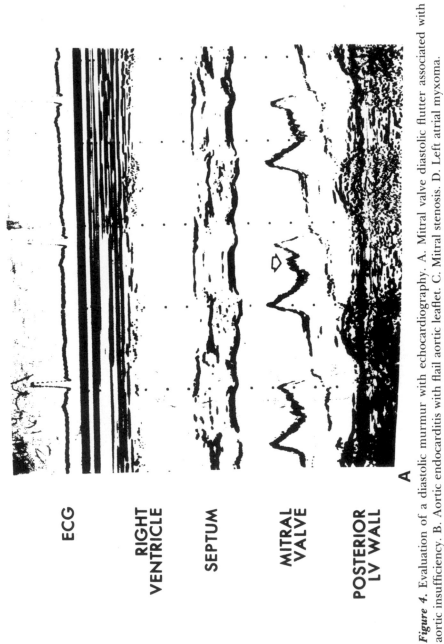

Figure 4. Evaluation of a diastolic murmur with echocardiography. A. Mitral valve diastolic flutter associated with aortic insufficiency. B. Aortic endocarditis with flail aortic leaflet. C. Mitral stenosis. D. Left atrial myxoma.

Illustration continued on the opposite page

ECG

RIGHT VENTRICLE

SEPTUM

MITRAL VALVE

POSTERIOR LV WALL

A

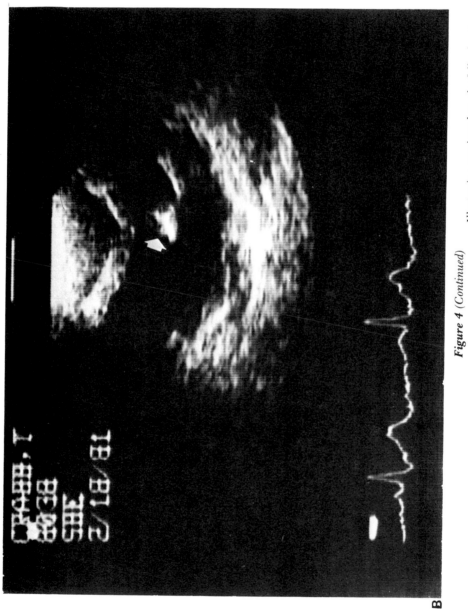

Figure 4 (*Continued*)

Illustration continued on the following page

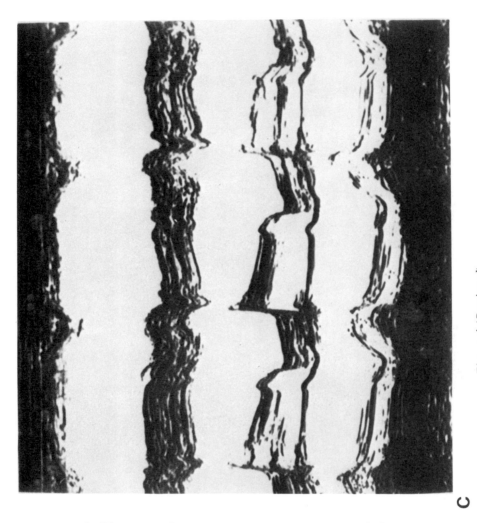

RIGHT
VENTRICLE

SEPTUM

MITRAL
VALVE

POSTERIOR
LV WALL

C

Figure 4 (Continued)

Illustration continued on the opposite page

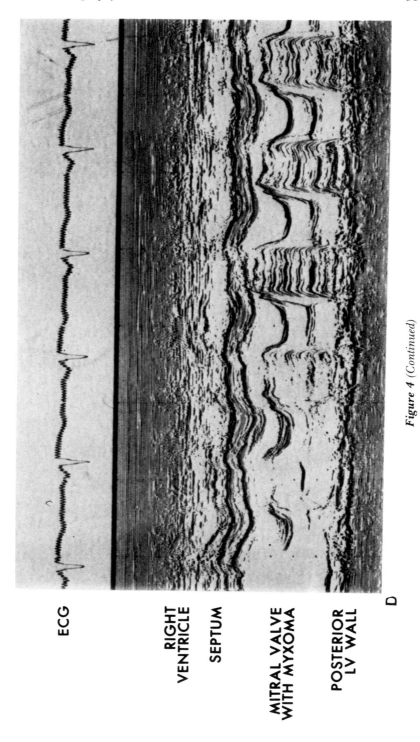

ECG

RIGHT
VENTRICLE

SEPTUM

MITRAL VALVE
WITH MYXOMA

POSTERIOR
LV WALL

D

Figure 4 (Continued)

(a result of the commissural fusion characteristic of rheumatic val-
vulitis). Edmiston et al.[4] evaluated the sensitivity, specificity, and
diagnostic limitations of several variables in 63 patients with mitral
stenosis confirmed by cardiac catheterization and 69 patients with
other confirmed cardiac defects eliciting physical or certain echocardiographic findings that may be mistaken for those of mitral
stenosis. An E–F slope of less than 40 mm/sec was 90% sensitive
for mitral stenosis and specificity was 93%. Anterior or flat posterior leaflet motion was 79% sensitive, but 100% specific. In contrast, a D–E excursion of less than 20 mm was only 78% sensitive
and had poor specificity (38%—that is many conditions other than
mitral stenosis reduce mitral valve excursion).

Although conventional single dimensional echocardiography is
a sensitive noninvasive method for documenting the presence of
rheumatic mitral valve disease, it is more limited in predicting its
severity. The hemodynamic severity of the lesion is estimated not
from the mitral valve, but from left atrial and right ventricular
enlargement and other indicators of pulmonary hypertension. As
with aortic stenosis, preliminary studies with two dimensional sector scanning have shown promising results for accurately determining orifice size.

Left atrial myxoma manifests a characteristic pattern and echocardiography is clearly the procedure of choice when that lesion
is suspected (Figure 4). Congenital heart diseases often have typical
echocardiographic features, but a detailed discussion is beyond the
scope of this chapter. The reader is referred to one of several good
textbooks available on that subject. One fairly common situation
in which echocardiography may be helpful is in the evaluation of
a soft systolic basal murmur. Although it can usually be concluded
from the clinical evaluation that the lesion is hemodynamically
mild, the question of bacterial endocarditis prophylaxis is raised.
If the murmur is felt to be a benign functional (innocent) murmur,
no prophylaxis is indicated; but, occasionally, the murmur of a
nonstenotic bicuspid aortic valve may be the cause, and here prophylaxis is utilized. About 70% of bicuspid valves will result in an
abnormality on echocardiography. Unfortunately, on occasion,
normal aortic valves will show echocardiographic abnormalities
similar to bicuspid valve so that clinical judgment remains the
mainstay in the decision for prophylaxis.

Chest Pain

When the diagnosis of chest pain is the question, several conditions exist in which echocardiography may be useful. If a cardiac murmur is present, valvular aortic stenosis, idiopathic hypertrophic subaortic stenosis, and mitral valve prolapse are considerations, and each has characteristic echocardiographic abnormalities. If careful examination fails to reveal a murmur, pericardial disease and coronary artery disease are possibilities. The echocardiogram is an extremely sensitive tool for diagnosing pericardial fluid (as little as 25–50 cc may produce an echo-free space between the pericardium and the epicardium). Of course, pericarditis can be present with no significant effusion, so one cannot with certainty rule this out if no pericardial fluid is seen.

The most common echocardiographic abnormality seen in coronary artery disease is abnormal motion of left ventricular wall segments. It is detected in up to 85% of patients with acute transmural myocardial infarction, and its location closely corresponds to the electrocardiographic site of infarction.[5] Thus, the left septal and/or anterior left ventricular wall echoes are abnormal with anterior infarction and the posterior left ventricular wall is abnormal with inferior infarction. The abnormal motion may be less than normal, absent or paradoxical, but motion pattern alone does not distinguish between acute and chronic coronary artery disease. Abnormal motion also occurs with subendocardial infarction, but is generally of a lesser degree. Compensatory hyperdynamic motion may be seen in adjacent normal myocardium. In addition to wall motion abnormalities are abnormalities in systolic wall thickening.[6] Thinning of the wall during systole has been reported to occur only in acute ischemia or infarction. Although abnormalities of motion are not specific for coronary artery disease, the fact that the abnormalities are nearly segmental does help to differentiate it from a congestive cardiomyopathy of other etiology, in which the abnormalities are more global. The major limitation in using echocardiography to diagnose coronary artery disease has been the technical difficulty of examining all of the left ventricle. Two-dimensional sector scanning has improved upon this limitation and has expanded its use in the evaluation of patients with suspected ventricular aneurysm.

Postoperative Fever

A special situation exists when postoperative fever occurs, particularly in patients with known cardiac structural defects. Here, of course, the question of endocarditis is raised. When a classic valvular vegetation is echocardiographically visualized (Figure 4), the diagnosis is clear, but it has been shown by a number of studies that echocardiographic vegetations are visualized in only 30–50% of patients with documented endocarditis (Table 3).[7-19] In addition, in patients with valvular disease, the diagnosis is rendered more difficult because the leaflets are already thickened and more dense, due to the associated fibrosis and calcification. Secondary findings of endocarditis are also more difficult to evaluate (e.g., diastolic mitral valve flutter suggesting aortic regurgitation could be due to endocarditits, but might also be the result of the original aortic valve disease). Here, a preoperative echocardiogram, if available for comparison, may prove valuable, but it probably is not cost-effective to obtain preoperative echocardiograms on all patients with valvular disease solely for this purpose.

Although the echocardiogram is a test commonly used to aid in the diagnosis of bacterial endocarditis, its independent diagnostic

Table 3

Echocardiographic Sensitivity in Previous Studies Reviewing Apparently Unselected Patients with Known Endocarditis

Principal Investigator	Patients	Vegetations Detected	Sensitivity
Wann, 1976[7]	65	22	34%
Roy, 1976[8]	84	27	84%
Young, 1977[9]	59	23	39%
Thomson, 1977[10]	20	11	55%
Naik, 1978[11]	9	9	100%
Hoche, 1978[12]	56	34	61%
Martin, 1978[13]	40	5	13%
Gura, 1978[14]	78	36	46%
Ibrahim, 1978[15]	9	6	67%
Mintz, 1979[16]	22	9	41%
Strom, 1979[17]	30	17	57%
Wann, 1979[18]	23	18	78%
Stewart, 1980[19]	87	47	54%
Total	582	264	45%

impact is often not considered. Woodrow et al.[20] assessed the utility
of the echocardiogram to diagnose or exclude bacterial endocarditis in 66 patients. Four patients with definite vegetations on M-
mode echocardiograms had endocarditis, while none of 26 patients
with entirely normal echocardiograms had endocarditis. Thus, in
30 of the 66 subjects, the echocardiogram was useful in ruling in
or out endocarditis. However, the overall sensitivity of the echocardiogram was only 39%, since failure to visualize vegetations on
otherwise abnormal valves (the most common result) had little diagnostic impact in excluding endocarditis.

Thus, the echocardiogram can be an invaluable aid in perioperative assessment. It is when the history and/or physical examination leave significant doubt as to the etiology or severity of the
cardiac problem, or symptoms and signs do not seem to correlate
with each other or with ancillary tests, such as the electrocardiogram or chest x-ray, that echocardiography should be considered.
Markiewicz et al.[21] asssessed the contribution of M-mode echocardiography to cardiac diagnosis in 1,000 successive subjects (Table
4). In 447 patients in which the clinician reached a diagnosis fol-

Table 4
Contribution to Diagnosis in Group A Patients (N = 447)

Clinical Diagnosis	Echocardiographic Findings (no.)		
	Unsuspected Diagnosis*	Confirmatory Diagnosis**	Normal
Valvular heart disease	23	124	17
Mitral valve prolapse	6	30	29
Pericardial disease	3	36	20
Congestive cardiomyopathy	8	24	6
Asymmetric septal hypertrophy	5	7	4
Endocarditis	—	4	9
	45 (10%)	225 (50%)	85 (19%)

*Refers to patients in whom the echocardiographic study demonstrated a dis-
ease, unsuspected clinically.
**Refers to patients in whom the echocardiographic diagnosis was similar to the
clinical diagnosis.
(Reprinted with permission of Dun-Donnelley Publishing Corporation and Walter
Markiewicz: Markiewicz W, Peled B, Hammerman H, et al: *American Journal of
Medicine* 65:803, 1976.)

lowing his initial evaluation, a disorder was unsuspected prior to echocardiography in 10%, and echocardiography confirmed the clinician diagnosis in 50%. In 19%, the echocardiographic findings were normal. Thus, although a normal echocardiogram does not rule out cardiac disease in all cases, it almost certainly mitigates against significant valvular disease, left ventricular dysfunction, and/or pericardial effusion, and is a valuable addition to the data base.

References

1. Harlan WR, Oberman A, Grimm R, et al.: Chronic congestive heart failure in coronary artery disease: Clinical criteria. *Ann Intern Med* 86:133, 1977.
2. Fortuin NJ, Pawsey CGK: The evaluation of left ventricular function by echocardiography. *Am J Med* 63:1, 1977.
3. Savage DD, Drayer J, Henry WL, et al.: Echocardiographic assessment of cardiac anatomy and function in hypertensive subjects. *Circulation* 59:623, 1979.
4. Edmiston WA, Kim SJ, Allen JW: Echographic diagnosis of mitral stenosis. *Cardiovasc Med* 3:59, 1978.
5. Kerber RE, Marcus ML, Ehrhardt J, et al.: Correlation between echocardiographically demonstrated segmental dyskinesis and regional myocardial perfusion. *Circulation* 52:1097, 1975.
6. Kerber RE, Marcus ML, Wilson R, et al.: Effects of acute coronary occlusion on the motion and perfusion of the normal and ischemic interventricular septum. *Circulation* 54:928, 1976.
7. Wann LS, Dillon JC, Weyman AE, et al.: Echocardiography in bacterial endocarditis. *N Engl J Med* 295:135, 1976.
8. Roy P, Tajik AJ, Giuliana ER, et al.: Spectrum of echocardiographic findings in bacterial endocarditis. *Circulation* 53:474, 1976.
9. Young DW, Guinones MA, Ishimori T, et al.: Prognostic significance of valvular vegetations identified by M-mode echocardiography in infective endocarditis. Circulation 58(Suppl II):41 (abstr), 1978.
10. Thomson KR, Nanda NC, Gramiak R: The reliability of echocardiography in the diagnosis of infective endocarditis. *Radiology* 125:473, 1977.
11. Naik DR, Ward C, Hardisty C: The role of echocardiography in suspected infective endocarditis. *Clinical Radiology* 29:381, 1978.
12. Hoche JP, King DL: Sensitivity and specificity of echocardiography in the diagnosis of infective endocarditis. In White D, Lyons EA (Eds.): *Ultrasound in Medicine*, Vol 4. New York, Plenum Press, p. 9, 1978.
13. Martin RP, Meltzer RS, Chia BL, et al.: The clinical utility of two-dimensional echocardiography in bacterial endocarditis. *Circulation* 58 (Suppl II):187 (abstr), 1978.

14. Gura GM, Tajik AJ, Seward JB: Correlation of initial echocardiographic findings with outcome in patients with bacterial endocarditis. *Circulation* 58 (Suppl II):232 (abstr), 1978.
15. Ibrahim MM, El-Said G: Echocardiographic findings in bacterial endocarditis. *Cardiovascular Disease,* Bulletin Texas Heart Institute 5:337, 1978.
16. Mintz GS, Kotler MN, Segal BL, et al.: Comparison of two-dimensional and M-mode echocardiography in the evaluation of patients with infective endocarditis. *Am J Cardiol* 43:738, 1979.
17. Strom J, Davis R, Frishman W, et al.: The demonstration of vegetations by echocardiography in bacterial endocarditis: An indication for early surgical intervention. *Circulation* 60 (Suppl II):37 (abstr), 1979.
18. Wann LS, Hallam CC, Dillon JC, et al.: Comparison of M-mode and cross-sectional echocardiography in infective endocarditis. *Circulation* 60:728, 1979.
19. Stewart JA, Silimperi D, Harris P, et al.: Echocardiographic documentation of vegetative lesions in infective endocarditis: Clinical implications. *Circulation* 61(2):374, 1980.
20. Woodrow TW, Glasser SP, Clark PI, et al.: The independent impact of M-mode echocardiography on the diagnosis of suspected endocarditis. *J Cardiovas Ultrasonography,* in press.
21. Markiewicz W, Peled B, Hammerman H, et al.: Contribution of M-mode echocardiography to cardiac diagnosis. *Am J Med* 65:803, 1978.

CHAPTER VII

Noninvasive Assessment of Peripheral Vascular Diseases

William M. Blackshear, Jr., M.D.
and Patricia Miscioscia, R.N.

The patient with atherosclerotic heart disease also often suffers from the effects of atherosclerosis in the peripheral arterial system. The association between coronary atherosclerosis and carotid artery occlusive disease is well documented, and many patients who present with severe ischemia of the lower extremities also have symptomatic coronary artery disease. Furthermore, patients with valvular disease, mural thrombus, or chronic atrial arrhythmias run the risk of peripheral arterial thromboembolic complications. In addition to arterial diseases, patients with chronic congestive heart failure are more prone to develop acute deep venous thrombosis, particularly in the postoperative period. In this section, we will review commonly available noninvasive techniques which can be used by a trained vascular laboratory technician for the diagnosis and quantitation of carotid artery disease, peripheral arterial occlusive disease, and acute deep venous thrombosis.

Carotid Artery Disease

Atherosclerotic disease of the internal carotid artery may produce symptoms by one of two basic mechanisms. First, hemispheric blood flow may be reduced ipsilateral to a high grade (>50% diameter reduction) stenosis or occlusion of the internal carotid artery. Second, thrombotic or atherosclerotic material present within an ulcerated plaque may embolize to the intracranial vessels producing a more localized area of ischemia. Lesions which reduce cerebral blood flow may produce transient episodes of ischemia (TIAs), completed strokes, or symptoms due to a generalized reduction in hemispheric blood flow, (vertigo, confusion, "vertebrobasilar" symptoms). Emboli to the intracranial circulation may also produce TIAs, amaurosis fugax, or strokes. The patient with symptomatic carotid occlusive disease is at increased risk for stroke and should be promptly evaluated so that appropriate therapy can be initiated.

An asymptomatic cervical bruit detected on routine physical examination may signify the presence of a previously unsuspected high grade internal carotid stenosis. Although only 60% of such bruits are in fact associated with potentially flow reducing internal carotid lesions, this finding is often a cause of concern, particularly if the patient is soon to undergo a major operation. The risk of stroke with an asymptomatic carotid stenosis is not well established and data on this point is often contradictory. Many authorities feel, however, that patients with high-grade internal carotid stenoses are prone to suffer spontaneous strokes, particularly during an episode of hypotension which may occur during a major surgical procedure.

Four vessel multiview angiography of the carotid bifurcation is an accurate method of detecting carotid occlusive disease; however, because of its expense and small but definite risk of complications, it cannot be used as a screening examination nor can it be used repeatedly to follow the course of previously documented plaques. In addition, many physicians are reluctant to recommend angiography for the patient with somewhat atypical symptoms or for the asymptomatic patient with a cervical bruit.

Because of the problems inherent with angiography, a variety of noninvasive examinations have been developed in recent years which are designed to detect carotid lesions. All of these studies are safe, painless, and can be performed on outpatients as well as inpatients. They can be repeated frequently to detect disease progression. For purposes of discussion carotid artery examinations may be divided into indirect and direct studies.

Indirect Studies

Indirect tests for carotid occlusive disease measure parameters in the periorbital region related to ophthalmic artery pressure and flow. The ophthalmic artery is the first branch of the internal carotid artery (ICA), originating shortly after the ICA enters the cranium. It gives rise to the retinal artery and to the supraorbital and frontal arteries which supply the periorbital tissues superior to the inner half of the globe. A high-grade (>50% diameter reduction) ICA stenosis or occlusion may reduce pressure and flow in the ipsilateral cerebral hemisphere and ophthalmic artery. Therefore a positive result with an indirect carotid examination suggests the presence of a flow reducing carotid lesion. These studies will not differentiate between high-grade stenosis, which is surgically treatable, and occlusion which is not surgically treatable in most cases. Neither will they detect an ulcerated plaque which does not compromise the lumen of the ICA enough to reduce hemispheric blood flow. Thus they cannot be used to evaluate the patient with symptoms due to intracranial emboli.

Oculoplethysmography

Oculoplethysmography (OPG) was initially developed by Kartchner and McRae. In brief, the technique utilizes fluid-filled cups applied to the anesthetized globes and photoplethysmographic clips placed on the earlobes. A wave form representing ocular filling is generated on a chart recorder with every pulse cycle. These wave forms are electronically compared as they are recorded. A unilateral delay in pulse arrival time compared to the contralateral eye suggests a flow reducing ICA lesion on the side of the delay. The ocular waves are also compared with ear tracings to detect bilateral ICA lesions.

Although this technique is simple and relatively easy to use, recent evidence suggests its accuracy is not sufficient. While it is frequently positive with extremely high-grade carotid stenosis or occlusion, it fails to detect many lesser lesions which are also potentially flow reducing. Furthermore, it is quite unreliable with bilateral ICA disease.

Oculopneumoplethysmography

Oculopneumoplethysmography, developed by Gee, utilizes an air-filled cup applied to the anesthetized globe. A high negative pressure is applied through the cup which obliterates ocular pulsations. As this pressure is slowly reduced, the point of return of pulsations is noted. This point has been demonstrated experimentally to correlate well with ophthalmic artery systolic pressure. A unilateral decrease in systolic pressure usually signifies a flow reducing carotid lesion. By comparing both ocular pressures with the brachial systolic pressure, bilateral internal carotid disease can be detected.

This technique is an accurate method for the detection of very high-grade ICA stenoses (>75% diameter reduction) or occlusion and is more accurate than oculoplethysmography in the identification of bilateral disease. However, its ability to detect lesser degrees of flow reducing stenosis is not good, and its value in the patient with hypertension is limited since the highest ophthalmic artery pressure detectable is 110 mm of mercury.

Supraorbital Doppler Examination

The supraorbital Doppler examination uses a directional Doppler probe to record flow direction in the supraorbital and frontal arteries as they emerge from the orbital rim. Flow in these vessels is normally antegrade, out of the orbit; however, if hemispheric blood pressure is reduced by a high grade ICA stenosis or occlusion, pressure in the external carotid artery (ECA) may be higher than that in the intracranial vessels. The ECA will then provide collateral flow through the supraorbital and/or frontal arteries to the intracranial vessels and the baseline flow direction in these periorbital arteries will be reversed. This reversal of flow can be identified and recorded with the directional Doppler. By successively compressing ECA branches, such as the superficial temporal or facial arteries, the source of the collateral flow can be identified.

The supraorbital Doppler examination is accurate when positive; however, a negative study does not exclude the presence of a significant carotid lesion. Associated external carotid stenosis is a frequent cause for false negative examinations.

Direct Studies

Direct studies for carotid occlusive disease utilize information gained directly from the carotid bifurcation in the neck. The earliest direct studies were forms of bruit analysis. Recently however, techniques utilizing various forms of ultrasound have made significant advances in the detection and quantitation of carotid lesions.

Carotid Phonoangiography

Carotid phonangiography (CPA) was initially developed by Kartchner and McRae for use in conjunction with their OPG unit. It utilizes a hand-held microphone to record bruits from the low, mid, and upper neck. A Polaroid photograph is made of each bruit in relation to the first and second heart sounds. Bruits which are loudest in the mid or upper neck are interpreted to reflect carotid artery disease, particularly if they extend into diastole. Conversely, bruits which are of equal intensity in all three positions or are loudest low in the neck are thought to be transmitted from intrathoracic or valvular lesions.

The utility of this technique for the detection of carotid stenoses is limited. Only 60% of cervical bruits originate from the internal carotid artery and there is no way to verify that bruits detected with the CPA arise from the ICA. Furthermore many carotid stenoses produce no bruit and thus cannot be detected.

Ultrasonic Imaging

Ultrasonic imaging techniques utilize gray scale ultrasound or Doppler flow mapping to image the bifurcation vessels. The common, external, and internal carotid arteries can thus be precisely identified and specific lesions localized.

Gray scale ultrasound scanners designed specifically for carotid artery imaging have recently been developed. These devices use high frequency (10mHz) ultrasound to produce real time images of the bifurcation vessels. Resolution with these instruments is excellent, permitting identification of many low grade (<50% stenosis) plaques as well as advanced lesions. The major shortcoming of B-mode carotid imaging is that thrombus and fatty plaque have an acoustic reflectivity similar to that of blood. It is therefore often difficult to distinguish the interface between fatty plaque or clot and flowing blood. Determination of the exact degree of diameter reduction can be difficult in these cases and identification of ICA occlusion may also be difficult. These problems have contributed to diagnostic errors in over one-third of cases in some series.

Doppler Flow Imaging

Doppler flow imaging, or ultrasonic arteriography, utilizes continuous wave or pulsed Doppler ultrasound to construct a flow map of the carotid bifurcation. The examination is performed by placing the Doppler transducer over the carotid artery low in the neck. At every point where the Doppler detects arterial flow a spot is registered and retained on a storage oscilloscope. By moving the transducer up the neck over the carotid bifurcation a flow map can be built up, identifying the common, external, and internal carotid arteries. The lumen is narrowed in the area of a plaque (Figure 1). ICA occlusion is identified by failure to detect flow in the normal position of the ICA adjacent to the internal jugular vein (Figure 2).

A single carotid bifurcation image can be constructed in five to ten minutes in most patients; however, it is imperative that the patient cooperate with the examiner by maintaining a steady position throughout. An additional problem is that calcification in the arterial wall may inhibit the transmission of ultrasound, making a precise delineation of the degree of luminal narrowing difficult. This problem can usually be overcome by analyzing the flow velocity signal distal to the stenosis (see below).

The continuous wave ultrasonic arteriograph detects flow from all vessels within the path of the ultrasound beam, although the carotid signal can usually be separated from adjacent vessels by use of directional flow capabilities. The pulsed Doppler has the ability to detect flow from a small area within tissue, called a sample volume. This sample volume can be placed in the central portion of the artery under study where the maximum fluctuations in flow

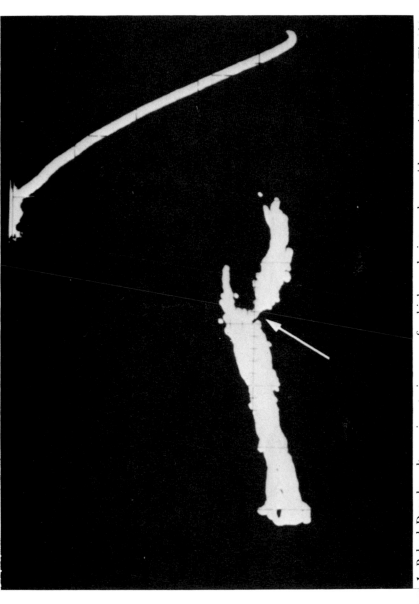

Figure 1. Pulsed Doppler ultrasonic arteriogram of a high-grade internal carotid stenosis (arrow). The lumen is narrowed at the site of the lesion and a high frequency Doppler signal was detected at this site.

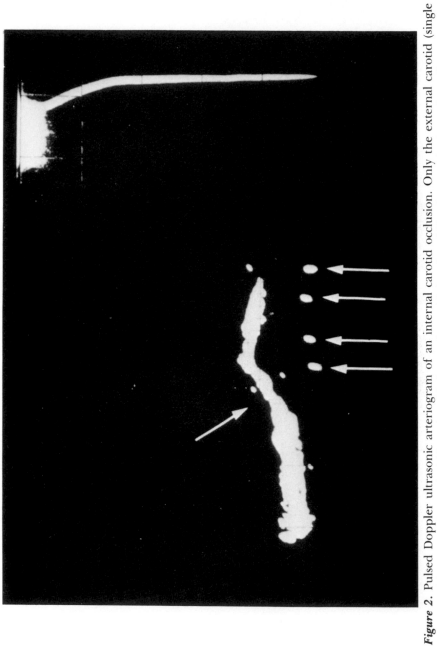

Figure 2. Pulsed Doppler ultrasonic arteriogram of an internal carotid occlusion. Only the external carotid (single arrow) could be imaged past the bifurcation. No internal carotid signal could be detected in the region adjacent to the internal jugular vein (multiple arrows).

velocity occur. Thus the device can be positioned to image only the vessel of interest.

Excellent results have been reported with both of these instruments in the detection of high-grade internal carotid stenoses and occlusions (Table 1). Over 90% accuracy compared with angiography has been reported from several centers. An important advantage of these techniques is that they can differentiate between a high-grade ICA stenosis and ICA occlusion, thus eliminating the need for angiography in some patients with occlusion. Ultrasonic arteriography can also detect many plaques which are not large enough to reduce hemispheric blood flow but may be potential sources of intracranial emboli. A sensitivity of 70–80% in the identification of these lesions has been reported.

Flow Velocity Analysis

Arterial stenoses which reduce the normal diameter of the lumen affect the flow velocity pattern in two ways, which can be detected by the Doppler. First, within the stenosis itself flow velocity is elevated in proportion to the degree of luminal narrowing. This produces a corresponding elevation in the frequency of the audible Doppler signal. Second, distal to the stenosis eddies generated by the plaque produce flow disturbances which also affect

Table 1
Pulsed Doppler Ultrasound in the Detection of High-grade Carotid Artery Stenosis

Series	Sensitivity (%)	Specificity (%)
Barnes, et al., 1976[19] (N = 47)	88	98
Blackshear, et al., 1979[5] (N = 62)	92	92
Sumner, et al., 1979[14] (N = 200)	86	90
Hobson, et al., 1980[20] (N = 172)	89	83
Barnes, 1977[3] (N = 82)	95	77

the Doppler signal. This effect can best be described as "harshening." Both ultrasonic arteriography and duplex scanning can provide diagnostically useful flow velocity data.

Ultrasonic Arteriography

Continuous wave and pulsed Doppler ultrasonic arteriography described in the preceding section can also be used for audible evaluations of flow velocity patterns. The flow map generated with either instrument can be used as a guide to precisely identify the vessel under examination. Doppler signals in and distal to an area of suspected pathology can then be evaluated. In addition, the signal distal to an area of calcification will also yield useful information relative to the presence of a proximal lesion. High-grade flow reducing stenoses produce a characteristic marked elevation of the Doppler frequency and a harsh, turbulent signal distal to the plaque. Lesser stenotic lesions elevate the Doppler frequency less than the high-grade stenoses, but turbulent flow is also detected. Therefore, using this technique normal vessels can frequently be distinguished from those with relatively minor disease. Furthermore, an estimate of the degree of stenosis is also possible.

Flow velocity analysis provides physiologic data which complements the anatomic data provided by ultrasonic imaging. This is particularly useful in the detection of low-grade stenotic lesions.

Duplex Scanning

The duplex scanner combines real time B-mode imaging of the carotid bifurcation vessels with a pulsed Doppler for flow velocity analysis. The instantaneous real time images can be used to rapidly identify the bifurcation vessels. The pulsed Doppler sample volume can then be placed within the lumen at any point for evaluation of the flow velocity pattern. The same alterations described for ultrasonic arteriography are detected with the duplex scanner. Occluded vessels are diagnosed by failure to detect flow with the sample volume positioned within the lumen of an imaged vessel. The accuracy of this technique in the identification of both high-

and low-grade ICA stenoses is comparable to that achieved with ultrasonic arteriography. In addition, the real time imaging capability greatly facilitates examinations.

Pulsed Doppler Spectrum Analysis

By passing a pulsed Doppler signal through a spectrum analyzer, a hard copy output of the frequency content of that signal is obtained. Precise quantification of the frequency content of the signal is then possible. This permits an objective evaluation of the flow velocity alterations within and distal to a plaque. The high peak systolic frequencies in high-grade stenoses can be easily identified (Figure 3). The harsh Doppler signal generated by turbulent flow can also be readily detected as a broadening of the normally narrow pulsed Doppler frequency spectrum.

High-grade ICA stenoses can be readily identified using audible analysis alone by noting the marked elevation of systolic frequency. Spectrum analysis permits identification of turbulent flow generated by minor plaques. The changes in the Doppler signal produced by these lesions are not always audible to the examiner's ear. Detection of ulcerated non-stenotic plaques is, therefore, feasible using this technique. Just as importantly, vessels with a normal flow pattern can also be clearly identified. Objective determination of flow velocity increase and flow disturbance permits quantification of the degree of luminal narrowing in many cases.

Summary

Recent advances in ultrasonic imaging techniques combined with qualitative audible flow velocity analysis or quantitative spectral flow velocity analysis permit accurate evaluation of patients with suspected carotid artery disease. The advantages and disadvantages of ultrasonic carotid artery imaging are listed in Table 2. Flow reducing lesions can be accurately identified and high-grade stenosis differentiated from ICA occlusion. Asymptomatic bruits can be localized as to the vessel of origin and an estimate of the degree of stenosis obtained. Many non-flow reducing stenoses

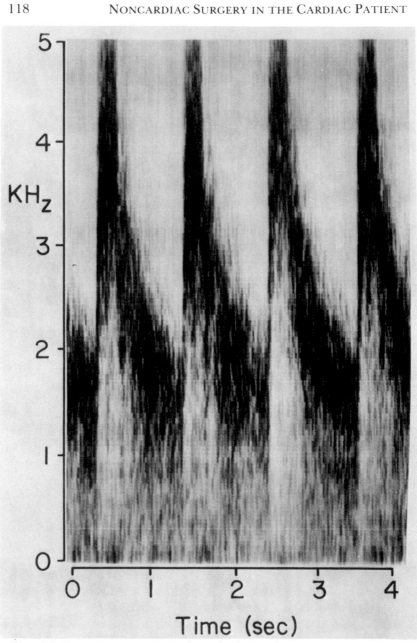

Figure 3. Frequency spectrum of a pulsed Doppler signal recorded from a high-grade internal carotid stenosis. The peak systolic frequency is markedly elevated (>5.0 mHz) and the area under the systolic peak is opacified, reflecting disturbed flow at this site.

Table 2
Ultrasonic Carotid Artery Imaging

Advantages	Disadvantages
Rapid	Experienced operator required
Repeatable	No intracranial or proximal images
Good patient acceptance	generated
Safe	Occasional misidentification of
Differentiate stenosis from	vessels
occlusion	Patient cooperation necessary
Quantitate degree of stenosis	
Inexpensive compared to	
angiography	

which are potential sources of intracranial emboli can also be identified as can vessels which are essentially normal. Proper use of these techniques will permit a more rational selection of patients for arteriography, and serial examinations of vessels with documented lesions can be used to identify disease progression.

Peripheral Arterial Occlusive Disease

Lower extremity arterial occlusive disease is best characterized by the arterial segment involved in the disease process: aortoiliac, femoropopliteal, or tibioperoneal. Multilevel disease in which two or more levels are involved is also common. Symptoms due to arterial insufficiency are usually manifest initially as intermittent claudication. This term refers to a specific symptom complex consisting of pain in an affected muscle group which occurs only after a specified degree of exercise and is relieved by rest in the erect position. It is due to a reduction in perfusion pressure within the small arteries and arterioles supplying the muscle group and is associated with proximal occlusive disease.

Vasodilatation is induced by the accumulation of metabolic products in the muscles during exercise. In the presence of proximal arterial obstruction flow to the exercising muscles cannot be increased to the degree required to maintain baseline pressure. When the pressure falls below a certain critical level (usually 50–60 mm of mercury) pain results. The pain persists until pressure rises above this critical level due to increased flow through collateral vessels. Aortoiliac disease characteristically produces hip and thigh claudication, femoropopliteal disease causes calf claudication, and tibioperoneal involvement produces symptoms in the foot. Multilevel disease may produce any combination of symptoms.

When the disease is more severe, the baseline perfusion pressure may be below this critical level continually. In this case the patient suffers from constant ischemic rest pain. This pain is usually described as a continual ache or burning, and it characteristically occurs distally in the limb in the ball of the foot or in the toes.

A careful history and physical examination will usually identify limbs with significant occlusive disease. Furthermore, lower extremity angiography does not carry the risk of carotid arteriography and can be used to identify suspected lesions. However, there are many circumstances in which the objective data provided by noninvasive vascular laboratory studies can be of value in the patient with lower extremity occlusive disease, particularly those with associated cardiac problems. First, physiologic data can assist in the assessment of the hemodynamic significance of a questionable lesion seen on angiography. Second, arterial occlusive disease often coexists with other causes of lower extremity pain, particularly in the older age group, e.g., arthritis, neuropathy, lumbosacral disc disease. Vascular laboratory studies can accurately determine whether the patient's symptoms are due to arterial disease. The risk of a major arterial reconstruction may therefore be avoided in those patients in whom noninvasive studies suggest that the arterial disease is not the primary factor producing leg pain.

Third, noninvasive studies can be safely repeated on numerous occasions to objectively document clinical improvement or to detect disease progression. Angiography cannot of course be repeated frequently for routine follow-up. Finally, in the patient whose claudication is truly disabling and requires operation or in the patient with ischemic rest pain threatening loss of limb, appropriate noninvasive studies can quantitate the severity of disease preoperatively and localize the involved segments. Postoperative studies can then be used to document the results of operation.

Since the symptoms of lower extremity atherosclerosis are due to reduced perfusion pressure, noninvasive pressure measurements form the basis for most vascular laboratory studies. In addition, Doppler flow velocity recordings can often supplement the information gained from pressure studies.

Pressure Studies

Noninvasive pressure studies of the lower extremity arterial circulation can be performed with a variety of instruments. The most common instrument used for systolic pressure measurements is the continuous wave Doppler flow velocity detector; however, similar information can be obtained with a strain gauge plethysmograph or a pulse volume recorder using a gauge positioned around the foot or toes. Systolic pressure is the most sensitive determinant of tissue perfusion. The Doppler measures systolic pressure by identifying the pressure at which distal arterial flow resumes as a blood pressure cuff is slowly deflated. Both the strain gauge plethysmograph and the pulse volume recorder measure systolic pressure by noting the point of return of oscillations as the limb expands and contracts with each cardiac cycle. Hereafter the technique of systolic pressure measurements using the Doppler will be discussed although the comments also apply to measurements obtained using the other two instruments.

Identification of limbs harboring arterial occlusive disease which is hemodynamically significant at rest is based on measurement of the ankle–arm index (AAI). It is important to note that for all arterial pressure measurements, the systolic pressure detected is that in the arteries at the site of the blood pressure cuff, not at the point of Doppler auscultation. First, the brachial systolic pressure is measured in both arms. The highest recording obtained is then used for future reference. With a blood pressure cuff placed just above the ankle, systolic pressures are measured in both the dorsalis pedis and posterior tibial arteries. The highest pressure recorded in either of these two vessels is then divided by the highest brachial pressure. This is the ankle–arm index. Normally the AAI should be greater than or equal to 1.0. A value lower than this is diagnostic of proximal arterial obstruction in the arteries supplying the limb. Rarely, severe medial calcification will preclude pressure measurements since the vessels cannot be compressed with the cuff inflated to maximum levels. In this circumstance flow velocity data (see below) can be most helpful. An example of the AAI is presented in Table 3.

If proximal obstruction is identified, the level of obstruction can be further localized with segmental pressure measurements. To perform these measurements narrow blood pressure cuffs are

Table 3
An Example of the Ankle–Arm Index (AAI) Calculation

Artery	Systolic Pressure (MM Hg)
Right Brachial	115
Left Brachial	120*
Right Dorsalis Pedis	90*
Right Posterior Tibial	75

*Right leg AAI = 90 ÷ 120 = 0.75

placed on the limb at the level of the upper thigh, the lower thigh above the knee, and below the knee. Systolic pressure is measured at each of these levels. Pressure at the upper thigh level should at least be equal to the highest brachial pressure and in most cases it is much higher due to cuff artifact caused by the thick upper thigh mass. An upper thigh pressure lower than the brachial pressure signifies the presence of hemodynamically significant aortoiliac disease. The gradient between any two adjacent levels in the limb should be less than 30 mm of mercury. A gradient of more than 30 mmHg is diagnostic of obstruction in the intervening segment. Thus, the upper thigh-above-knee gradient reflects superficial femoral artery flow, the above knee-below knee gradient reflects popliteal artery flow, and the below knee–ankle gradient reflects tibioperoneal flow.

A normal AAI or a systolic ankle pressure of 90 mm of mercury or above effectively rules out the diagnosis of ischemic rest pain. However, it does not eliminate the possibility of intermittent claudication. To evaluate the patient with suspected claudication, a treadmill exercise tolerance test is performed. The patient is placed on a treadmill at a rate of two miles per hour with a 12% uphill grade. He is asked to walk for a maximum of five minutes or until he is forced to stop by leg pain. Immediately after the cessation of exercise the patient is placed in the supine position and the ankle pressures are repeated bilaterally. A normal response is no change or an increase in the highest ankle pressure (Figure 4). With a significant proximal arterial obstruction, the systolic ankle pressure will fall. If a drop in ankle pressure is detected, the pressure is repeated every two minutes for 15 minutes or until it returns to baseline levels. The severity of claudication can be quantitated by

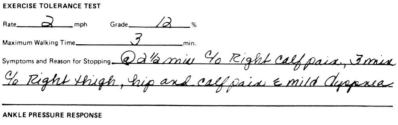

EXERCISE TOLERANCE TEST

Rate_____ 2 _____ mph   Grade_____ 12 _____ %

Maximum Walking Time_____ 3 _____ min.

Symptoms and Reason for Stopping_____ @ 2½ min % Right calf pain, 3 min
% Right thigh, hip and calf pain & mild dyspnea

_____

ANKLE PRESSURE RESPONSE

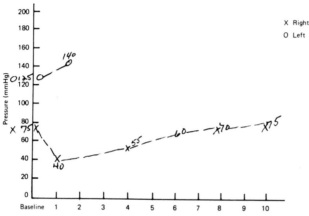

Figure 4. Treadmill exercise tolerance test on a patient with right leg claudication. After three minutes of exercise the ankle pressure dropped significantly on the right and required ten minutes to return to baseline levels. The response on the left was normal.

noting the maximum walking time, the magnitude of the initial pressure drop, and the time required for recovery. The patient with lower extremity pain or exercise due to arterial occlusive disease will exhibit an initial pressure drop after exercise in the symptomatic limb which is below the critical level of 50–60 mm of mercury.

Flow Velocity Analysis

Continuous wave directional Doppler velocity wave forms from a chart recorder can provide additional information relative to the severity and locale of lower extremity occlusive disease. A normal directional Doppler wave form is triphasic, exhibiting a large systolic forward flow component followed by a brief reversal of flow in early diastole. A much smaller forward flow component is then present in mid-diastole with no flow in late diastole. With arterial obstruction proximal to the site of recording, the reverse flow component is lost. When this obstruction becomes quite severe, flow is continuous in the forward direction well above the baseline.

Resting Doppler wave forms recorded from the common femoral arteries and from the pedal vessels can provide useful confirmatory information relative to the presence of aortoiliac or distal disease. An abnormal common femoral wave form suggests proximal disease and this will also be manifest in an abnormal pedal wave form. Conversely, a normal common femoral wave form combined with an abnormal pedal recording suggests disease distal to the inguinal ligament. Post-exercise Doppler wave forms can also be used to detect occult aortoiliac disease, which is only manifest after exercise. A normal resting common femoral wave form which becomes abnormal after exercise strongly suggests proximal obstruction.

Plethysmographic wave forms recorded with a strain gauge plethysmograph or with a pulse volume recorder can also identify arterial obstruction. A normal wave form exhibits a sharp upward systolic sweep and a rapid downslope with a prominent dicrotic notch on the midportion of the downslope. With obstruction proximal to the site of recording, the wave form becomes blunted with a slower systolic upsweep and loss of the dicrotic notch.

Acute Deep Venous Thrombosis

Epidemiologic studies suggest that the patient with cardiac disease is at increased risk for the development of acute deep venous thrombosis (DVT) in the veins of the lower extremities. This is particularly true in the post-operative cardiac patient. A prior history of chronic venous disease further increases the risk of DVT.

Although contrast venography will identify venous thrombosis in most cases, it cannot be used as a routine screening examination. Noninvasive studies are quite useful to detect thrombosis in the major deep veins of the lower extremity, reducing the need for venography to those limbs with equivocal test results. These studies can also be used to identify patients with pre-existent venous disease who may benefit from some form of prophylaxis to prevent the development of this potentially serious complication.

The most useful instruments for the evaluation of the lower extremity veins are the Doppler flow velocity detector, the phleborrheograph, and the impedance or strain gauge plethysmograph.

Doppler Flow Velocity Detector

A hand-held 5 megaHerz Doppler flow velocity detector can be utilized to examine major lower extremity deep veins. With the patient in the supine position the knee is flexed approximately 20° and supported so that the limb bears no weight. The posterior tibial, popliteal, superficial femoral, and common femoral veins are routinely examined. When indicated, the greater and lesser saphenous veins can also be studied. The deep veins are localized by identifying the corresponding artery and listening for the low velocity venous signal immediately adjacent to the pulsatile arterial signal. At each location several characteristics of venous flow are evaluated. It is important to note whether the signal is *phasic,* that is, does it vary normally with the respiratory cycle implying a relatively direct connection with the abdominal veins or is the signal *absent,* implying thrombosis, or *continuous,* implying steady flow through high resistance collateral vessels around a thrombosed main channel. *Augmentation* of venous flow in response to distal limb compression is also assessed as is cessation of and resumption of venous flow in response to alternate compression and release of the limb proximal to the site of auscultation. An abnormality in one of these augmentation maneuvers suggests the possibility of obstruction in the intervening deep venous segment. With proximal compression or with a Valsalva maneuver the *competence* of venous valves can also be qualitatively assessed. Finally, a *pulsatile* venous flow signal suggests elevated right heart pressures due to congestive failure or fluid load.

In many clinical series the Doppler has proven to have a sensitivity of well over 90% in the detection of acute deep venous thrombosis involving the veins proximal to and including the popliteal vein (Table 4). Its accuracy in the detection of isolated calf vein thrombosis is not as great, but in experienced hands a sensi-

Table 4
Sensitivity of Doppler and Plethysmography in the Detection of Acute
DVT Proximal to Calf

Series	Doppler (%)	Plethysmography (%)
Strandness and Sumner (1975)[13]	93	
Nicholos et al. (1977)[22]	78	83 (SPG)
Zielinsky et al. (1978)[23]	92	92 (IPG)
Barnes et al. (1977)[17]		90 (SPG)
Yao et al. (1974)[21]	89	89 (IPG)
Hull et al. (1976)[8]		93 (IPG)
Wheeler et al. (1980)[18]		96 (IPG)
Raines (1978)[15]		98 (PVR)

SPG—Strain gauge plethysmograph
IPG—Impedance plethysmograph
PVR—Pulse volume recorder

tivity approaching 80% can be expected. An additional feature of clinical importance is that when the Doppler examination is not totally diagnostic of venous thrombosis, many patients will exhibit minor abnormalities which are interpreted as possibly indicative of disease. These patients can be appropriately referred for venography. The use of this technique is thus limited to those patients who truly benefit from the injection of contrast material.

The venous Doppler examination is quick, reliable, and can easily be performed in virtually any clinical setting including office, emergency department, or hospital bedside. The one shortcoming of the technique is that it requires an experienced examiner to achieve reliable and reproducible results.

Phleborrheography

Phleborrheography, originally developed by Cranley, utilizes several air-filled cuffs placed about the lower extremity at multiple levels. These cuffs are each connected to transducers which measure limb expansion and contraction in response to respiratory movements and also in response to inflation of cuffs proximal and distal to the site of recording. This information is printed on a chart recorder for later analysis. As the foregoing indicates, the parameters measured and the functions studied with phleborrheography are similar to those measured qualitatively with the venous Doppler examination; however, the hard copy output provided by the phleborrheograph is more suitable for objective analysis by an interpreter other than the examiner. In addition, the examination can be reliably performed by a technician with a much shorter period of training than is required for the venous Doppler examination. The accuracy reported for phleborrheography is similar to that obtained with the Doppler both with regard to the calf veins and to the proximal deep veins.

Venous Outflow Plethysmography

Venous outflow plethysmography provides a semi-quantitative measurement of the rate of emptying of the major lower extremity deep veins after occlusion of venous outflow at the thigh levels for a standard period of time (usually two minutes). The examination is performed by placing the patient in the supine position and elevating the limbs to a predetermined height with the legs supported at the heel and thigh. The large thigh cuff is inflated to approximately 50 mm of mercury pressure which effectively occludes venous outflow. Arterial inflow is unimpeded, however, and during the two-minute occlusion period the calf veins distend with blood. The relative increase in calf volume during this period of time is referred to as venous capacitance. After instantaneous deflation of the thigh cuff, the rate of venous emptying can be recorded (venous outflow).

The impedence plethysmograph measures these changes in calf volume by detecting alterations in a current passed between two electrodes positioned on the calf. Blood is an excellent conductor and an increase or decrease in the amount of blood contained in the calf will be reflected on a recorder as an increase or decrease in the current flow between these electrodes. The strain gauge plethysmograph measures these changes directly utilizing a small mercury-filled silastic tube placed around the calf. Distention of this gauge alters the electrical conductivity of the mercury and this alteration can also be recorded on a chart recorder.

Limbs with significant outflow obstruction due to thrombosis will exhibit a markedly reduced rate of venous outflow at one-half, one, and two seconds after cuff deflation (Figure 5). The ratio of

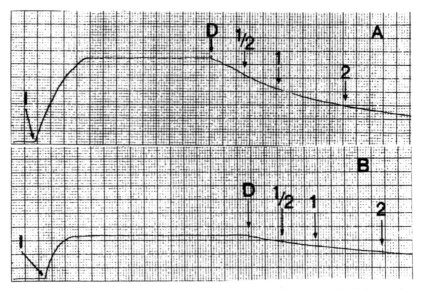

Figure 5. Venous capacitance and outflow recorded from both legs of a patient with acute DVT of the left superficial femoral vein. The normal limb (A) exhibits a rapid rise in venous volume over two minutes after inflation of the thigh cuff (I). At this point the recording speed is increased and the cuff is instantaneously deflated (D). Venous outflow is measured at one-half, one, and two seconds (62.5cc, 51.0cc, 44.8cc). The diseased limb (B) exhibits a markedly reduced venous outflow at all three times of measurement (23.5cc, 18.5cc, 15.2cc).

outflow to venous capacitance will also be markedly depressed. Venous plethysmography thus provides a quantitative measurement of the adequacy of the venous drainage system. Both of these techniques have been demonstrated to have a sensitivity of over 90% in the detection of acute deep venous thrombosis proximal to the calf (Table 3). The reliability in the detection of calf vein thrombosis is much less, however.

The results of venous outflow plethysmography often correlate well with the clinical status of the limb in the recovery period after an episode of DVT. Limbs which exhibit a rapid return of venous outflow to the normal range seldom have significant problems with chronic edema and ulceration. Conversely, limbs with severe persistent obstruction by plethysmography often go on to develop symptoms of chronic deep venous insufficiency, the post-phlebitic syndrome.

An important additional advantage of venous plethysmography is in the patient with documented prior DVT. These patients often present with recurrent bouts of lower extremity pain and/or swelling and the decision as to whether these current symptoms represent development of new thrombosis is often difficult. Both the Doppler examination and venography are usually abnormal; however, the abnormalities detected can often not be definitely identified as new. If a deterioration in venous outflow can be identified compared to a prior study, it is quite likely that significant progression of thrombosis has occurred. However, if the venous outflows are essentially the same as the earlier study, recurrent DVT is unlikely.

Summary

The judicious use of noninvasive tests of peripheral arterial and venous function can provide important diagnostic information for the detection and quantitation of peripheral arterial and venous diseases. The physiologic information thus obtained is often quite useful in the evaluation of existing vascular lesions or in assessing potential risks. These important studies should not be neglected in the patient with cardiac disease and significant peripheral arterial or venous disorders. Proper use and interpretation of noninvasive physiologic data can facilitate patient evaluation and properly select those patients who will benefit from more invasive procedures.

Suggested Reading

1. Alexander RH, et al.: Thrombophlebitis and thromboembolism: Results of a prospective study. *Ann Surg* 180:883, 1974.
2. Barnes RW, et al.: Noninvasive quantitation of maximum venous outflow in acute thrombophlebitis. *Surgery* 72:971, 1972.
3. Barnes RW, et al.: Doppler cerebrovascular examination: Improved results with refinements in technique. *Stroke* 8:468, 1977.
4. Blackshear WM, et al.: A prospective evaluation of oculoplethysmog-

raphy and carotid phonoangiography. *Surg Gynecol Obstet* 148:201, 1979.

5. Blackshear WM, et al.: Detection of carotid occlusive disease by ultrasonic imaging and pulsed doppler spectrum analysis. *Surgery* 86:698, 1979.

6. Cranley JJ, et al.: Phleborrheographic technique for diagnosing deep venous thrombosis of the lower extremities. *Surg Gynecol Obstet* 141:331, 1975.

7. Gee W, Mehigan JT, Wylie EJ: Measurement of collateral hemispheric blood pressure by ocular pneumoplethysmography. *Am J Surg* 130:121, 1975.

8. Hull R, et al.: Impedance plethysmography using the occlusive cuff technique in the diagnosis of venous thrombosis. *Circulation* 53:696, 1976.

9. Kartchner MM, McRae LP, Morrison FD: Noninvasive detection and evaluation of carotid occlusive disease. *Arch Surg* 106:528, 1973.

10. Mercier LA, et al.: High resolution ultrasound angiography: A comparison with carotid angiography. In Bernstein EF (Ed.): *Noninvasive Diagnostic Techniques in Vascular Disease.* St. Louis, C V Mosby Co, 1978.

11. O'Donnell JA, Lipp J, Hobson RW: New methods of testing for deep venous thrombosis. *Am Surg* 44:121, 1978.

12. Rutherford RB (Ed.): *Vascular Surgery.* Philadelphia, WB Saunders Co, 1977.

13. Strandness DE, Sumner DS: *Hemodynamics for Surgeons.* New York, Grune & Stratton, 1975.

14. Sumner DS, et al.: Noninvasive diagnosis of extracranial carotid arterial disease. A prospective evaluation of pulsed Doppler imaging and oculoplethysmography. *Arch Surg* 114:1222, 1979.

15. Raines JK, Darling RC, Buth J, et al.: Vascular laboratory criteria for the management of peripheral vascular disease of the lower extremities. *Surgery* 79:21, 1976.

16. Barnes RW, Shanik GD, Slaymaker EE: An index of healing in below-knee amputation: Leg blood pressure by Doppler ultrasound. *Surgery* 79:13, 1976.

17. Barnes RW, Hokanson DE, Wu KK, et al.: Detection of deep vein thrombosis with an automatic electrically calibrated strain gauge plethysmograph. *Surgery* 82:219, 1977.

18. Wheeler HB: A modern approach to diagnosing deep venous thrombosis. *Journal of Cardiovascular Medicine* 5(3):217, 1980.

19. Barnes RW, Bone GE, Runerston J, et al.: Noninvasive ultrasonic carotid angiography: Prospective validation by contrast arteriography. *Surgery* 80:328, 1976.

20. Hobson RW, Berry SM, Katocs AS Jr, et al.: Comparison of pulsed doppler and real-time B-mode echo arteriography for noninvasive imagery of the extracranial carotid arteries. *Surgery* 87:286, 1980.

21. Yao JST, Herekin RE, Bergan JJ: Venous thromboembolic disease. Evaluation of a new methodology in treatment. *Arch Surg* 109:664, 1974.

22. Nicholas GG, Miller FJ Jr, DeMuth WE Jr, et al.: Clinical vascular laboratory diagnosis of deep venous thrombosis. *Ann Surg* 186:213, 1977.
23. Zielinsky A, Hull R, Hirsh J, et al.: Comparative study of doppler ultrasound (DP) and impedance plethysmography (IPG) in the diagnosis of symptomatic and asymptomatic deep vein thrombosis (DVT). *Circulation* 57 & 58 (II):117, 1978.

CHAPTER VIII

Pulmonary Function

Keith W. Chandler, M.D.
and David A. Solomon, M.D.

Interdependence of Heart and Lungs

In his review of the development of respiratory physiology, Perkins[1] emphasized the close ties which exist between the cardiovascular and respiratory systems. In the fifth century B.C., blood vessels were hypothesized to be the route whereby air, "the chief cause of life," was conducted through the body. Adherents to Hippocratic doctrines avowed that the innate heat generated by the fiery processes of the heart was cooled by respiration with atria pumping air received from the lungs to the ventricles. Subsequent intellectual challenges and experimental investigations led to the refinement of these dim notions. The particular relationship between the heart and lungs has been redefined, yet the existence of a high degree of interdependence has never been questioned.

The evaluation of a patient with heart disease for coexistent pulmonary disease acknowledges the connection between these two organ systems. Heart disease is frequently accompanied by lung disease as a result of the coincident occurrence of two separate diseases, or as a result of exposure to single causative agents effecting disease in both organs or, finally, as a result of antecedent disease of one organ leading to dysfunction of the other.

Both chronic obstructive lung disease and many types of heart disease (hypertensive, arteriosclerotic, valvular, myopathic) commonly manifest their symptoms in the fifth through the seventh decades of a person's life, and the conjoint appearance of lung disease in a patient with heart disease is often encountered. The primary agent incriminated in the development of chronic obstructive pulmonary disease undeniably is cigarette smoking. Likewise, association between cigarette smoking and the development of coronary heart disease is emphasized by long-term epidemiological studies[2] and the evidence for the independent relationship of cigarette smoking to premature ischemic heart disease recently was well reviewed.[3] Elevated carboxyhemoglobin levels of the magnitude encountered after smoking impair maximal exercise performance in patients with chronic obstructive pulmonary disease[4] and in patients with angina pectoris.[5] Not surprisingly, then, cigarette smokers are vulnerable to the development of both heart and lung diseases.

Pulmonary Sequelae of Heart Disease

Heart disease has well defined pulmonary sequelae. The effect of pulmonary vascular congestion on the function of the lung has been investigated most thoroughly in patients immediately following myocardial infarction. Following myocardial infarction, all major subdivisions of lung volume are reduced subsequent to acute elevations of mean left atrial pressure. With pulmonary vascular congestion following myocardial infarction, the vital capacity may be reduced to fifty percent of its predicted value.[6] A subsequent fall in the functional residual capacity (the amount of air remaining within the lungs at the end of a normal breath) leads to arterial hypoxemia since basal alveoli are not then well ventilated relative to their perfusion (ventilation-perfusion inequality). Additional arterial desaturation occurs from an increase in the magnitude of intrapulmonary shunting, which in turn is caused by elevation of left atrial pressure leading to congestive atelectasis and pulmonary vasoconstriction.[7] If elevations of pulmonary capillary pressure are chronically maintained, irreversible alterations in pulmonary function may ensue. These alterations result from long-standing pulmonary vascular engorgement and interstitial edema or fibrosis with the magnitude of abnormalities paralleling the severity of the heart failure.

Whether lung disease in turn leads to the development of cardiovascular disease (apart, for example, from the appearance of cor pulmonale as a result of obliteration of the pulmonary vascular bed or of pulmonary hypertension as a result of arterial hypoxemia) is a controversial subject.[8] Few current studies support an independent role for chronic lung disease in the development of left ventricular failure. In one postmortem study, 28% of 72 patients with severe obstructive lung disease had left ventricular hypertrophy.[9] In these patients, hypertensive, arteriosclerotic, or valvular heart disease rather than the lung disease seemed to be responsible for the left ventricular hypertrophy. Additional studies in patients with chronic lung disease have confirmed the impression that left ventricular function in the majority of such patients is normal.[10,11] When left ventricular performance is abnormal, intrinsic heart disease is usually responsible.

In view of the mutual coexistence of an interaction between heart disease and lung disease, a well-considered approach to patients with cardiac disease is mandatory prior to the performance of any surgical procedures.

Preoperative Risk Factors

Although the symptoms of episodic breathlessness, exertional dyspnea, orthopnea, chronic cough, wheezing, hemoptysis, and recurrent pulmonary infections may figure prominently in the medical history of patients with heart disease, such symptoms are nonspecific and also may occur as a result of lung disease. Certain additional information may be more useful in indicating the presence of underlying pulmonary disease. Such information, when obtained, may be important in identifying patients at higher risk for the development of postoperative pulmonary complications (Table 1).

Table 1
Preoperative Risk Factors for Postoperative Pulmonary Complications*

Cigarette smoking (10 cigarettes/day)	Airflow obstruction
Recent upper respiratory tract infection	Obesity
Age	

*Fever, atelectasis, pneumonia, hypoxemia, pleurisy, pleural effusion

Cigarette Smoking

Statistical proof that cigarette smoking is a factor in the development of postoperative pulmonary complications was offered in 1944 by Morton.[12] In prospectively monitoring the hospital courses of 1,257 consecutive patients who were to undergo a variety of abdominal operations, he described an incidence of postoperative bronchitis, bronchopneumonia, and atelectasis of 58% in men who smoked greater than ten cigarettes per day. In the comparable group of nonsmoking men, the postoperative course was complicated by such pulmonary events in only 7% (five of sixty-six). The light smoking group (less than ten cigarettes per day) experienced an intermediate incidence of complications. Morton postulated that cigarette smoking was an "etiological factor of great importance" in the genesis of such complications because of the *catarrhe des fumeurs* so commonly associated with cigarette smoking. Such chronic tracheobronchitis during the post-laparotomy period would then dispose to the "stagnation of bronchial secretion" and acute decompensation. More recently, reported studies confirm the finding of a greatly increased risk of pulmonary complications following abdominal surgery in cigarette smokers[13] and that the degree of increased risk correlates with the number of cigarettes smoked daily.[14] Chalon et al. found that the pulmonary morbidity following general endotracheal anesthesia for elective surgery is 8 percent in nonsmokers, is 9 percent in smokers of less than ten cigarettes per day, and climbs to 30 percent in smokers of greater than ten cigarettes per day.[14] As was also suggested by Morton, the increased incidence of pulmonary complications in moderate or heavy cigarette smokers following surgery may in turn be related to the presence of tracheobronchitis, defined as a history of sputum production in the preoperative period.[15-17] A history of moderate or heavy cigarette smoking accompanied by dyspnea, chronic cough, or sputum production should alert the physician to be particularly watchful for postoperative pulmonary complications.

Upper Respiratory Tract Infection

Acute lung disease as manifested by a recent viral upper respiratory tract infection may be an identifiable factor in the onset of subsequent postsurgical respiratory problems. Such infections induce inflammatory changes in the airways, enhance sensitivity of airway reflexes to inhaled irritants, and alter regulation of bronchiolar smooth muscle tone.[18] Normal adults during naturally acquired respiratory tract infections demonstrate deterioration of airways function.[19] Even in the absence of symptoms or signs of airways disease, respiratory tract involvement is spirometrically demonstrable, and may persist for at least three weeks following a seemingly uncomplicated viral infection. The only reported investgation confirming the clinical importance of a recent upper respiratory tract infection in the development of roentgenographically apparent pulmonary complications dealt with children undergoing repair of congenital cardiovascular defects.[20] Forty-five percent (seven of sixteen) of children who reported the presence of upper respiratory tract infections within the two weeks prior to surgery developed postoperative pulmonary abnormalities. In the absence of a history of recent infection, abnormalities developed in twenty percent (eight of forty) of children following surgery.

Age

Although advanced age has been proposed as a factor relating to a greater risk for the appearance of postoperative pulmonary disease,[17,21] there is no uniform agreement on this issue. While a greater incidence of impaired pulmonary function with advanced age is apparent,[22] apart from postoperative hypoxemia, no increased incidence of pulmonary complications with aging was documented in a prospective study of patients undergoing elective upper abdominal surgery.[13] Cited studies purporting to demonstrate a correlation of age with postoperative respiratory events fail to segregate age as a variable independent of other known risk factors for postoperative pulmonary complications such as a history of cigarette smoking or the site of the patient's surgical incision.

Airflow Obstruction

Signs of airways obstruction are generally nonspecific, insensitive, and subject to such interobserver variability that the conclusion is warranted "that no sign is infallible and that most of them have a repeatability about midway between that due to chance and the maximum possible."[23] Jugular venous filling during expiration, loss of the movement of upper ribs, diminished breath sounds, and reduced length of trachea palpable above the sternal notch, although once described as physical signs of airways obstruction and lung distension, are misleading.[24] Other findings may be more suggestive of airways obstruction. Pursed lip breathing and expiratory grunting are often noted in patients with severe obstructive airways disease. Inspiratory excavation of the suprasternal and supraclavicular fossae and employment of scaleni and sternocleidomastoid muscles during inspiration can also reliably indicate the presence of severe airways obstruction.[24-26] Paradoxical inward motion of the abdomen during inspiration is a physical finding of great importance. Patients with chronic obstructive lung disease whose abdominal walls move inward during inspiration and outward during expiration have more severe lung disease than those patients with chronic obstructive pulmonary disease whose breathing movements are synchronous with the anterior abdominal wall (moving outward during the inspiratory descent of the diaphragm and inward during exhalation).[27] Inward movement of the abdomen during inspiration is a very specific and frequently disregarded sign of the diaphragmatic dysfunction present in patients with severe airflow obstruction.

Early inspiratory rales or crackles (those which appear shortly after the start of inspiration and which do not continue beyond the first half of inspiration) strongly suggest the presence of chronic obstructive lung disease.[28] This early crackling is low pitched, often audible at the mouth, and presumably results from the passage of air through an intermittently occluded airway.[29] Late inspiratory crackles extend into the second half of inspiration. They suggest the presence of a restrictive or interstitial lung disorder such as pulmonary fibrosis or pulmonary congestion as a result of heart failure.[28] These crackles are usually profuse, are best heard over the lower lung zones, are only rarely transmitted to the mouth, and probably represent the explosive reopening of closed peripheral airways.[29,30] Although wheezing correlates poorly with the severity of airways disease,[24] the presence of intense wheezing during deep unforced exhalation usually signified moderate to severe airflow obstruction.[31]

The forced expiratory time is the most direct sign of airways obstruction.[25] The patient is instructed to forcefully exhale through a widely opened mouth from full inspiration. The duration of audible expiration is timed with the second hand of a watch while listening at the mouth or over the trachea with a stethoscope. A forced expiratory time less than five seconds predicts at worst a mild obstructive impairment while a forced expiratory time of greater than six seconds predicts moderate or severe obstructive lung disease.[32] Whether a patient with any of the aforementioned physical findings is at higher risk for the development of pulmonary complications following thoracic or abdominal surgery has not been adequately investigated, but the presence of such findings should heighten one's suspicion that chronic pulmonary disease is present to a moderate or severe degree.

Obesity

The only other physical finding for which a correlation has been sought with the development of postoperative pulmonary complications is obesity. A preoperative weight 10 percent greater[13] or 15 percent greater[33] than normal has been defined as carrying an increased risk of pulmonary complications following upper abdominal surgery. Although suggestive, studies which propose to identify obesity as a risk factor for postoperative pulmonary morbidity have failed to segregate the risk of complications as a result of obesity from those related to other known risk factors such as chronic pulmonary disease.

Pulmonary Function Studies

Not everyone finds pulmonary function testing a useful component of the preoperative pulmonary evaluation. Graven and colleagues[34] confirmed that patients with a history of "chronic respiratory disease" were at greater risk for the development of bronchitis, pulmonary collapse, or pulmonary consolidation following upper abdominal surgery, but were unable to correlate this risk with results of preoperative pulmonary function testing. Cain, Stevens and Adaniya[35] retrospectively reviewed the clinical courses of 106 patients who had major thoracic or upper abdominal surgery and abnormal pulmonary function tests (66% complained of pulmonary symptoms preoperatively). They were unable to correlate pulmonary complications following surgery with the degree of preoperative pulmonary function testing abnormalities.

Most proponents who advocate obtaining preoperative pulmonary function studies prior to thoracic or abdominal surgery emphasize that abnormal tests are predictive of *groups* of patients who are subject to a higher incidence of pulmonary complications. However, individual patients with abnormal preoperative studies are capable of tolerating surgery in many situations without the appearance of postoperative morbidity. Normal preoperative pulmonary function generally means that the post-abdominal surgery period will not be complicated by untoward pulmonary events, while abnormal preoperative function will identify patients most at risk for complications.

Hence, patients scheduled to undergo elective thoracic or abdominal surgery are the primary candidates for preoperative pulmonary function testing so that the magnitude of pulmonary impairment may be objectively assessed. Patients scheduled to undergo nonabdominal-nonthoracic surgical procedures under general anesthesia who are suspected of having severe lung disease should also be considered candidates for preoperative testing. In these patients, if severe lung disease is documented, arterial blood gases should be drawn to permit the detection of hypercapnia, a highly significant risk factor for the development of postoperative ventilatory failure.

The performance of spirometry is the most widely employed pulmonary function study in the management of patients with respiratory disease. For the purpose of identifying those at risk for postoperative pulmonary problems, it is superior to all other tests. Indications for obtaining spirometry in the preoperative patient are found in Table 2. The timed spirogram is performed by a subject who inhales maximally and subsequently exhales as rapidly, as forcefully, and as completely as possible into a spirometer which records volume of air expired in relationship to time. Diminished expiratory flow usually is a reflection of increased airways resistance. The most useful spirometric parameter is the volume of air expired in the first second, the forced expiratory volume or FEV_1. To allow for ease of interpretation, the FEV_1 is at times expressed as a percentage of the forced vital capacity (FEV_1/FVC). The mean forced expiratory flow during the middle half of the forced vital capacity, $FEF_{25\%-75\%}$, is an example of a measurement which relates

Table 2
Indications for Preoperative Spirometry

History
Cigarette smoking, even if asymptomatic
Chronic cough
Asthma
Recurrent pneumonia
Previous or planned chest surgery
Dyspnea
Physical Examination
Wheezes
Early inspiratory rales
Prolonged expiratory time
Decreased breath sounds

expiratory flow to volume. Since the FEV_1 and $FEF_{25\%-75\%}$ are abnormal in patients with airways obstruction, some observers recommend the routine calculation of both[36] so that technical errors leading to variation in the measurements of the spirogram[37] may be made more apparent. Although additional information may be derived from an analysis of the forced vital capacity curve, the FEV_1, FVC, FEV_1/FVC and $FEF_{25\%-75\%}$ provide the most clinically relevant information. Normal reference values for these functions are available so that any patient may be compared with subjects of the same age, gender, body size, and race. In patients with evidence of airflow obstruction, a repetition of spirometry can be performed following inhalation of a bronchodilator in order to assess bronchodilator responsiveness.

Obstructive Lung Disease

An obstructive ventilatory defect exists when expiratory flows are diminished, as indicated by low FEV_1/FVC ratio ($<75\%$) or from the observed FEV_1 expressed as a percentage of the predicted reference value. When the observed FEV_1 is 65–79% of predicted in a patient with airways obstruction, mild impairment is suggested. Moderate impairment is suggested by an FEV_1 50–64% of that predicted; and an FEV_1 less than 50% of predicted indicates a severe impairment. Other features indicative of obstructive lung disease include a fifteen percent post-bronchodilator improvement in FVC or FEV_1. The absence of this degree of improvement should not lead one to conclude that a clinical response to a therapeutic trial of bronchodilators will necessarily be lacking, since some patients who ultimately respond to bronchodilatory therapy may fail to demonstrate a response to aerosolized bronchodilators. A restrictive ventilatory defect exists when an abnormally low vital capacity (less than 80% of predicted) is found in the absence of airflow obstruction (FEV_1/FVC greater than 75%). The severity of restrictive disease may be graded on the basis of observed vital capacity relative to the predicted vital capacity.

Preoperative spirometry identifies a group of patients who are at greater risk of postoperative pulmonary complications following thoracic or abdominal surgery. Patients with moderate or severe obstructive lung disease should have elective surgery postponed until maximal improvement of airways obstruction is obtained. Preoperative spirometry also allows for the prediction of the need for ventilatory support in the post-operative period. Miller and his colleagues were among the first to propose that preoperative spirometry could allow the separation of patients into groups composed of those who would be expected to tolerate thoracic or abdominal surgery and those for whom surgery might be expected to be attended by postoperative respiratory failure.[38] Patients with marginal pulmonary reserve can be identified preoperatively by spirometry, and decisions regarding postoperative weaning from mechanical ventilation as opposed to routine extubation following general endotracheal anesthesia may be formulated based largely on its results. Importantly, no degree of ventilatory impairment should absolutely preclude surgery once the patient has been found to otherwise be a surgical candidate. This is so because mortality is not excessive and hospitalization is not necessarily prolonged for surgical patients with severe pulmonary obstructive disease,[35,39] provided careful and adequate support is given. Mortality and postoperative pulmonary morbidity are not excessive if perioperative care is well-directed.[40,41] Although there is no prohibitive degree of pulmonary impairment which alone contravenes elective surgery, the presence of severely impaired pulmonary function, preoperative hypercapnia, or cor pulmonale should alert the patient's physicians to the possibility of an increased risk of postoperative pulmonary morbidity and, in particular, to an increased incidence of ventilatory failure.

Heart Disease

As previously noted, the presence of heart disease often results in a clinical picture suggestive of pulmonary disease. Exertional dyspnea, wheezing, chronic cough, frequent respiratory infections, and hemoptysis are signs and symptoms which are common to diseases affecting both the cardiovascular and respiratory systems. Since pulmonary and cardiovascular diseases commonly coexist, the ability to quantify separately the contribution of each to a patient's symptoms would be clinically valuable.

Chest roentgenograms may be useful in the detection of pulmonary and cardiac disease. Although experience teaches that the role of the chest roentgenogram in the diagnosis of chronic obstructive lung disease is limited,[42] a large retrosternal airspace, depression of the right diaphragmatic dome to the level of the anterior seventh rib, or a transverse diameter of the heart less than 11.5 cm all suggest the presence of chronic airway obstruction.[43] Similarly, while such findings as cardiac enlargement, azygos vein dilatation, and vascular redistribution of blood to the upper lobes are useful roentgenographic signs of congestive heart failure, left ventricular failure can occur in the presence of a roentgenographically unenlarged heart.[44] Moreover, the selective parenchymal and vascular damage to both lower lobes in a variety of diseases, including emphysema, may produce a shift in perfusion to the upper lobes roentgenographically mimicking early heart failure.

As might be expected, myocardial and valvular heart disease may result in abnormalities of pulmonary function tests. Initially, such abnormalities may be subtle. Following a seemingly uncomplicated myocardial infarction, ventilation of the lung bases is impaired, ventilation-perfusion imbalance occurs, and hypoxemia results.[45] With greater degrees of cardiac disease, more pronounced abnormalities of pulmonary function become apparent, possibly leading to the misdiagnosis of concomitant pulmonary disease. Acute and chronic left ventricular failure cause diminished vital capacity, and the magnitude of the diminution correlates with the severity of the left ventricular dysfunction. Gray et al.,[6] in performing pulmonary function studies on eighteen patients within five days of an acute myocardial infarction, described a depression of the vital capacity. A close correspondence existed between day-to-day changes in vital capacity and pulmonary artery diastolic pressures. The vital capacity of patients with normal cardiovascular hemodynamics was seventy-five percent of the predicted value, while in patients with pulmonary vascular congestion, the vital capacity was diminished to fifty percent of its predicted value. When a vital capacity measurement was obtained two weeks to fourteen weeks following the initial determinations, the mean vital capacity was restored to the normal range. These findings unequivocally support the conclusion that following myocardial infarction, when pulmonary vascular congestion is present, the vital capacity is reduced. With resolution of the left ventricular dysfunction, the vital capacity normalizes. Similar conclusions are substantiated by serial pulmonary function studies in patients with chronic left ventricular failure and mitral stenosis.[46]

Because of alterations in vital capacity induced by left ventricular or mitral valvular disease, a single determination of vital capacity, if diminished, may not allow for the separation of dyspnea on the basis of cardiac disease from dyspnea as a result of lung disease. Patients who are dyspneic with minimal exertion or while at rest may have vital capacities that are depressed to surprisingly similar degrees, whether due to cardiac disease or chronic airways obstruction.[47] Other pulmonary function studies may allow for a more correct assignment of the cause of breathlessness to lung disease or to heart disease. For example, the FEV_1 is diminished in patients with heart disease in proportion to the diminished FVC[47,48] so that the FEV_1/FVC ratio is virtually normal. Patients with disabling chronic airway obstruction demonstrate a disproportionately low FEV_1. In fact, patients with severe effort intolerance resulting from obstructive airway disease almost always have an FEV_1 of less than one liter.[49]

When congestive heart failure and obstructive pulmonary disease coexist, serial pulmonary function studies must be interpreted with caution. Not uncommonly, with amelioration of the congestive heart failure, the vital capacity remains unchanged, and the parameters of airflow obstruction in the timed expiratory spirogram may paradoxically worsen. Presumably, with clearing of interstitial edema, elastic recoil pressure, once augmented by the presence of lung water, declines, yielding lower expiratory flow rates.

Means exist, then, for the assessment of a patient's possible pulmonary compromise when cardiac disease coexists. When the vital capacity is diminished by either lung or heart disease, serial improvement with treatment directed toward the latter suggests a causative role for congestive failure. Furthermore, greater degrees of airways obstruction suggest a primary role for pulmonary disease. When better understanding is crucial, preoperative pulmonary function testing in patients with both heart and lung disease may permit a clearer appreciation of the relationship of these diseases to symptomatic complaints.

References

1. Perkins JF Jr.: Historical development of respiratory physiology. In Fenn WO and Rahn H (Eds.): *Handbook of Physiology, section 3, Respiration, vol. 1.* Baltimore, Waverly Press, Inc., 1964.
2. Dyer AR, Stamler J, Ubell E, et al.: A self-scoring five-question risk test for coronary heart disease. *Circulation* 60:914, 1979.
3. Kannel WB: Update on the role of cigarette smoking in coronary artery disease. *Am Heart J* 101:319, 1981.
4. Aronow WS, Ferlinz J, Glauser F: Effect of carbon monoxide on exercise performance in chronic obstructive pulmonary disease. *Am J Med* 63:904, 1977.
5. Aronow WS, Rokaw SN: Carboxyhemoglobin caused by smoking non-nicotine cigarettes effects in angina pectoris. *Circulation* 44:782, 1971.
6. Gray BA, Hyde RW, Hodges M, et al.: Alterations in lung volume and pulmonary function in relation to hemodynamic changes in acute myocardial infarction. *Circulation* 59:551, 1979.
7. Stanley TH, Lunn JK, Liu W, et al.: Effects of left atrial pressure on pulmonary shunt and the deadspace/tidal volume ratio. *Anesthesiology* 49:128, 1978.
8. Berger HJ, Matthay RA: Noninvasive radiographic assessment of cardiovascular function in acute and chronic respiratory failure. *Am J Cardiol* 47:950, 1981.
9. Murphy ML, Adamson J, Hutcheson F: Left ventricular hypertrophy in patients with chronic bronchitis and emphysema. *Ann Intern Med* 81:307, 1974.
10. Steele P, Ellis JH Jr, Van Dyke D, et al.: Left ventricular ejection fraction in severe chronic obstructive airways disease. *Am J Med* 59:21, 1975.
11. Christianson LC, Shah A, Fisher VJ: Quantitative left ventricular cine angiography in patients with chronic obstructive pulmonary disease. *Am J Med* 66:399, 1979.
12. Morton HJV: Tobacco smoking and pulmonary complications after operation. *Lancet* 1:368, 1944.
13. Latimer RG, Dickman M, Day WC, et al.: Ventilatory patterns and pulmonary complications after upper abdominal surgery determined by preoperative and postoperative computerized spirometry and blood gas analysis. *Am J Surg* 122:622, 1971.

14. Chalon J, Tayyab MA, Ramanathan S: Cytology of respiratory epithelium as a predictor of respiratory complications after operation. *Chest* 67:32, 1975.
15. Schlenker JD, Hubay CA: Colonization of the respiratory tract and postoperative pulmonary infections: The value of intraoperative endotracheal aspirate cultures. *Arch Surg* 107:313, 1973.
16. Schlenker JD, Hubay CA: The pathogenesis of postoperative atelectasis: A clinical study. *Arch Surg* 107:846, 1973.
17. Laszlo G, Archer GG, Darrell JH, et al.: The diagnosis and prophylaxis of pulmonary complications of surgical operation. *Br J Surg* 60:129, 1973.
18. O'Connor SA, Jones DP, Collins JV, et al.: Changes in pulmonary function after naturally acquired respiratory infection in normal persons. *Am Rev Respir Dis* 120:1087, 1979.
19. Little JW, Hall WJ, Douglas RG Jr, et al.: Amantadine effect on peripheral airways abnormalities in influenza: A study in fifteen students with natural influenza A infection. *Ann Intern Med* 85:177, 1976.
20. Steward DJ, Sloan AJ: Recent upper respiratory infection and pulmonary artery clamping in the aetiology of postoperative respiratory complications. *Canad Anaesth Soc J* 16:57, 1969.
21. Modell JH, Moya F: Postoperative pulmonary complications: Incidence and management. *Anesth Analg* 45:432, 1966.
22. Asley F, Kannel WB, Sorlie PD, et al.: Pulmonary function: Relation to aging, cigarette habit, and mortality: The Framingham study. *Ann Intern Med* 82:739, 1975.
23. Godfrey S, Edwards RHT, Campbell EJM, et al.: Repeatability of physical signs in airways obstruction. *Thorax* 24:4, 1969.
24. Godfrey S, Edwards RHT, Campbell EJM, et al.: Clinical and physiologic associations of some physical signs observed in patients with chronic airways obstruction. *Thorax* 25:285, 1970.
25. Campbell EJM: Physical signs of diffuse airways obstruction and lung distension. *Thorax* 24:1, 1969.
26. Forgacs P: The functional significance of clinical signs in diffuse airway obstruction. *Br J Dis Chest* 65:170, 1971.
27. Ashutosh K, Gilbert R, Auchincloss JH Jr, et al.: Asynchronous breathing movements in patients with chronic obstructive pulmonary disease. *Chest* 67:553, 1975.
28. Nath AR, Capel LH: Inspiratory crackles—early and late. *Thorax* 29:223, 1974.
29. Forgacs P: The functional basis of pulmonary sounds. *Chest* 73:399, 1978.
30. Nath AR, Capel LH: Inspiratory crackles and mechanical events of breathing. *Thorax* 29:695, 1974.
31. Marini JJ, Pierson DJ, Hudson LD, et al.: The significance of wheezing in chronic airflow obstruction. *Am Rev Respir Dis* 120:1069, 1979.
32. Lal S, Ferguson AD, Campbell EJM: Forced expiratory time: A simple test for airways obstruction. *Br Med J* 1:814, 1964.

33. Hansen G, Drablos PA, Steinert R: Pulmonary complications, ventilation, and blood gases after upper abdominal surgery. *Acta Anesthesiol Scand* 21:211, 1977.
34. Craven JL, Evans GA, Davenport PJ, et al.: The evaluation of the incentive spirometer in the management of postoperative pulmonary complications. *Br J Surg* 61:793, 1974.
35. Cain HD, Stevens PM, Adaniya R: Preoperative pulmonary function and complications after cardiovascular surgery. *Chest* 76:130, 1979.
36. Bates DV, Macklem PT, Christie RV: *Respiratory function in disease.* Philadelphia, WB Saunders Co, 1971.
37. Snider GL, Rieger RA, Demas T, et al.: Variations in the measurement of spirograms. *Am J Med Sci* 254:679, 1967.
38. Miller WF, Wu N, Johnson RL Jr: Convenient method of evaluating pulmonary ventilatory function with a single breath test. *Anesthesiology* 17:480, 1956.
39. Boutros AR, Weisel M: Comparison of effects of three anesthetic techniques on patients with severe pulmonary obstructive disease. *Canad Anaesth Soc J* 18:286, 1971.
40. Milledge JS, Nunn JF: Criteria of fitness for anaesthesia in patients with chronic obstructive lung disease. *Br Med J* 3:670, 1975.
41. Williams CD, Brenowitz JB: "Prohibitive" lung function and major surgical procedures. *Am J Surg* 132:763, 1976.
42. Felson B: *Chest Roentgenology.* Philadelphia, WB Saunders Co, 1973.
43. Burki NK, Krumpelman JL: Correlation of pulmonary function with the chest roentgenogram in chronic airway obstruction. *Am Rev Respir Dis* 121:217, 1980.
44. Harlan WR, Oberman A, Grimm R, et al.: Chronic congestive heart failure in coronary artery disease: Clinical criteria. *Ann Intern Med* 86:133, 1977.
45. Hales CA, Kazemi H: Pulmonary function after uncomplicated myocardial infarction. *Chest* 72:350, 1977.
46. Richards DGB, Whitfield AGW, Arnott WM, et al.: The lung volume in low output cardiac syndromes. *Br Heart J* 13:381, 1951.
47. Frank NR, Cugell DW, Gaensler EA, Ellis LB: Ventilatory studies in mitral stenosis. *Am J Med* 15:60, 1953.
48. Friedman BL, Macias J DeJ, Yu PN: Pulmonary function studies in patients with mitral stenosis. *Am Rev Tuberc* 79:265, 1959.
49. Capel LH, Smart J: Obstructive airway disease. *Lancet* 1:960, 1959.

CHAPTER IX

Invasive Testing

Eric E. Harrison, M.D.
and Sheldon S. Sbar, M.D.

Introduction

In patients who undergo general anesthesia and surgery, the presence of cardiovascular disease is associated with increased morbidity and mortality.[1-13] Coronary artery disease has been the most intensively studied risk factor for noncardiac surgery.[1-10] On the other hand, patients with valvular heart disease are less well studied but also appear to have a greater cardiovascular risk, with a higher mortality rate noted in patients with aortic valve disease than in patients with mitral valve disease.[11] Clinically severe aortic stenosis has been specifically implicated as a risk factor in noncardiac surgical patients.[5] Morrison noted a slight increase in surgical risk in patients with mitral valve disease.[8] Other forms of heart disease, such as hypertension and that associated with pulmonary disease, have not been linked independently of atherosclerosis or pulmonary disease as causes of increased surgical risk.[11] However, there is evidence that congestive heart failure imparts a significant increase in surgical risk.[5] Although these associations have been demonstrated in many studies, few studies have correlated the distribution and quantification of coronary artery disease,[1] the hemodynamic severity of aortic and mitral valve disease, and left ventricular end-diastolic pressure and angiographically defined ejection fraction with noncardiac surgical risk. In some cases, a precise anatomic and hemodynamic definition at rest and during stress might be useful information in making decisions as to noncardiac surgical risk in the cardiovascular patient and in defining

149

risk subsets. This information would have to be considered along with other factors affecting surgical risk, such as the type of surgery, duration of surgery, surgical skill, type of anesthesia, the anesthesiologist's skill, risk of hypotension, previous cardiac events, cardiac symptoms, available postoperative care, elective versus emergent surgery, age of the patient, and previous palliative or corrective cardiac surgery.

Coronary Anatomy

There is extensive data relating coronary artery anatomy and left ventricular function to long-term prognosis in patients with coronary artery disease.[15] Consideration has been given to relating these same factors to noncardiac surgical risks, particularly in view of the low risk of cardiac catheterization, but prospective angiographic studies have not been reported. In one retrospective report,[1] a group of patients who had angiographic evidence of coronary artery disease were studied. Forty-nine patients underwent 58 noncardiac operations, with three patients suffering perioperative myocardial infarctions. Fifteen of the 49 patients studied had three vessel coronary artery disease, and the three patients with myocardial infarctions were from this group (a 20% incidence of perioperative myocardial infarctions in patients with severe three vessel coronary artery disease). Unfortunately, because of the small numbers involved, it is difficult to draw general conclusions from this study concerning the noncardiac surgical risk of patients with one, two, and three vessel coronary artery disease. The suggestion is, however, that three vessel disease is associated with a high perioperative infarction rate in patients undergoing prolonged major surgery. One group uses coronary angiography and ventriculography to separate high and low risk patient groups for elective abdominal aortic aneurysmectomy or surgical correction of aortoiliac occlusive disease.[16] However, the natural history of these groups was not evaluated.

Coronary Artery Bypass

It has been proposed that patients with coronary artery disease who have had coronary artery bypass surgery or who have simultaneous coronary artery bypass grafting and noncardiac surgery have a low risk of perioperative cardiac mortality following noncardiac surgical procedures.[11,17-30] The implication of this hypothesis is that patients with coronary artery disease who are being considered for certain noncardiac surgical procedures should first be evaluated invasively and subsets selected for coronary artery bypass surgery prior to or simultaneously with the noncardiac surgery.[16,20,31]

Although an invasive evaluation of coronary pathoanatomy has been proposed for many patients about to undergo noncardiac surgery, the greatest experience reported in the recent literature has pertained to elective abdominal aortic aneurysm resection, lower extremity revascularization procedures, and carotid vascular surgery (see Chapter XIII). Extensive data are available as to the cardiac mortality of patients undergoing operations for these conditions, but cardiac morbidity data have not been uniformly compiled and no randomized studies performed. Nonetheless, these conditions will be discussed and summarized from chapters XII and XIII since it represents the majority of information available.

Elective Abdominal Aortic Aneurysm Resection

Some authors have recommended routine coronary angiography in all patients considered for abdominal aortic aneurysm resection or aortoiliac reconstruction.[16] This approach has been suggested because of the high prevalence of coronary artery disease in patients with peripheral vascular disease (15–54%),[32] and because myocardial infarction accounts for 40% of all early postoperative deaths following abdominal aortic aneurysmectomy and 67% of all those following aorto-femoral bypass. The value of this approach may be tested by a comparison of cardiac morbidity and mortality in patients with similar disease who have not had prior coronary artery bypass grafting.

Cardiac mortality figures vary in elective abdominal aortic aneurysm resection.[32] In three separate but very similar *early* series of unselected cases, Young reported a 15.6% overall mortality rate[34] (Table 1), Szilagyi reported a 13% overall mortality rate,[34] and Baker reported a 9.5% overall mortality rate.[36] Combining these three studies, the mean mortality rate was 12% for 704 patients. In four more *recent* series of unselected cases, overall mortality

Table 1
Mortality in Elective Abdominal Aortic Aneurysm Repair
(unselected cases)

Author	Patient Number	Overall Mortality	M.I.* Mortality
Early studies:			
Young[33]	64	15.6%	—
Szilagyi[34]	400	13.0%	—
Baker[35]	240	9.5%	—
TOTAL	704	12.0% Mean	
Recent studies:			
Thompson[36]	108	5.5%	4.8%
Young[33]	111	6.3%	—
Szilagyi[34]	111	7.2%	—
Yashar[37]	105	5.6%	2.0%
TOTAL	435	6.2% Mean	3.3% Mean

*Mortality rate from myocardial infarction

ranged from 5.5% to 7.2% (Table 1) with a mean of 6.2% in 435 patients. Thus, the mortality rate of unselected cases has decreased by half in recent years. However, when patients with known un-operated coronary artery disease are studied, the mortality rate remains high, ranging from 8.1% to 13% (almost all from myocardial infarctions), giving a mean mortality rate of 11.6% for 671 cases[33,34,37–39] (Table 2). The high cardiac mortality rate in these patients may be explained by the hypotension, blood loss, duration of surgery, and afterload changes due to aortic cross clamping. In contrast, patients without known coronary artery disease experienced mortality ranging from 0–4.4%,[16,33,34,38,39] giving a combined mortality rate in 661 patients of 2.6% (Table 2).

More recent experiences of elective abdominal aortic aneurysm resection from 1978 to 1981 report much lower mortality rates in patients with no known coronary artery disease and in patients with a history of prior infarction or angina. Brown et al. report a 0.8% mortality from myocardial infarction in 249 patients without a history consistent with coronary disease, and a 3% mortality from myocardial infarction in 167 patients with a history of coronary disease.[40] Improvement of survival was attributed to better moni-

Table 2
Mortality in Elective Abdominal Aortic Aneurysm Repair

Author	Patient Number	Overall Mortality	M.I.* Mortality
Without Evidence of Heart Disease			
Young[33]	60	0%	—
Yashar[37]	68	4.4%	—
Hicks[38]	68	0%	—
DeBakey[32]	465	3.0%	—
TOTAL	661	2.6% Mean	—
Without Heart Disease			
Hertzer	30	3.3%	0%
With Heart Disease			
Yashar[37]	37	8.1%	—
Young[33]	59	12.0%	—
DeBakey[32]	418	13.0%	—
Hicks[38]	157	9.0%	—
TOTAL	671	11.6% Mean	—

*Mortality rate from myocardial infarction

toring and better care before, during, and after aneurysm operation.

In patients who have had coronary artery bypass surgery prior to abdominal aortic aneurysm resection, the mortality rate is also relatively low and interestingly similar to that seen in patients without coronary artery disease. In groups of bypassed patients, Hertzer reported a 4% (1/26) mortality rate for coronary artery bypass grafting and no mortality rate for abdominal aortic aneurysm resection.[16] Edwards, Crawford, and McCollum in separate series reported no mortality for abdominal aortic aneurysm resection in bypassed patients.[17-19] But, to these figures must be added the mortality rate of coronary artery bypass surgery. Simultaneous coronary artery bypass grafting and abdominal aortic aneurysm resection has been undertaken in three patients by Reis and Hannah with no mortality (Table 3).[21]

In conclusion, patients with abdominal aortic aneurysms appear to have a high prevalence of coronary artery disease. Those with

Table 3

Elective Abdominal Aortic Aneurysm Repair Mortality in Prior CABG*
or Simultaneous CABG

Author	Patient Number	Overall Mortality
Hertzer[28]	21	0%
McCollum[19]	17	0%
Crawford[18]	49	0%
Edwards[17]	8	0%
Reis[21]	3	0%
TOTAL	98	0%

*Coronary artery bypass grafting

coronary artery disease have a higher operative mortality rate than those without coronary disease. Coronary arteriography is useful in separating out these two populations. Those with severe coronary artery disease who are deemed operable for coronary artery bypass and survive coronary artery bypass grafting, and are still considered candidates for abdominal aortic aneurysm resection have a low operative risk for the latter. Thus, inoperable cardiac patients with severe cardiac disease might be managed conservatively, or if they have symptomatic expanding abdominal aortic aneurysms, might be operated on with an awareness of enhanced risk and additional precautions taken.

Lower Extremity Revascularization

The approach for patients with abdominal aortic aneurysms has been applied to patients in need of aortoiliac, ilio-femoral, and femoro-popliteal bypass. These patients also have a high prevalence of coronary disease. Tomatis et al. demonstrated that significant (75–100% obstruction of a major vessel) coronary disease was present in 47% of those with aortoiliac disease and 48% of those with femoro-popliteal disease.[32] Hertzer et al. showed that even without symptoms or EKG evidence of cardiac disease, 15 of 45 (33%) patients with aortoiliac disease had significant coronary artery disease.[16] These same authors studied another group of 26 patients *with* symptoms or EKG evidence of coronary disease and

Table 4
Mortality in Elective Lower Extremity Revascularization

Author	Patient Number	Overall Mortality	M.I.* Mortality	Operation
		Unselected Cases		
Inahara[39]	180	4.5%	—	Aorto-iliac endartetectomy
Malone[40]	180**	2.5%	1.0%	Aorto-femoral grafting
Pilcher[41]	69	—	0.0%	Aorto-iliac endarterectomy
TOTAL	429	3.3% Mean	0.8% Mean	
		No Heart Disease		
Hertzer	39	—	0.0%	Aorto-bifemoral bypass
	Prior CABG or Simultaneous CABG			
Hertzer[16]	6	—	0.0%	Aorto-bifemoral bypass
Edwards[17]	25	—	3.8%	Various procedures
Crawford[18]	53	—	0.0%	Aorto-femoral revascularization
McCollum[19]	31	—	0.0%	Aorto-iliac femoral-popliteal
Reis[21]	1	—	0.0%	Aorto-femoral bypass
TOTAL	116	—	0.9% Mean	

*Mortality from myocardial infarction
**104/180 (58%) had evidence of coronary artery disease

found 22 (85%) with significant coronary disease. Aortoiliac and lower extremity vascular disease, then, are markers for coronary artery disease, but the influence of bypass grafting may not be great since the operative mortality of lower extremity revascularization is low, ranging from 0–4.5%[16–19,41–43] (Table 4). Thus, despite the high prevalence of cardiac disease in patients with peripheral vascular disease who have lower extremity revascularization procedures, the overall operative mortality rate is so low that coronary bypass grafting prior to lower extremity revascularization would not be expected to significantly affect the operative risk.

Carotid Endarterectomy

The overall mean mortality rate of unselected patients having carotid endarterectomy is 2.7%, and the mean myocardial infarction mortality rate is 0.94% (Table 5).[44–51] In contrast, patients having carotid endarterectomy who also had a history of coronary artery disease, have mortality rates ranging from 1.8%–16%[23,25,30,42,50,51] (Table 6). Combining the studies, 456 patients had a mean mortality rate of 5.9%, mostly due to perioperative myocardial infarction. On the other hand, operative mortality rates are generally much lower in patients who have coronary artery bypass grafting prior to carotid endarterectomy, and range from 0–4%[17,19,23,31] (Table 7). It should again be noted, however, that these figures do not take into consideration the mortality rate of coronary artery bypass surgery.

Because of the information presented above, some authors have advocated simultaneous coronary and carotid surgery, citing a decrease in both cardiac and cerebrovascular morbidity and mortality. Morris[23] demonstrated no cardiac mortality in 44 patients; Hertzer[28] demonstrated a 2% cardiac mortality rate in 115 patients with a 10% myocardial infarction rate; Urschel[31] demonstrated no cardiac mortality in eight patients; and Bernhard reported no car-

Table 5

Mortality in Elective Carotid Endarterectomy (unselected cases)

Author	Patient Number	Overall Mortality	M.I.* Mortality
DeWeese[43]	103	—	0.97%
Thompson[44]	592	—	0.85%
Nunn[45]	234	—	1.20%
Javid[46]	56	—	1.78%
Lefrak[47]	34	—	2.90%
Fields[48]	169	3.5%	—
Keshishian[49]	200	2.0%	—
Riles[42]	683	—	0.80%
TOTAL	2,071	2.7%	0.94%

*Mortality rate from myocardial infarction

Table 6
Mortality in Elective Carotid Endarterectomy

Author	Patient Number	Overall Mortality	M.I.* Mortality
	History of Coronary Disease		
Riles[42]	284	—	1.8%
Morris[23]	35	—	9.0%
Bernhard[50]	15	—	13.0%
Urschel[30]	8	—	0.0%**
Rubio and Guin[51]	37	—	16.0%
Ennix[53]	77	—	14.0%
TOTAL	456	—	5.9% Mean
	No History of Coronary Disease		
Riles[42]	399	—	0.0%

*Mortality rate from myocardial infarction
**12% sustained nonfatal M.I.

Table 7
Mortality in Carotid Endarterectomy (prior to CABG or simultaneous CABG)

Author	Patient	Overall Mortality	M.I.* Mortality
Ennix[53]	135	3.0%	0.8%
Reis[21]	4	—	0.0%
Okies[24]	6	—	0.0%
Morris[23]	44	4.5%	0.0%
McCollum[19]	5	0.0%	0.0%
Crawford[18]	97	2.0%	0.0%
Edwards[17]	25	—	4.0%
Bernhard[50]	15	0.0%	0.0%
Urschel[30]	8	0.0%	0.0%
Urschel[29]	17	0.0%	0.0%
TOTAL	356	2.5% Mean	0.6% Mean

*Mortality from myocardial infarction

diac mortality in 15 patients.[49] Ennix et al.[55] reported an operative mortality rate of 0.8%. Combining the studies of patients with simultaneous or prior coronary bypass and carotid endarterectomy, 356 patients had a mean overall mortality rate of 2.5% and a mean myocardial infarction mortality rate of 0.6%.

In conclusion, patients with symptomatic carotid vascular disease frequently have symptomatic coronary artery disease. In one study by Marzewski et al., when stenosis of an intracranial internal carotid artery (greater than 50%) was present, 58% of the patients had concomitant severe coronary artery disease.[56] Their cardiac mortality rate ranges from 2–16% after carotid endarterectomy— in patients with coronary disease. Cardiac mortality rates during carotid endarterectomy are very low in patients without evidence of cardiac disease. In patients with symptomatic cardiac disease who have been selected for coronary bypass surgery prior to or concomitant with carotid endarterectomy, the operative mortality may approach the operative mortality of patients without symptomatic cardiac disease, but controlled studies are needed to validate this approach.

Coronary Artery Bypass Grafting Prior to Heterogeneous Noncardiac Surgical Procedures

Other studies have investigated the operative cardiac morbidity and mortality rate in patients with prior coronary artery bypass grafting who have undergone heterogeneous noncardiac surgical procedures (Table 8). Mahar et al.[1] reported 49 patients with an angiographically documented coronary artery disease who underwent various surgical procedures and contrasted this group with another group of 99 patients who had undergone prior coronary artery bypass grafting. There was a lower incidence of perioperative myocardial infarction in the latter group. However, it should be noted that there had been six perioperative myocardial infarctions during bypass grafting so that when the staged procedures are considered in sequence, the myocardial infarction rate for this group of patients was the same as the unbypassed coronary artery disease group.

Crawford et al.[18] have reviewed their experience with 358 patients who had had prior coronary artery bypass grafting and 484

Table 8

Mortality and M.I. Incidence of Various Noncardiac Surgical
Procedures

Author	Patient Number	CABG M.I. Rate	Overall Mortality	M.I. Mortality	Noncardiac Surgery M.I. Incidence
In Patients With Prior CABG					
Mahar[1]	99	6%	0%	0%	0.0%
Crawford[18]	358	unknown	0%	0%	1.2%
McCollum[19]	60	unknown	0%	0%	0.0%
TOTAL	517		0%	0%	0.77% Mean
No Prior CABG					
Mahar[1]	49	N/A	0%	2%	6.0%

subsequent various noncardiac surgical procedures (mostly major procedures). In this large group of patients, there were no deaths of cardiac origin and only six perioperative myocardial infarctions. McCollum[19] reported 60 patients who had coronary artery bypass grafting. These patients underwent 77 subsequent noncardiac major operations without cardiac mortality or myocardial infarctions. Akl et al.[30] reported on 35 patients who had earlier myocardial revascularization and a total of 44 noncardiac operations under general[40] or spinal[4] anesthesia. There was one cardiac death (thought to be arrhythmic) and three postoperative complications.

Thus, it appears that patients selected by angiography and other factors, who survive coronary artery bypass grafting and are selected for other major subsequent surgical procedures, have a low operative cardiac morbidity and mortality.

Recent Myocardial Infarction

It has been demonstrated that patients with recent myocardial infarctions have a high perioperative mortality and myocardial infarction rate when submitted to noncardiac surgical procedures (see Chapter XIII). This broad statement needs to be examined in terms of the supporting data. Large retrospective case study reviews from large centers over the last forty years have contributed this data. When these studies are reviewed and compiled, the final analysis reveals that the data is inadequate. This is because sample sizes are small (mortality within six months of a myocardial infarction was evaluated in a total of only 82 subjects, and reinfarction was evaluated in a total of only 99 subjects). Also, these patients comprise a heterogeneous group undergoing heterogeneous surgical procedures. Finally, the cause of death, incidence, and kind of complications, and whether the surgery was elective or emergent is not generally given. It has been postulated that subendocardial myocardial infarctions are unstable incomplete infarctions which carry an even higher risk of subsequent cardiac events. But, this hypothesis has not been well tested in surgical patients undergoing noncardiac surgery. Steen et al. did report 33 patients with preoperative subendocardial infarction, but the infarction to surgical interval was not given for this specific group of patients.[6] Two (6%) sustained new postoperative infarctions with no deaths. This infarction rate in this same study was no different than that of patients with prior transmural infarctions. An earlier study in 1964 by Arkins et al. did not have available more recent CPK-MB and myocardial scan tests for defining subendocardial infarction.[2] However, of 14 patients with recent subendocardial infarction, who underwent noncardiac surgery, the mortality rate was only 7% (1/14). These numbers of patients are not adequate to draw conclusions regarding the noncardiac surgical risk of patients with prior subendocardial infarction. Our own group has observed in the catheterization laboratory that subendocardial infarctions, defined by clinical, electrocardiographic, enzymatic, and nuclear criteria represent a heterogeneous group. At one end of the spectrum is the patient with single right coronary artery disease and a non-Q wave postero-basilar infarction which is transmural, small, and electrocardiographically silent; at the other end of the angiographic spectrum is the patient with three vessel coronary artery disease, and antero-apical hypokinesis with a high grade left anterior descending lesion. Subsets of patients such as these would have a different prognosis and, conceivably, would present different noncardiac surgical risks.

It has been recommended that noncardiac surgery be delayed six months to a year after myocardial infarctions.[5] This is in fact a "survivors" test, whereby the high risk patients will not survive the interval and the low risk patients will survive to be considered for surgery. Recent studies have shown that the mortality rate after acute myocardial infarction decreases with time. Cardiac mortality rates during the six months after infarction have been reported as high as 15%. This is almost four times the death rate of the subsequent six months.[59] Furthermore, the role of post myocardial infarction stress testing and cardiac cathetherization has not been defined in this group of patients.[59,60] Assessment of left ventricular function and coronary artery anatomy as well as exercise testing offers a reasonable approach to assessing the extent of damage and disease in a patient who is considered for noncardiac surgery after a recent myocardial infarction. In addition, the role of coronary artery bypass surgery has also not been assessed as an approach to altering the subsequent risk of noncardiac surgery in some patients who have had myocardial infarctions within three months.

In conclusion, recent myocardial infarction has been demonstrated as a risk factor for postoperative myocardial infarction and death. However, which subsets of those patients with recent myocardial infarctions are at greatest risk during subsequent noncardiac surgery have not been identified. Many questions remain. How many of the patients reported in the literature were operated on, despite a recent myocardial infarction because of a serious life-threatening emergency and, therefore, had a high mortality rate because of the seriousness of the emergency surgery? Also, in how many was surgery delayed because of a recent myocardial infarction until it was used as a last resort? Did these patients have major life-threatening surgical procedures? How many of these patients had unstable infarctions, postinfarction angina, unstable angina, or congestive heart failure? What is the cause of death in patients with recent myocardial infarctions who undergo noncardiac surgery? Are the complications related to a new separate infarction, extension of infarction, congestive heart failure, or arrhythmias? The mortality rate is high in those patients who have a second infarction, but is it in excess of patients having second infarctions who have not undergone noncardiac surgery (greater than 50%)? There are more questions than answers about this group of patients.

Congestive Heart Failure

Congestive heart failure has been implicated as an independent risk variable for the development of cardiac complications in the postoperative period after noncardiac surgery (see Chapter XVI). Of 35 patients with either a third heart sound or jugular venous distention, Goldman et al. reported that 14% (5/35) developed life-threatening but nonfatal cardiac complications and an additional 20% (7/35) died from cardiac causes.[5] Del Guercio and Cohn assessed by Swan-Ganz catheterizations an elderly group of 148 consecutive patients who had been previously cleared for noncardiac surgery.[60] Serial pressure measurements were measured in the right atrium, right ventricle, pulmonary artery, and pulmonary capillary wedge positions. Cardiac output was measured by thermodilution or indocyanine green, and by oximetry. Primary and derived hemodynamic data included cardiac index, pulse rate, stroke index, left ventricular stroke work, peripheral vascular resistance, right ventricular stroke work, pulmonary vascular resistance, and a Sarnoff ventricular function curve. Based on these studies, patients were classified into four levels of perioperative management and risk from Group I, those of little risk through Group IV, high risk. Thirteen patients were placed in Group III or IV on the basis of pulmonary capillary wedge pressures greater than 15 mmHg. Group I patients who had surgery experienced no mortality. Group II and III patients (intermediate pressure data and output levels) experienced an 8.5% mortality. Group IV patients who had gross physiologic aberrancies were managed in three ways. Of 34 patients, 19 were managed conservatively, seven were sent to lesser operations under local anesthesia, and eight had major surgery. All eight having major surgery died.

In conclusion, congestive heart failure is a significant risk factor for major noncardiac surgery, and hemodynamic parameters may be useful in defining low risk and high risk subsets.

Valvular Heart Disease

It has been reported that patients with valvular heart disease tolerate noncardiac surgery better than those with atherosclerotic disease.[11] However, there are not many studies of noncardiac surgical outcomes in patients with valvular heart disease. Morrison reported a 4.8% mortality rate for 108 patients with mitral valve disease undergoing 147 procedures and concluded that there was a slight increase in surgical risk.[8] Important risk factors were mitral stenosis, cardiac enlargement, and the presence of atrial fibrillation, which was probably indicative of advanced longstanding disease. The mortality rates were generally higher in patients in higher functional classifications using the New York Heart Association Classification. A higher mortality was noted in patients with aortic valve disease compared with mitral valve disease.[11] Morrison's studies were done between 1933 and 1943 and, therefore, prior to the era of cardiac catheterization and echocardiography. Thus, specific valve lesions were not well defined.

Goldman et al.[5] followed 12 patients with aortic insufficiency, 14 patients with mitral stenosis, 54 patients with mitral regurgitation, and 23 patients with aortic stenosis through noncardiac surgery to assess valvular heart disease as a risk factor. Only aortic stenosis was correlated as presenting an increased surgical risk with cardiac deaths occurring in 13% (3/23). In this study, signs of congestive heart failure, such as an S_3 or jugular venous distention, were analyzed separately from valvular heart disease and found to be an independent variable directly related to cardiac risk.

Cardiac catheterization along with echocardiography should play a central role in evaluating the severity of valvular heart disease at rest and during stress, left ventricular function, and the presence of concomitant coronary artery disease. Because of the advances of modern cardiac surgery, the demonstration of severe disease is more than academic (See also Chapter XIV).

Other Cardiac Diseases

Other types of cardiac diseases such as idiopathic hypertrophic subaortic stenosis, nonrheumatic mitral insufficiency, congestive cardiomyopathy, and forms of congenital heart disease have not been related specifically to noncardiac surgical risk.[5] A reasonable approach to defining an individual's surgical risk would be to take into consideration the clinical classification, the severity of the lesion or lesions, and the cardiac reserve.

Conclusion

Cardiac disease increases noncardiac surgical risk. Significant coronary artery disease, left ventricular dysfunction, and severe valvular heart disease, especially aortic stenosis, have been specifically identified as risk factors.[2–5,11] Very few studies have related anatomical and hemodynamic data to surgical outcomes. Recent literature examines the distribution and extent of coronary artery disease and its relationship to morbidity and mortality. Some low risk and high risk subsets can, perhaps, be selected by cardiac catheterization. Some patients may tolerate abdominal aortic aneurysm resection, lower extremity revascularization, carotid endarterectomy, and heterogeneous noncardiac surgical procedures better with than without prior coronary artery bypass grafting. Patients in whom left ventricular function is in question can be investigated by Swan-Ganz catheterization, and risk categories may be defined. Further studies are needed to relate cardiac catheterization and stress test data to noncardiac surgical risk in those patients expe-

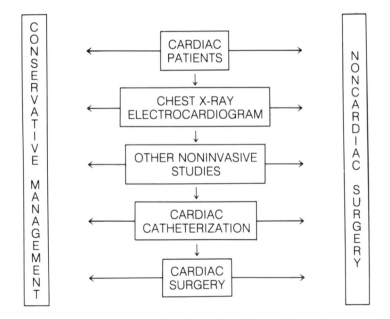

Figure 1. Scheme for the evaluation of cardiac patients for noncardiac surgery.

riencing recent myocardial infarctions, subendocardial infarction, and the various angina syndromes.

A diagrammatic scheme for the approach to the cardiac patient considered for noncardiac surgery is offered in Figure 1. The surgical procedure being considered may in itself be a low risk procedure, even for a cardiac patient. Thus, in cases of simple inguinal hernia repair or transurethral prostatectomy, the patient may undergo surgery without in-depth evaluation. When higher cardiac risk surgery is considered, some patients on the basis of history, physical examination, chest x-ray, and electrocardiogram may be found to occupy a low risk or high risk category and may be assigned to noncardiac surgical treatment or to conservative management on the basis of this information. Others may require extensive noninvasive studies to determine left ventricular function or perfusion, while others may go on to cardiac catheterization for complete assessment and may be considered for subsequent cardiac surgery to reduce noncardiac surgical risk, go on and have noncardiac surgery, or be managed conservatively without any surgery. Further refinement of this general approach will have to await larger preoperative angiographic studies.

References

1. Mahar LJ, Steen PA, Tinker JH, et al.: Perioperative myocardial infarction in patients with coronary artery disease with and without aorto-coronary artery bypass grafts. *J Thorac Cardiovasc Surg* 76:533, 1978.
2. Arkins R, Smessaert AA, Hicks RG: Mortality and morbidity in surgical patients with coronary artery disease. *JAMA* 190:485, 1964.
3. Topkins MJ, Artusio JF Jr: Myocardial infarction and surgery. *Anesth Analg* 43:716, 1964.
4. Tarhan S, Moffitt EA, Taylor WF, et al.: Myocardial infarction after general anesthesia. *JAMA* 220:1451, 1972.
5. Goldman L, Caldera DL, Nussbaum SR, et al.: Multifactorial index of cardiac risk in noncardiac surgical procedures. *N Engl J Med* 297:845, 1977.
6. Steen PA, Tinker JH, Tarhan S: Myocardial reinfarction after anesthesia and surgery. *JAMA* 239:2566, 1978.
7. Nachlas MM, Abrams SJ, Goldberg MM: The influence of arteriosclerotic heart disease on surgical risk. *Am J Surg* 101:447, 1961.
8. Morrison DR: The risk of surgery in heart disease. *Surgery* 23:561, 1948.

9. Hannigan CA, Wroblewski F, Lewis WH Jr, et al.: Major surgery in patients with healed myocardial infarction. *Am J Med Sci* 222:628, 1951.
10. Etsten BE, Weaver DC, Li TH, et al.: Appraisal of the coronary patient as an operative risk. *NY J Med* 54:2065, 1954.
11. Skinner JF, Pearce ML: Surgical risk in the cardiac patient. *J Chron Dis* 17:57, 1964.
12. Fraser JG, Ramachandra PR, Davis HS: Anesthesia and recent myocardial infarction. *JAMA* 199:96, 1967.
13. Alexander S: Surgical risk in the patient with arteriosclerotic heart disease. *Surg Clin N Am* 48:513, 1968.
14. Pupello DF, Spoto E Jr: Long-term results of coronary bypass surgery. *J Florida M A* 66:1044, 1979.
15. Sones FM Jr: Complications of coronary arteriography and left heart catheterization. *Cleve Clin Quar 45:21, 1978.*
16. Hertzer NR, Young JR, Kramer JR, et al.: Routine coronary angiography prior to elective aortic reconstruction. *Arch Surg* 114:1336, 1979.
17. Edwards WH, Mulherin JL Jr, Walker WE: Vascular reconstructive surgery following myocardial revascularization. *Ann Surg* 187:653, 1978.
18. Crawford ES, Morris GC, Howell JF, et al.: Operative risk in patients with previous coronary artery bypass. *Ann Thorac Surg* 26:215, 1978.
19. McCollum GH, Garcia-Rinaldi R, Graham JM, et al.: Myocardial revascularization prior to subsequent major surgery in patients with coronary artery disease. *Surgery* 81:302, 1977.
20. Scher KS, Tice DA: Operative risk in patients with previous coronary artery bypass. *Arch Surg* 111:807, 1976.
21. Reis RL, Hannah H III: Management of patients with severe, coexistent coronary artery and peripheral vascular disease. *J Thorac Cardiovasc Surgery* 73:909, 1977.
22. Diethrich EB, Zamorano C, Ravindranath K: Simultaneous surgical correction of coronary and peripheral vascular arterial lesions. *Chest* 68:409, 1975.
23. Morris GC, Ennis CL Jr, Lawrie GM, et al.: Management of coexistent carotid and coronary artery occlusive atherosclerosis. *Cleve Clin Quar* 45:125, 1978.
24. Okies JE, MacManus Q, Starr A: Myocardial revascularization and carotid endarterectomy: A combined approach. *Ann Thorac Surg* 23:560, 1977.
25. Check W: Simultaneous coronary bypass and carotid endarterectomy advocated. *JAMA* 240:725, 1978.
26. Shore RT, Johnson WD: Combined surgical treatment for coronary artery surgery complicated by extracranial carotid disease. *Chest* 66:336, 1974.
27. Okies JE, MacManus Q, Starr A: Myocardial revascularization and carotid endarterectomy—a combined approach? *Chest* 68:422, 1975.

28. Hertzer NR, Loop FD, Taylor PC, et al.: Staged and combined surgical approach to simultaneous carotid and coronary vascular disease. *Surgery* 84:803, 1978.
29. Urschel HC Jr: Management of concomitant coronary and carotid artery obstructive disease. *Clev Clin Quar* 45:128, 1978.
30. Akl BF, Talbot W, Neal JF, et al.: Noncardiac operations after coronary revascularization. *West J Med* 136:91, 1982
31. Urschel HC, Razzuk MA, Gardner MA: Management of concomitant occlusive disease of the carotid and coronary arteries. *J Thorac Cardiovasc Surg* 72:829, 1976.
32. Tomatis LA, Fierens EE, Verbrugge GP: Evaluation of surgical risk in peripheral vascular disease by coronary arteriography: A series of 100 cases. *Surgery* 71:429, 1972.
33. DeBakey ME, Crawford ES, Cooley DA, et al.: Aneurysm of abdominal aorta, analysis of results of graft replacement therapy one to eleven years after operation. *Ann Surg* 160:622, 1964.
34. Young AE, Sandberg GW, Couch NP: The reduction of mortality of abdominal aortic aneurysm resection. *Am J Surg* 134:585, 1977.
35. Szilagyi DE, Smith RF, Franklin J, et al.: Contribution of abdominal aortic aneurysmectomy to prolongation of life. *Ann Surg* 164:678, 1966.
36. Baker AG, Roberts B: Long-term survival following abdominal aortic aneurysmectomy. *JAMA* 212:445, 1970.
37. Thompson JE, Hollier LH, Patman RD, et al.: Surgical management of abdominal aortic aneurysm-factors influencing mortality and morbidity: a 20 year experience. *Ann Surg* 181:654, 1975.
38. Yashar JJ, Indeglia RA, Yashar J: Surgery for abdominal aortic aneurysms. *Am J Surg* 123:398, 1972.
39. Hicks GL, Eastland MW, DeWeese JA, et al.: Survival improvement following aortic aneurysm resection. *Ann Surg* 181:863, 1975.
40. Brown OW, Hollier LH, Pairolero PC, et al.: Abdominal aortic aneurysm and coronary artery disease. *Arch Surg* 116:1484, 1981.
41. Inahara T: Evaluation of endarterectomy for aortoiliac and aortoiliofemoral occlusive disease. *Arch Surg* 110:1458, 1975.
42. Malone JM, Moore WS, Goldstone J: Life expectancy following aortofemoral arterial grafting. *Surgery* 81:551, 1977.
43. Pilcher DB, Barker WF, Cannon JA: An aortoiliac endarterectomy case series followed 10 years or more. *Surgery* 67:5, 1970.
44. Riles TS, Kopelman I, Imparato AM: Myocardial infarction following carotid endarterectomy: A review of 683 operations. *Surgery* 85:249, 1979.
45. DeWeese JA, Robb CH, Satran R, et al.: Results of carotid endarterectomies for transient ischemic attacks five years later. *Ann Surg* 178:258, 1973.
46. Thompson JE, Austin DJ, Patman RD: Carotid endarterectomy for cerebrovascular insufficiency, long-term results in 592 patients followed up to thirteen years. *Ann Surg* 172:663, 1970.

47. Nunn DB: Carotid endarterectomy: An analysis of 234 operative cases. *Ann Surg* 182:733,1975.
48. Javid H, Ostermiller WE, Hengesh JW, et al.: Natural history of carotid bifurcation atheroma. *Surgery* 67:80, 1970.
49. Lefrak EA, Guinn GA: Prophylactic carotid artery surgery in patients requiring a second operation. *South Med J* 67:185, 1974.
50. Fields WS, Maslenikov V, Meyer JS, et al: Joint study of extracranial arterial occlusion progress report of prognosis following surgery or nonsurgical treatment for transient cerebral ischemic attacks and cervical carotid artery lesions. *JAMA* 211:1993, 1970.
51. Keshishian JM: Carotid endarterectomy: Mortality rate. *Stroke* 9(2):172, 1978.
52. Bernhard VM, Johnson WD, Peterson JJ: Carotid artery stenosis. *Arch Surg* 105:837, 1972.
53. Rubio RA, Guinn GA: Myocardial infarction following carotid endarterectomy. *Cardiovasc Dis* 2:402, 1975.
54. Szklo M, Goldberg R, Kennedy HL, et al.: Survival of patients with nontransmural myocardial infarction: A population based study. *Am J Cardiol* 42:648, 1978.
55. Ennix C, Morris G, Lawrie G, et al.: Simultaneous coronary bypass and carotid endarterectomy advocated. *JAMA* 240:725, 1978.
56. Marzewski D, Furlan A, Little J, et al.: Prognosis grim for internal carotid stenosis. *JAMA* 247:1920, 1982.
57. The Anturane Reinfarction Trial Research Group: Sulfinpyrazone in the prevention of sudden death after myocardial infarction. *N Engl J Med* 302:250, 1980.
58. Markiewicz W, Houston N, Debusk RF: Exercise testing soon after myocardial infarction. *Circulation* 6:26, 1977.
59. Smith JW, Dennis CA, Gassman A, et al.: Exercise testing three weeks after myocardial infarction. *Chest* 75:1, 1979.
60. Del Guercio LRM, Cohn JD: Monitoring operative risk in the elderly. *JAMA* 243:1350, 1980.

The Perioperative Management

In this Section, specific types of problems are discussed with emphasis on the effect of that problem on the risk of noncardiac surgery. As persons are living longer, the elderly patient's response to surgery has assumed increasing importance. A discussion of what aging is, and the expected cardiopulmonary–renal changes with aging precedes the final assessment that age has on surgical risk. The discussion on arrhythmias and conduction disturbances emphasizes those situations most likely to be encountered in cardiac patients. For example, the use of temporary pacemakers during surgery in patients with bundle branch blocks is discussed. This is followed by discussions on the risk and management of patients undergoing noncardiac surgery who have coronary artery disease, peripheral and cerebrovascular disease, valvular heart disease, hypertension, and congestive heart failure due to these or any cardiac condition. Three special situations are discussed in the final chapters—namely, the assessment and risk of the pregnant patient with cardiac disease, the cardiac patient with pulmonary disease, and, finally, the management and treatment of dental disease in the cardiac patient. This last subject is included because of its commonness, its importance in patients with all types of heart disease (but, particularly, valvular disease), and because most physicians have limited knowledge in this area.

CHAPTER X

The Elderly Patient

Patricia P. Barry, M.D.

Introduction

Aging in living tissues is a phenomenon of universal importance and currently unexplained cause; numerous theories are presently under investigation. According to a recent review by Morris Rockstein,[1] any acceptable theory must meet three criteria:
- It must be evident in all members of a given species.
- It must be progressive with time.
- It must be deleterious, leading to failure of the organ or system. Hayflick[2] is a proponent of the genetic hypotheses, which include:
- The existence of "aging genes" which code for senile changes.
- The exhaustion of the supply of genetic information by the organism.
- The accumulation of inaccurate information or erroneous genetic material by somatic mutation, which occurs due to random events.[3]

Rockstein refers to these as the "Gene Theory," the "Running-Out of Program Theory," and the "Somatic Mutation Theory," respectively.

Hayflick[2] points out that support for these genetic theories comes from several observations which have been made concerning the growth of human cells *in vitro*. It has been noted that only *abnormal* cells are capable of unlimited multiplication; normal cells have a finite life span, which varies according to the species of origin in most cases.

171

Other intriguing theories reviewed by Rockstein[1] include the following:

"Cross-Linkage Theory": Increasing cross-linkage, in proteins such as collagen and essential molecules such as DNA, are responsible for failure of tissues and organs.

"Free-Radical Theory": Free radicals accumulate in cells and cause damage to cell membranes and chromosomes.

"Clinker Theory": Aging represents an accumulation of deleterious substances (somatic mutations, cross-linkages, free radicals) within the body's cells. Some, such as lipofuscin, are inert but displace other, more important components. Others, such as free radicals and histones, produce changes in cell components.

"Error Theory": As cells function, random errors occur in protein synthesis, especially enzyme synthesis, leading to failure of the cell.

"Wear and Tear Theory": Cells continuously "wear out," aggravated by internal and external stress factors, such as accumulation of deleterious substances. This seems particularly applicable to post-mitotic cells such as brain and muscle.

"Autoimmune Theory": Walford[4] postulates that defects occur with aging of the immune system, leading to increases in the production of autoantibodies.

Many of these theories apply directly to specific organs or systems, but none adequately explains the total complex process of aging, which is accompanied not only by increasing incidence of pathology, but also by physiologic changes due to loss of body tissues and other aging phenomena. The result of these changes is a steady decline in the functional capacity of most organ systems. It is important to note that there is great individual variation in the process, due to factors other than chronological age: genetic, environmental, and constitutional. It is also critical to realize that aging of tissues within each individual is a differential process which may be identified at varying times in specific organs, as indicated in Figure 1.[5]

The organs of special concern in the elderly patient being evaluated preoperatively include cardiovascular, pulmonary, and renal systems. Even in the absence of identified disease states, the natural changes that occur as the human body ages create altered physiology. It is critical that the health practitioner be aware of these declining functions and allow for their effects in the care of the older patient. Although this book specifically addresses the prob-

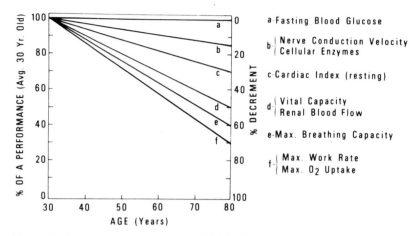

Figure 1. Age decrements in physiological performance (Reprinted with permission of MacMillan Publishing Co., Inc.: Timiras PS: *Developmental Physiology and Aging*, 1972, p. 419.)

lems of the cardiac patient undergoing non-cardiac surgery, it will become apparent that the elderly patient, due to the altered physiology which accompanies the aging process, must be considered as having significant limitations in the cardiovascular system. These must be evaluated and considered in planning the pre- and post-operative management, just as the altered physiology resulting from disease states must be a prime consideration in patient care in the peri-operative period.

Physiologic Changes of Aging

General Body Changes

There appears to be an age-related impairment in the function of the autonomic nervous system, reflected in such clinically significant problems as greater liability to hypothermia, and increasing susceptibility to postural hypotension.[6]

Some general changes have also been noted, as aging progresses, which may have relevance. The amount of adipose tissue increases, and the amount of muscle mass decreases. However, the total body weight, as well as the lean body mass, tend to decrease with age.

Table 1
Some Physiologic Changes of Aging

Organ	Impaired Function
General body	autonomic system
Cardiovascular	decreased MHR ↓ cardiac output ↑ TPR altered blood flow distribution
Pulmonary	↓ compliance ↓ vital capacity ↑ FRC and RV ↓ FEV_1 ↑ $\dot{V}/\dot{Q}$ mismatching ↓ pO_2 ↓ defense mechanism
Renal	↓ GFR ↓ RPF ↓ tubular function ↓ concentrating and diluting ability

↓	= decrease	$\dot{V}/\dot{Q}$	= ventilation perfusion
↑	= increase	GFR	= glomerular filtration rate
TPR	= total peripheral resistance	RPF	= renal plasma flow
FRC	= functional residual capacity		
RV	= residual volume		
FEV_1	= forced expiratory volume in 1 second		

The adipose tissue tends to assume a centripetal distribution: increased on trunk and decreased on limbs. Total body water decreases with age, as does density of bone.[7]

Cardiovascular

The following cardiovascular functions have been studied for age-related changes: heart rate; left ventricular function; peripheral resistance and blood pressure; and distribution of blood flow.

Heart Rate

The resting heart rate appears to be unchanged with age. However, in response to a maximal load, the heart rate increase is impaired,[8,9] blunted by such factors as increased vagal tone, increased connective tissue in the conducting system, and decreased catecholamine influence. The time required to return to normal after increased rate is also prolonged.[10]

During the cardiac cycle, there is progressive prolongation of the period of isovolumic relaxation, relatively independent of heart rate. This may be an important factor in the inability of older persons to tolerate tachyarrhythmias. A rate of 120 or more in a person over 70 appears to be a critical limiting factor.[11]

Left Ventricular Function

Cardiac output is decreased approximately 1% per year after age 50, chiefly due to the decrease in stroke volume per unit of body size (stroke index). A decrease in body size as well as heart rate also appears to play a role.[12] The left ventricular ejection fraction is abnormal in response to exercise in the aged. This change is unrelated to differences in end-diastolic volume or blood pressure, but does seem to be related to wall-motion abnormalities.[13]

The Frank-Starling mechanism appears to be intact—an increase in myofibrillar length, as end-diastolic ventricular volume is increased, results in improved ventricular performance.

Peripheral Resistance and Blood Pressure

Total peripheral resistance (mean arterial pressure/cardiac output) is increased by about 1% per year (corresponding to the decrease in cardiac output of 1% per year).[14] The incidence of hypertension, here defined as systolic pressure greater than 159, with or without diastolic greater than 94, increases with age. However, the prevalence of "classical" (systolic-diastolic) hypertension remains relatively stable, whereas the incidence of pure systolic hypertension continues to rise.[15] Both types have been shown to be associated with increased risk of stroke, heart failure, and ischemic heart disease in elderly subjects. It has been shown that treatment of "classical" hypertension significantly reduces morbidity and mortality; unfortunately, no such controlled prospective studies have been carried out for pure systolic hypertension.[16] Pure systolic hypertension is known to be associated with atherosclerotic cardiovascular disease; however, cause and effect have not been proven. Thus the benefits of treatment can only be assumed.[17]

Distribution of Blood Flow

Decreased cardiac output results in asymmetrically reduced flow to various organ systems. Flow to the kidney and splanchnic bed is reduced proportionately more than flow to other tissues such as brain and coronary vessels.[18]

Pulmonary

It is somewhat unclear which respiratory changes found in the elderly are due exclusively to the effects of aging, and which may be due to other factors, such as smoking, environmental exposure, or physical activity. The following characteristics of lung function have been evaluated[10,19,20]: compliance, lung volumes, air flow, ventilation, arterial blood gases, and defense mechanisms.

Compliance

According to Murray,[19] the most significant effect of aging on pulmonary function is the change in compliance of both chest wall and lung. There is progressive kyphosis and ossification, with increased anteroposterior diameter of the chest, resulting in a significant reduction in the mobility and compliance of the chest wall, as well as a reduction in the force of the expiratory muscles.[10] In addition, there appears to be slightly decreased compliance of the lung tissue itself, with increased distensibility and decreased recoil.[19] This is probably less significant than the chest wall changes.

Lung Volumes

Anatomical as well as compliance changes cause an alteration in lung volumes. Thus, there is increased functional residual capacity and residual volume, with decreased vital capacity, while total lung capacity, as well as tidal volume, are virtually unchanged.[19,20]

Air Flow

The Forced Expiratory Volume (FEV_1) declines, as does the Forced Vital Capacity (FVC), with age.[21] (The FEV_1 appears to decline at about 30 cc/year in the absence of pulmonary disease.) In addition, relatively consistent changes have been shown in the Maximum Voluntary Ventilation (MVV) and the Maximum Mid-Expiratory Flow (MMF).[20]

Ventilation

There appears to be an increase in apical ventilation, with a decrease in basal ventilation, leading to an increase in ventilation–perfusion mismatching. In elderly subjects, the opening and closing volumes are higher, due not only to decreased elastic recoil, but also to increased opening and closing pressures as well. The $\dot{V}/\dot{Q}$ abnormality appears to be greatest in the lower lung fields; in the upper lung fields increased perfusion has been described, which would tend to reduce $\dot{V}/\dot{Q}$ mismatching in this area.[22]

Arterial Blood Gases

The elderly have a reduced partial pressure of arterial oxygen, which appears to represent a decline of about 0.40 mm/Hg per year after age 20,[20] probably due to the ventilation–perfusion mismatching described above. No change in the arterial carbon dioxide partial pressure has been described, nor can a change in pH be regarded as a normal accompaniment of aging, suggesting that alveolar hypoventilation is not a significant factor in the aged lung.[19]

Defense Mechanisms

Decreased compliance and air flow can result in loss of effectiveness of the cough reflex.[23] Accumulation of secretions thus predisposes to development of respiratory infections. It is not known whether pulmonary macrophages or mucociliary clearance is affected by age; the hypothesis is that both mechanisms are diminished.[19]

B-cell function is altered with aging; antibody response to foreign antigens such as pneumococcus is reduced, whereas the production of autoantibodies is increased, resulting in increased incidence of antinuclear, antithyroid, and rheumatoid antibodies.[24] This alteration in B-cell function may actually reflect a decrease in T-cell regulatory function, rather than a primary B-cell abnormality. Evidence of T-cell compromise is evident in tests of delayed hypersensitivity; decreased responses also correlate with increased mortality.[25] The increased incidence of tumors and infections reflects this immunological impairment, not only in the lung, but in the rest of the body.

Renal

The influence of age on several indices of renal function were reviewed by Lindeman[26]: glomerular filtration rate (GFR); renal plasma and blood flow; maximum tubular transport capacity; concentrating and diluting ability; and glomerular permeability.

Glomerular Filtration Rate

As shown by Davies and Shock,[27] a decrease of 46% in creatinine clearance occurred with age in 70 males between 20 and 90 years of age and free of history or clinical evidence of renal, cerebrovascular, or cardiac disease, or essential hypertension. Longitudinal studies have confirmed those observations.[28,29]

Renal Plasma and Blood Flow

Davies and Shock[27] also demonstrated a decrease of 53% in the effective renal plasma flow in the same subjects. This was slightly greater than the decrease in GFR. These findings may be related to decreased cardiac output and reductions in the renal vascular bed.[29]

Maximum Tubular Transport Capacity

Davies and Shock[27] also found a decrease of 43% in the tubular maximum for diodrast, which measures the ability of the tubules to secrete diodrast when the tubular transport capacity is saturated. The correlation of the reduction in GFR with the reduction in tubular function suggests a reduced number of functioning nephrons. However, changes at the cellular level have been demonstrated and are undoubtedly involved as well.[26]

Concentrating and Diluting Ability

Lindeman et al.[30] have demonstrated a decline in maximum osmolality from 1040 mOs/L to 750 mOs/L between ages 20 and 80. The ability to form a dilute urine is also impaired, from 52 mOs/L in the young to 90 mOs/L in the old.[31] However, when the diluting ability is corrected for the solute load per nephron, it is found that this clinical impairment (and possibly that of concentrating, as well) is due to the decreased number of functioning nephrons and not to a defect in the capacity of the nephron itself.[26]

Glomerular Permeability

Lowenstein et al.[32] could find no evidence of altered glomerular permeability with age.

Assessment of Pre-Operative States in the Elderly Patient

The elderly exhibit many modifications of disease presentation, compared with younger adults and, indeed, with each other. The assessment of the older patient is complicated by two major problems[33]:

Multiple disease: Most elderly patients do not unify all their findings into one convenient diagnosis, but rather accumulate many chronic conditions which require careful treatment and are complicated by significant physiologic decline in function, in addition to interactions among the diseases themselves.

Altered response to illness: Especially important are altered pain and temperature responses which mask many significant illnesses such as myocardial infarction and acute abdomen (which may be painless), and severe infections (which may be afebrile). The elderly also have increased susceptibility to hypothermia.

History

Obtaining the necessary information is the first concern. It cannot be stressed too often that patience and kindness are absolutely imperative in dealing with the elderly patient. Such problems as hearing and visual impairment, confusion, poor memory, and easy fatigability may present major obstacles to the taking of an adequate medical history. Some useful techniques mentioned in an excellent book by Caird and Judge[34] include:

• Practice careful communication in a manner which can be understood. Do not raise the voice more than is absolutely necessary, looking directly at the patient.

• Ask simple and direct questions.

• If there is confusion or memory impairment, obtain a history from a reliable other person, usually a relative.

• Ask which problems are most disturbing to the patient, and which are most disturbing to the other person.

Elderly patients often present with nonspecific symptoms or complaints. It may be more helpful to evaluate changes in status by duration and sequence of events, rather than to try to elicit more specific information about the symptom complex.[34]

The past history is extremely important, as it often provides valuable information concerning previous illness (which may affect present status). Records of previous hospitalizations and procedures should be acquired to obtain information about previous surgeries, complications, and the patient's experience in stressful situations.[34]

Drug ingestion is critical and must include not only prescription medications, but also proprietary medications, which may be taken in large amounts; specific inquiry must be made into the dosage and frequency of use.[35] It is often helpful to request the patient or family bring in all medications in bottles. Smoking history should also be determined in any patient.

Nutritional history should be obtained not only by specific inquiry about dietary components, but by indirect questioning concerning the number of hot meals, cost of groceries, and source of food preparation. Old people are particularly susceptible to dietary inadequacies due to financial problems, physical limitations, loneliness, food fads, and inadequate information or skills in food purchasing or preparation. Alcohol consumption may be a critical factor in dietary adequacy.[35]

The social history will be extremely important in formulating the patient's post-operative discharge plans. It should be obtained during the initial evaluation, in order to begin adequate preparations for follow-up care.

A careful and thorough review of systems is essential to bring out problems which the older patient may have forgotten, ignored, or attributed to "getting old."

The classic symptoms of cardiac disease may *not* be present in the elderly. The clinician should, to be sure, seek to elicit the classic complaints, such as retrosternal chest pain; however, cardiac ischemia may present as dyspnea, nausea, slight discomfort, or chest tightness; myocardial infarction may be painless in the elderly as well as in diabetics; and congestive heart failure may be manifested as wheezing, fatigue, lethargy, weakness, confusion, anorexia, or simply a cough. Arrhythmias may also present as fatigue, syncope, weakness, or dizziness. Old people may simply "take to bed" with such problems as congestive heart failure and emphysema.[36,37]

Elderly patients may manifest classic respiratory symptoms such as dyspnea, cough, or pleuritic chest pain. However, nonspecific complaints such as anorexia, lethargy, fatigue, and weight loss may be the only presenting symptoms of chronic respiratory diseases such as emphysema and tuberculosis, and confusion may be the only symptom of pneumonia or acute bronchitis, in which fever, pleuritic pain, and cough may be entirely absent.[36]

Genitourinary problems may be identified by the usual complaints of dysuria, incontinence, frequency or inability to urinate; however, urinary obstruction or urinary tract infections, or uremia may be asymptomatic or result only in anorexia, confusion, or fatigue.

Physical

The physical examination must be conducted with gentleness and concern for the patient's modesty, dignity, and fatigability. Examination of the cardiovascular system requires careful attention to the cardiac rate and rhythm, and the blood pressure (supine and erect). As noted, blood pressures up to 160/95 have been found in normal elderly persons, and should not require anti-hypertensive therapy, especially when evidence of end-organ disease is lacking.[38] Kyphoscoliosis may displace the apical impulse, and render it unreliable as an indication of cardiac size. Presence of a gallop rhythm or murmur is extremely important, and usually has the same significance as in the young. Systolic murmurs, however, are common and frequently benign, especially if they are the soft and ejection-type. They are often due to sclerotic changes of the aortic valve.[34] Ankle edema is often due to venous insufficiency, and is an unreliable sign of failure in the absence of other findings.

Examination of the chest may be difficult due to kyphoscoliosis, which may obscure clinical findings on physical examination, and may increase the anteroposterior diameter in the absence of underlying pulmonary disease.[37]

Evaluation of the vascular system may reveal the presence of atherosclerotic disease. Special note should be made of the carotid pulsations, and presence or absence of bruits, as well as the peripheral pulses in the arms and legs and the presence of bruits in the abdomen. Thin, shiny skin and loss of hair on the feet also suggest chronic ischemia.[34]

Nutritional adequacy can be vital to the success of an elective surgical procedure. Physical measurements such as weight, triceps skin fold, and arm circumference may be of value.[39]

Laboratory Evaluation

The routine studies of complete blood count, urinalysis, blood chemistries, chest x-ray and ECG are probably essential in the elderly patient. The physiologic changes of aging do not alter the normal values of the CBC, urinalysis, or blood chemistries significantly; thus, abnormal findings should be carefully evaluated.

The typical chest x-ray in the older patient may show changes of hyperinflation, increased A-P diameter, and increased lung markings. Heart size should remain normal, although calcification and bony changes of osteoporosis are often evident, as is degenerative joint disease of the vertebrae.[10]

The typical resting ECG shows several changes with advancing age, many of which may be due to the concomitant effect of atherosclerosis. In general, the observed changes have less association with increased mortality than in younger subjects. P-wave notching, ST depression, and T-wave flattening, or even inversion, are more frequently noted. The axis shifts leftward, and voltage tends to decrease due to increasing A-P diameter of the chest and decreased myocardial mass. In addition to the above, there is increased frequency of bundle-branch and hemiblocks, as well as first-degree block, often due to degenerative disease of the conducting system.[40]

It may be advisable to evaluate pulmonary function in the preoperative period with a determination of arterial pO_2, pCO_2, and pH, as well as an FEV_1, bearing in mind that pO_2 declines approximately 0.40 mm/Hg/year after age 20, and that normal values for FEV_1 are age-dependent.

Laboratory values of serum albumin, red cell indices, white cell count, and transferrin level will assist in the evaluation of nutritional status.[39] Laboratory indices of renal function which are applicable in younger patients may be less reliable in the elderly. The major difficulty occurs with the use of the serum creatinine alone as an index of GFR, particularly if it is used to calculate drug dosages; it is not reliably predictable.

Cockcroft and Gault[41] have demonstrated that the excretion of creatinine (in mg/kg/24 hr) decreases about 50% from the third to the ninth decades, probably due to a decrease in muscle mass with aging. This tends to alter the relationship between serum creatinine (in mg/100 ml) and creatinine clearance (in ml/min). The authors of this study evaluated a formula:

$$C_{cr} = \frac{(140 - age)\ (wt.\ kg)}{72 \times S_{cr}}$$

used to calculate estimated creatinine clearance, to be compared with that actually measured in the same elderly patients. They concluded that the correlation between the formula value and measured value was equal to that between two measured values. A nomogram developed by Siersback-Nielsen et al.[42] was also evaluated and found to be as reliable as the above formula in estimating the alteration in creatinine clearance which has been observed with age. However, it should be pointed out that Rowe, Adres, Tobin, Norris, and Shock studied the age-related decrease in creatinine clearance, and concluded that it is not predictable in individual patients, based upon age and weight. They therefore recommend actual measurement of creatinine clearance in elderly patients to determine the status of renal function.[43]

This same group also established a nomogram which provides normative standards for creatinine clearance, corrected by age. It provides an age-adjusted percentile rank in creatinine clearance for individuals with known age and measured creatinine clearance.[29]

Clinical Significance of Age-Related Changes

The above-noted changes in the critical body systems result in serious compromise of the elderly person's ability to tolerate stress. Disturbances of the internal and external milieu may lend to failure of compensatory mechanisms necessary to maintain homeostasis. Attention must be directed specifically to the following critical areas of management: oxygenation; fluid and electrolyte balance; mobilization; and drug therapy.

Oxygenation

Decreased cardiac output and the likely presence of atherosclerotic disease of the coronary and cerebral vessels result in compromise of the circulation to these vital areas. Hypoxemia may thus lead to infarction of myocardium or cerebrum. Conducting system disease predisposes to cardiac arrhythmias. Existing alterations in pulmonary function decrease the reserve potential for maintaining adequate oxygenation; thus, the clinician must assume responsibility for ensuring an adequate airway, promoting coughing and deep breathing, avoiding aspiration, treating pulmonary infection promptly, and maintaining adequate fluid intake to mobilize secretions without precipitating fluid overload.[23] Frequent attention to the examination of the chest is essential, and arterial blood gases and chest x-rays may be needed, especially to evaluate nonspecific symptoms such as confusion or lethargy.

Fluid and Electrolyte Balance

Compromised left ventricular function, increased vagal tone, and decreased renal function result in an increased risk of fluid overload leading to edema and congestive heart failure. Conversely, inadequate hydration may have serious consequences such as hypotension, inability to mobilize secretions, pre-renal azotemia, and even renal failure. Rapid adjustments of renal concentrating mechanisms are often not possible in the elderly person, and fluid status should be carefully followed by intake and output records, daily weights, and, if necessary, even Swan-Ganz catheterization. Skin turgor and the status of mucous membranes may not be reliable as indicators of fluid balance.

Electrolyte abnormalities may be precipitated by intravenous solutions, medications, and over- or under-hydration. Homeostatic mechanisms may be inadequate to compensate for such stress, and severe problems may occur, particularly with sodium, potassium, and chloride. Careful attention to electrolyte determinations is essential, especially in patients receiving intravenous solutions, on diuretics, or with renal compromise.

Mobilization

Prolonged bed rest can result in atelectasis and pneumonia, pressure sores, venous thrombosis, weakness, and loss of confidence. Early ambulation is important, with adequate assistance to prevent falls. In addition, adequate pulmonary toilet is essential to aid in clearing of secretions. Proper use of physical and respiratory therapists is to be encouraged. Diseases such as arthritis and Parkinson's may add to the problem of encouraging mobilization; nevertheless, it is of critical importance in the post-operative period.

Drug Therapy

Decreased renal function and reduced plasma volume, among other changes, may seriously compromise the elderly person's ability to tolerate average doses of many medications. The presence of multiple medical problems necessitates multiple medications; in addition, there may be particular drug therapy related to the perioperative period. Caution must be exercised and, where possible, levels determined when using many medications. Particular problems may be related to digoxin, aminoglycoside antibiotics, antihypertensives, diuretics, sedative-hypnotics, analgesics, antidepressants, and anti-Parkinson medications.[44] All of these have serious toxicities and/or side effects which are more common in elderly persons. A judicious review of medications is indicated during the preoperative evaluation, and frequently during the perioperative period, particularly in the presence of confusion, somnolence, cardiac arrhythmias, electrolyte abnormalities, azotemia, or postural hypotension.

Other

One concern relevant to the older patient is that of orientation, especially in the presence of sensory deprivation such as blindness or deafness. Frequent reorientation to place, time, and situation by staff can aid greatly in the prevention of confusion.

Nutrition is of great importance, and should receive appropriate attention during the perioperative period. The elderly patient may lack the reserves of the young, and a prolonged period of intravenous fluids, without oral alimentation, may rapidly deplete body stores. Parenteral hyperalimentation should be considered, if necessary, to promote adequate wound healing, essential energy for mobilization, and immunologic competence.

Effect of Aging on Surgical Mortality

Numerous studies have been performed attempting to relate surgical mortality to age, and these have shown a significant increase in perioperative morbidity and mortality as the patient's age increases. Cole[45] reviewed six reports in the medical literature and found an operative mortality of 2.6% under age 60 for major surgery, compared to 7.2% over age 60. For emergency surgery, the mortality increased from 6.5% to 18.5% over age 60. One major cause of death in patients in four studies reviewed was cardiac disease, which accounted for an average of 21.6% of all deaths, second only to inoperable cancer. In a study by Glenn and Hayes,[46] the mortality rate of patients over 65 increased markedly in the presence of major degenerative diseases, from 3.2%, to 33% in the presence of cirrhosis. Hypertensive heart disease conferred a mortality rate of 6.1% and atherosclerosis, 7.6%.

A review of 599 patients over age 80 in Vienna[47] included those with trauma and both emergency and elective surgery. The mortality rate for nontraumatic surgery in 211 patients was 11.8%. Death occurred most often after major surgery of the gastrointestinal tract, and cardiovascular diseases, cerebrovascular diseases, and renal insufficiency were the most frequent causes. In contrast, a study from Australia[48] reported a mortality rate of 9.2% (excluding terminal cancer) in 608 patients over age 70, with the major cause of death in these patients being respiratory, especially broncho-pneumonia. Significant risk factors appeared to be: pre-existing lung disease, cigarette smoking, and immobility. It appears from the multitude of studies that age constitutes a major risk factor for perioperative mortality. One cannot determine, however, from these studies, the significance of age as an *independent* risk factor, apart from its association with an increasing incidence of cardiopulmonary, renal, and gastrointestinal disease.

Two articles by Southwick and associates[49,50] reviewed risk factors for cardiac death in non-cardiac surgery. In both of these studies, age over 70 was found to be a statistically significant risk factor for postoperative cardiac mortality, contributing 5 out of a possible 53 "points." However, *all* patients in their cardiac death group had documented ischemic heart disease, congestive heart failure, abnormal cardiac rhythm, valvular heart disease or other evidence of major heart disease. Although 16 of the 19 patients who died of cardiac causes in the postoperative period were over 70 years of age, they could not have been considered "otherwise healthy" in any sense.

Two recent articles attempt to address the problem of predicting the effects of surgery in the elderly. Del Guercio and Cohn[51] performed elective Swan-Ganz catheterization in 148 patients over age 65, measuring pressures in the right atrium, right ventricle, and pulmonary artery, in addition to mixed venous blood gases, cardiac output, and pulmonary capillary wedge pressure. The Automated Physiologic Profile described by Cohn et al.[52] was used to devise four levels of perioperative management: Stage 1—no deficits; Stage 2—mild deficits (no delay in surgery, monitored by Swan-Ganz catheters perioperatively); Stage 3—moderate deficits (surgery delayed for preoperative stabilization, monitored perioperatively); and Stage 4—moderate to advanced deficits, not correctable (major surgery not recommended). In 86.5% of patients the authors felt that information not otherwise available was obtained; they had no major complications of the monitoring technique. They also noted good correlation with the staging criteria used by the American Society of Anesthesiologists; however, the anesthesiologists had difficulty in separating Stages 3 and 4 on a clinical basis. These results appear to offer a useful and safe evaluation system; however, in less experienced hands, one would have to consider the potential morbidity of the invasive monitoring procedure as being considerably more significant.

Djokovic and Hedley-Whyte[53] used the American Society of Anesthesiologists criteria to evaluate 500 patients over 80. Mortality in Class 2 was less than 1%; Class 3, 4%; and Class 4, 25%. The perioperative deaths (within 48 hours) were caused by mesenteric infarction; myocardial infarction was the leading cause of postoperative death (over 48 hours). In this study age *alone* did not appear to be a factor (up to 95 years old). Further studies are needed to document the usefulness of noninvasive versus invasive preoperative evaluation of the geriatric patient, and to establish the significance of age alone as a risk factor for perioperative mortality.

In conclusion, it is important to emphasize that elderly patients have a significant life expectancy. At age 70 a man has an average of 10+ years remaining, a woman, 13+. At age 80, 6+ years more are a definite possibility.[45] The clinician must bear in mind that elective surgical procedures to prevent major emergencies and to improve quality of life should be definitely considered as feasible, especially in the absence of evidence of serious systemic disease. Careful preoperative evaluation, considering the normal changes of aging, and cautious, prudent perioperative management, respecting the altered physiology of the aged, can lead to improved surgical morbidity and mortality, and an optimal chance for survival with an unimpaired lifestyle.

Acknowledgment

The author wishes to express appreciation to Knight Steel, M.D., Associate Professor and Chief, Geriatrics Section, Boston University Medical Center, for his constructive criticism and suggestions.

References

1. Rockstein M, Susman M: *Biology of Aging*. Belmont, Wadsworth Publishing Company, 1979.
2. Hayflick L: Biology of human aging. *Am J Med Sci* 265:432, 1973.
3. Curtis HJ, Miller K: Chromosome aberrations in liver cells of guinea pigs. *J Gerontol* 26:292, 1971.
4. Walford RL: *The Immunological Theory of Aging*. Baltimore, Williams & Wilkins Co., 1969.
5. Timiras PS: *Developmental Physiology and Aging*. New York, MacMillan Co., 1972.
6. Exton-Smith AN, Overstall PW: *Geriatrics. Guidelines in Medicine*. Vol. 1. Baltimore, University Park Press, 1979.
7. Rossman I: The anatomy of aging. In Rossman I (Ed.): *Clinical Geriatrics*. Philadelphia, JB Lippincott, 1979.
8. Norris AH, Shock NW, Yiengst MJ: Age changes in heart rate and blood pressure responses to tilting and standardized exercise. *Circulation* 8:521, 1953.
9. Montoye J, Willis PW III, Cunningham DA: Heart rate response to submaximal exercise: Relation to age and sex. *J Gerontol* 23:127, 1968.
10. Goldman R: Decline in organ function with aging. In Rossman I (Ed.): *Clinical Geriatrics, Ed. 2*. Philadelphia, JB Lippincott, 1979.
11. Harrison TR, Dixon K, Russell RO Jr, et al.: The relation of age to the duration of contraction, ejection, and relaxation of the normal human heart. *Am Heart J* 67:189, 1964.
12. Brandfonbrener J, Landowne M, Shock NW: Changes in cardiac output with age. *Circulation* 12:557, 1955.
13. Port S, Cobb FR, Coleman RE, Jones RH: Effect of age on the response of the left ventricular ejection fraction to exercise. *N Engl J Med* 303:1133, 1980.
14. Landowne M, Brandfonbrener J, Shock NW: The relation of age to certain measures of performance of the heart and circulation. *Circulation* 12:567, 1955.
15. Dyer AR, Stamler J, Shekelle RB, et al.: Hypertension in the elderly. *Med Clin NA* 61:513, 1977.
16. *Statement on Hypertension in the Elderly*. National High Blood Pressure Education Program Coordinating Committee, National Heart, Lung and Blood Institute, National Institutes of Health, Bethesda, Maryland, revised April 1980.
17. O'Malley K, O'Brien E: Management of hypertension in the elderly. *N Engl J Med* 302:1397, 1980.
18. Bender AD: The effect of increasing age on the distribution of peripheral blood flow in man. *J Am Geriatr Soc* 13:192, 1965.
19. Murray JF: Aging. In *The Normal Lung*. Philadelphia, WB Saunders Co., 1976.
20. Muiesan G, Sorbini CA, Grassi V: Respiratory function in the aged. *Bull Physiopath Resp* 7:973, 1971.
21. Milne JS, Williamson J: Respiratory function tests in older people. *Clinical Science* 42:371, 1972.

22. Holland J, Milic-Emili J, Macklem PT, Bates DV: Regional distribution of pulmonary ventilation and perfusion in elderly subjects. *J Clin Invest* 47:81, 1968.
23. Duncalf D, Kepes ER: Geriatric anesthesia. In Rossman I (Ed.): *Clinical Geriatrics, Ed. 2.* Philadelphia, JB Lippincott, 1979.
24. Rowley M, Buchanan H, Mackay IR: Reciprocal change with age in antibody to extrinsic and intrinsic antigens. *Lancet* 2:24, 1968.
25. Roberts-Thomson IC, Youngchaiyud U, Whittingham S, Mackay IR: Aging, immune response, and mortality. *Lancet* 2:368, 1974.
26. Lindeman RD: Age changes in renal function. In Goldman R, Rockstein M (Eds.): *The Physiology and Pathology of Human Aging.* New York, Academic Press, 1975.
27. Davies DF, Shock NW: Age changes in glomerular filtration rate, effective renal plasma flow, and tubular excretory capacity in adult males. *J Clin Invest* 29:496, 1950.
28. Shock NW: Current trends in research on the physiologic aspects of aging. *J Am Geriatr Soc* 15:995, 1967.
29. Rowe JW, Andres R, Tobin JD, et al.: The effect of age on creatinine clearance in man. A cross-sectional and longitudinal study. *J Gerontol* 31:155, 1976.
30. Lindeman RD, Van Buren HC, Raisz LG: Osmolar renal concentrating ability in healthy young men and in hospitalized patients without renal disease. *N Engl J Med* 262:1306, 1960.
31. Lindeman RD, Lee TD Jr, Yiengst MJ, Shock NW: Influence of age, renal disease, hypertension, diuretics, and calcium on the antidiuretic response to suboptimal infusions of vasopressin. *J Lab Clin Med* 68:206, 1966.
32. Lowenstein J, Faulstick DA, Yiengst MJ, Shock NW: The glomerular clearance and renal transport of hemoglobin in adult males. *J Clin Invest* 40:1172, 1961.
33. Hodkinson HM: *Common Symptoms of Disease in the Elderly.* Oxford, Blackwell, 1980.
34. Caird FI, Judge TG: *Assessment of the Elderly Patient, Ed. 2.* Philadelphia, JB Lippincott Co., 1979.
35. Steinberg FU: The evaluation and treatment of the geriatric patient. In Cowdry: *The Care of the Geriatric Patient, Ed. 5.* St. Louis, Mosby, 1976.
36. Sheehy T: Assessing the surgical risk in the elderly patient. *Medical Times* July 1980, p. 37.
37. Harris R: *The Management of Geriatric Cardiovascular Disease.* Philadelphia, JB Lippincott, 1970.
38. Russek HI, Rath MH, Tohman BL, Miller I: The influence of age on blood pressure. *Am Heart J* 32:468, 1946.
39. Blackburn GL, Bristrian BR, Maini BS, et al.: Nutritional and metabolic assessment of the hospitalized patient. *J of Parent and Ent Nutrition* 1:11, 1977.
40. Rodstein M: The ECG in old age: Implications for diagnosis, therapy, and prognosis. *Geriatrics,* February 1977, p. 76.

41. Cockcroft D, Gault MH: Prediction of creatinine clearance from serum creatinine. *Nephron* 16:31, 1976.
42. Siersback-Nielsen K, Molholm J, Hansen J, et al.: Rapid evaluation of creatinine clearance. *Lancet* 1:1133, 1971.
43. Rowe JW, Andres R, Tobin JD, et al.: Age-adjusted standards for creatinine clearance. *Ann Intern Med* 84:567, 1976.
44. Drugs in the elderly. *Med Letter* 21:43, 1979.
45. Cole WH: Medical differences between the young and aged. Effect of aging on surgical mortality. *J Am Geriatr Soc* 18:589, 1970.
46. Glenn F, Hayes DM: The age factor in the mortality rate of patients undergoing surgery of the biliary tract. *Surg Gynecol Obstet* 100:11, 1955.
47. Kohn P, Zekert F, Vormittag E, Grabner H: Risks of operation in patients over 80. *Geriatrics*, November 1973, p. 100.
48. Burnett W, McCaffrey J: Surgical procedures in the elderly. *Surg Gynecol Obstet* 134:221, 1972.
49. Southwick FS, Krogstad D, Murray B, et al.: Multifactorial index of cardiac risk in non-cardiac surgical procedures. *N Engl J Med* 297:845, 1977.
50. Goldman L, Caldera DL, Southwick FS, et al.: Cardiac risk factors and complications in non-cardiac surgery. *Medicine* 57:357, 1978.
51. Del Guercio LRM, Cohn JD: Monitoring operative risk in the elderly. *JAMA* 243:1350, 1980.
52. Cohn JD, Engler PE, Del Guercio LRM: The automated physiologic profile. *Crit Care Med* 3:51, 1975.
53. Djokovic JL, Hedley-Whyte J: Prediction of outcome of surgery and anesthesia in patients over 80. *JAMA* 242:2301, 1979.

CHAPTER XI

Arrhythmias and Conduction Disturbances

H. David Friedberg, M.D.

For any arrhythmia, there are five fundamental aspects, namely: *the clinical substrate.* Is there, for example, acute myocardial ischemia or infarction with risk of fibrillation? Is there a low serum potassium or, perhaps, an excess of digitalis? Or, is the patient symptom-free and, apparently, healthy? *the effect upon cardiac output* either at rest or on stress? Many an arrhythmia that does not interfere with the hemodynamic function of the heart is best left alone; *the site of origin* (sinus node, atrium, AV junction or ventricle); *the mode of impulse discharge* (for example: bradycardia, extrasystole, fibrillation, etc.); *the manner of impulse conduction* (normal, complete or incomplete block, etc.). Normal conduction is often not stated, but left implicit.

The primary aim of the treatment of the heart is to ameliorate the underlying cardiac condition. The primary aim of the treatment of arrhythmia is to *establish a suitable ventricular rate.* It is a truism, but one often forgotten, that it is the patient and not the arrhythmia that needs treatment.

Preoperative Evaluation

History

Cardiac arrhythmias occur in over 60% of patients in the perioperative period. The probability of developing a serious arrhythmia during or after surgery is greater if there is some disturbance

193

of rhythm in the preoperative electrocardiogram. Therefore, patients who give a history of disturbances of heart rythm need particular care in their assessment before general anesthesia and major surgery. It is usually possible to form an accurate idea of the probable rhythm disturbance if the history is well taken.

Particular attention should be paid to the following features: circumstances under which attacks happen; mode of onset—whether abrupt or gradual; mode of offset—whether abrupt or gradual; frequency of attacks; regularity of the heart beat during attacks; the patient may be asked to beat time with a pencil to indicate this; patients often have difficulty in estimating the rate. A metronome is a useful device—ask the patient, "Is it as fast as this, or faster?"; associated symptoms such as angina, shortness of breath, or symptoms suggesting anxiety; possible provoking factors such as anxiety, tobacco, or caffeine; a history of pounding of the heart suggests compensatory pauses occasioned by extrasystoles. One cannot use this method to determine whether the beats are ventricular or supraventricular, as both types may be followed by a compensatory pause.

Some Common Problems

Ventricular Extrasystoles

Ventricular premature beats are obvious: they stick out like a sore thumb. Their presence in the preoperative electrocardiogram should lead to a diligent search for underlying factors, such as ischemic heart disease or, indeed, any structural heart disease; for possible provoking stimuli such as anxiety, caffeine, tobacco, coronary disease, or digitalis toxicity. It should be remembered that although ventricular premature beats are often of the most serious import, the vast majority are benign. It should also be realized that the usual precursors to more serious ventricular arrhythmia (frequent, R on T, multiform) apply *primarily to the acutely ischemic* myocardium and not nearly so to otherwise well individuals.

Management. The serum potassium level should be kept near the higher limit of normal. Ventricular ectopic activity is often diminished if the serum potassium level is kept between 4.5 and 5.0 mEq/L. The patient must be monitored during anesthesia. If the premature beats become troublesome, the drug of choice is lidocaine followed by procainamide.

Supraventricular Extrasystoles

These beats are usually benign, but may indicate atrial stretch due to mitral valve disease or an increased left ventricular end-diastolic pressure. Thyrotoxicosis and chronic lung disease are also associated with supraventricular premature beats. They may presage atrial fibrillation or other paroxysmal tachyarrhythmia. Consideration should be given to prophylactic preoperative digitalization.

Atrial Fibrillation

Common causes of atrial fibrillation include mitral valve disease, left ventricular failure, and thyrotoxicosis. Patients with atrial fibrillation who are fully digitalized can usually tolerate surgery very well. If frequent atrial premature beats are present in a patient with a past history of atrial fibrillation, the patient should be digitalized. This will prevent an excessively rapid ventricular response from occurring, should atrial fibrillation or atrial flutter occur as a complication after surgery.

Management. It is usually sufficient to achieve control of the ventricular rate. Digitalis and propranolol are the drugs of choice and are usually very effective in controlling excessive tachycardia. Cardioversion is usually not necessary unless the patient has great need of the atrial transport function. An external shock of 200 to 400 Joules is needed and is not always successful.

Recurrent Paroxysmal Tachycardia

Patients who give a history of repeated attacks of paroxysmal tachycardia of supraventricular origin may cause some concern. Such attacks can often be prevented by the use of digitalis or propranolol. Attacks may be terminated by vagotonic maneuvers such as carotid sinus massage, by raising the blood pressure with neosynephrine or Aramine, and by Verapamil digitalis and/or propranolol. One should try to control these preoperatively.

Patients with Permanent Pacemakers

A special problem is the patient presenting for surgery who has had a permanent pacemaker implantation. It is estimated that over 250,000 persons now have permanent pacemakers, and surgery unrelated to the pacemaker may be necessary. The overall operative mortality does not seem to be affected in such individuals when the pacemaker function is normal. With the advancing pacemaker technology, the types and complexity of these units are increasing but, still, most pacemakers work on ventricular stimulation and are either demand or fixed rate. Demand pacemakers present two problems in patients about to undergo surgery. First, if the patient's own inherent rhythm is faster than the pacemaker rate, the unit, appropriately, does not pace. One needs, then, to place a magnet over the pacemaker, thereby converting it to a fixed rate pacemaker so that one can now evaluate its function. The other problem relating to its demand function is inappropriate sensing of electromagentic forces (such as electrocautery) which would inhibit pacemaker output despite the fact that the patient's intrinsic heart rate may be inadequate. This problem is particularly important in patients undergoing transurethral prostatectomy because of the routine need for electrocautery during this procedure. Although improved shielding and input filters have reduced this risk, caution is warranted; helpful precautions include changing the pacemaker to the fixed mode during surgery (possible in some models) placing an indifferent diathermy plate under the patient, away from the pacemaker site, limiting the duration of electrocautery, and carefully monitoring cardiac rhythm throughout the procedure.

Indications for Temporary Pacing

Sinus Bradycardia

This may be normal in athletes, or may reflect an increased vagal tone. It may also be a manifestation of S-A nodal disease. In a clinical study of 515 cases of sinus bradycardia by Kirk and Kvorn-ing,[1] symptoms of any sort occurred in less than 25%. The most common expected symptoms—syncope and dizziness occurred in less than 1%. Agruss et al.[2] studied a small group of elderly men (age 67–79) with chronic sinus bradycardia. Normal cardiac per-formance was found in all as was normal autonomic nerve func-tion. Thus, symptoms are not expected with this arrhythmia and treatment is rarely indicated. A temporary pacemaker should be considered for sinus bradycardia if there is other evidence of sinus nodal disease (such as S-A block or paroxysmal tachycardia) (Fig-ure 1); if the sinus rate cannot increase to 80 beats per minute on simple exercise; or if operations involving the eyes or carotid ar-teries are planned (see below). In the postoperative situation, sinus bradycardia usually reflects an increased vagal tone, perhaps ac-centuated by drugs such as morphine. Intravenous injection of Atropine 0.5 to 1.0 mgm is usually adequate to control this. Intra-venous infusion of Isoprenaline or the institution of temporary pacing is rarely needed.

Second-Degree AV Block, Type I, with Narrow QRS Complexes

In Type I AV block, (also called Wenckebach block) the P-R intervals are not all constant, but the P-R intervals increase in suc-cessive beats until one fails to be conducted to the ventricle. The next P-R interval is the shortest of the sequence. Permanent pacing is not necessarily indicated if there is no evidence of subnodal disease, or of episodic syncope or asystole. However, the operating room is not the place to discover that a pacemaker is indicated. It may be wise to place a temporary system before surgery, particu-larly if the block does not improve following Atropine.

Bifascicular Block

What should be done if right bundle branch block (RBBB) and left anterior hemiblock (LAHB) are present together in the pre-operative electrocardiogram? In the absence of other evidence of significant conduction system disease, it is rare that this conduction progresses in the postoperative state. Such other evidence might be a prolonged P-R interval, second-degree AV block, or a history

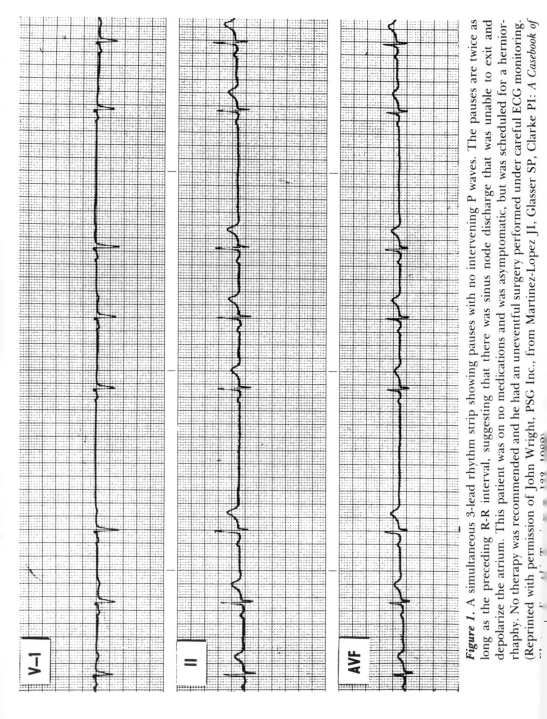

Figure 1. A simultaneous 3-lead rhythm strip showing pauses with no intervening P waves. The pauses are twice as long as the preceding R-R interval, suggesting that there was sinus node discharge that was unable to exit and depolarize the atrium. This patient was on no medications and was asymptomatic, but was scheduled for a herniorrhaphy. No therapy was recommended and he had an uneventful surgery performed under careful ECG monitoring. (Reprinted with permission of John Wright, PSG Inc., from Martinez-Lopez JI, Glasser SP, Clarke PI: *A Casebook of*

of syncope. If these conditions are absent, then watchful expectancy is indicated. This common finding, by itself, does not warrant pacing or His Bundle studies (Table 1).[3–10]

What should be done if RBBB and left posterior hemiblock (LPH) are present together in the preoperative electrocardiogram? This combination cannot be produced by a single localized lesion in the conducting system and, therefore, it suggests a more serious degree of involvement. The integrity of the anterior fascicle is then the determining factor in the safety of conduction. Authorities disagree whether a standby temporary pacemaker should be placed if no other evidence of conduction system disease is present, and this should be weighed against the fact that the introduction of a temporary pacing lead is a simple and generally safe maneuver. There is meager data in the literature, so that no firm rec-

Table 1

Perioperative Incidence of Atrioventricular Block in Subjects with Preoperative Bifascicular Block

	RBBB + LAH	RBBB + LPH	RBBB, LAH or LPH + 1° AVB	% Developing Complete AVB	LBBB	% Developing Complete AVB
Berg and Kotler[3]	26	—	—	0	4‡	0
Kunstadt, et al.[4]	21	—	—	0	3‡	0
Venkataraman, et al.[5]	38	—	6	1*	—	—
Pastore, et al.[6]	44	—	8	1†	—	—
Bellocci, et al.[7]	48	10	—	0	40	0
Rooney, et al.[8]	27	—	—	0	—	—
Gertler, et al.[9]	—	—	—	0	10	0
Goldman, et al.[10]	23	2	7	0	20	0
Totals	227	12	21	2	77	0

*Mobitz II block existed preoperatively
†transient complete heart block; Six subjects with preoperative temporary pacemakers had no heart block, but two developed ventricular irritability responding to electrode removal
‡patients with LBBB and PR prolongation

RBBB	= right bundle branch block	LPH	= left posterior hemiblock
LAH	= left anterior hemiblock	AVB	= atrioventricular block
		1° AVB	= with first degree AV block

ommendation can be made. Bellocci et al.[7] studied 98 patients with electrocardiographic evidence of bifascicular block, who had undergone general anesthesia. Forty-eight had RBBB with LAHB, ten had RBBB and LPH, and forty had left bundle branch block. None of the patients developed complete heart block in the perioperative, or one week postoperative, period, indicating that prophylactic pacing for this group is not warranted.

His Bundle Electrography

When a temporary pacing electrode is positioned within the heart, consideration should be given to record a His bundle electrogram. It is usually quite simple to test the integrity of the His-Purkinje system and the reliability of any subsidiary pacemakers by rapid atrial and rapid ventricular pacing. If the integrity of the His-Purkinje system is found to be impaired or if a subsidiary pacemaker is found to be unreliable, or if the H-V interval is found to be prolonged, the decision regarding later permanent pacing may be influenced.

In the study of Bellocci et al.,[7] referred to before, His bundle electrograms were performed in all patients with evidence of bifascicular block prior to surgery. Two groups were identified, forty-seven patients with normal HV times and fifty-one patients with prolonged HV times. As mentioned, none of the patients developed perioperative atrioventricular block. Three intraoperative and three postoperative episodes of ventricular tachycardia or ventricular fibrillation occurred, and these occurred only in the patients with prolonged HV intervals. Further analysis suggested that these episodes were confined to the patients with marked HV prolongation (greater than 75 msec) and that the prolonged HV interval group presented a significantly greater incidence of organic heart disease and cardiac symptoms. Finally, the HV duration was a more accurate predictor of major cardiac perioperative complications than the surface recordings, but only in patients with symptomatic heart disease—patients who were identifiable clinically.

His bundle tracings and other intracardiac electrical studies may be indicated for the evaluation of some types of A-V conduction disturbances and also in some cases of recurrent tachycardia.

Pharmacology

Anesthetic Agents

Many anesthetic agents produce arrhythmias. Chloroform was recognized as dangerous soon after its introduction. It sensitizes the ventricle to the development of catecholamine-induced ventricular fibrillation by reducing the fibrillation threshold. Cyclopropane has a similar but much smaller effect. Halopropane and teflurane are also arrhythmogenic at the customary concentrations used. Trichloroethylene has a similar effect. Other anesthetic agents do not usually provoke arrhythmias (See Chapter 2).

Lidocaine. The initial dose should be 100 to 200 mgms by intravenous bolus spaced over twenty minutes, followed by an infusion of 2–3 mgms per minute. This *must* be controlled by an infusion pump. The dose can be increased for short periods to 4 mgm per minute, should ventricular extrasystoles not be controlled.

Procainamide. Procainamide can be used if lidocaine fails to control ventricular irritability. An infusion of 2 to 6 mgm per minute is used. A loading dose of 100 to 300 mgm as a slow intravenous injection can be given. An intramuscular injection should not be used during surgery, as delayed hypotensive effects may cause problems.

Potassium. Serum potassium levels should be measured frequently during surgery. Every 20 minutes is not too frequent in difficult cases. Potassium chloride can be given at a rate of 0.5 to 1.0 mEq/minute into a large central vein with careful monitoring. Larger doses may be lethal.

Magnesium. Magnesium sulphate—1 gram to 2 grams intravenously—may control ventricular irritability in certain cases.

Reflex Arrhythmias

There are two important reflex arcs that may provoke arrhythmias: the *oculo-cardiac pathway* (Aschner-Dagnini reflex); this is provoked by pressure on the eyeball or traction on the extra-ocular muscles. It results in sinus bradycardia and in ventricular extrasystoles, especially in cases in which premature beats were previously present. It is potentiated by a high vagal tone, by digitalis, and by anesthetic agents; the *carotid sinus reflex* is provoked by pressure or other stimulation upon the carotid sinus or the carotid body, and is important in operations around the neck. This is again potentiated by digitalis, by vagal tone, and by anesthetic agents. It also results in a slowing of the S-A node and AV block and in ventricular arrhythmias. Both these reflexes have cardio-inhibitory and cardio-excitatory features.

Postoperative Arrhythmias

Sinus Tachycardia

Sinus tachycardia is the expression of the need for an increased cardiac output. It is not, per se, an indication of heart disease. It is commonly found with fever, anemia, or pain; indeed, some sinus tachycardia is the norm in the acute postoperative state. A rate faster than 120 per minute suggests *hypovolemia*. It is unwise to treat sinus tachycardia with cardiac-slowing drugs such as propranolol because it simply reflects the response of the sinus node to some stimulus which is usually extracardiac.

Sinus Bradycardia

Sinus bradycardia postoperatively may be normal (see discussion under "Preoperative Assessment of Sinus Bradycardia") or it may be the result of excessive vagal tone, perhaps the result of drugs such as morphine. If the slow sinus rate limits the cardiac output—hemodynamic interference—one may use atropine or isoprenaline (Isuprel®). In resistant cases, temporary atrial or ventricular pacing may be needed. As in the preoperative setting, if the patient is asymptomatic, no therapy is indicated.

Supraventricular Premature Beats

In the postoperative state, the development of supraventricular premature beats is a significant abnormality. This indicates fresh atrial stretch. Causes include left ventricular failure, acute cor pulmonale, or hypoxemia. If a supraventricular premature beat falls at the time of the vulnerable phase of the atrium, an atrial tachyarrhythmia may result (Figure 2).

Supraventricular Tachyarrhythmias

Supraventricular tachyarrhythmias occur relatively frequently after thoracic operations, but few studies have looked at its overall incidence after noncardiac surgery. Goldman noted 4% (35/916) developing new onset supraventricular tachycardia frequently occurring in the setting of concurrent medical problems[10] (Figure 3).

Atrial Flutter

Characteristically, atrial flutter has an atrial rate of about 300 beats per minute. There is 2:1 AV response and a ventricular rate of about 150 beats per minute. This rate is excessive and not well tolerated. Cardioversion with a small synchronized countershock (10 to 20 Joules) is nearly always successful in terminating the arrhythmia and is well tolerated without anesthesia. Since atrial flutter may be quite surreptitious, a heart rate of 150 beats per minute should be considered as due to atrial flutter until proved otherwise. Vagal maneuvers may be diagnostically useful. If the ventricular rate during atrial flutter is 75 to 100 beats per minute, the cardiac output may be satisfactory. Immediate elective cardioversion is, then, not necessary.

Atrial Fibrillation

The most important question in atrial fibrillation is the ventricular rate. Digitalis and propranolol are usually very effective in controlling excessive tachycardia. Compared to atrial flutter, cardioversion will generally require a much larger countershock (200 to 400 Joules) and is not always successful.

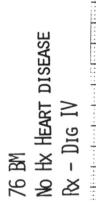

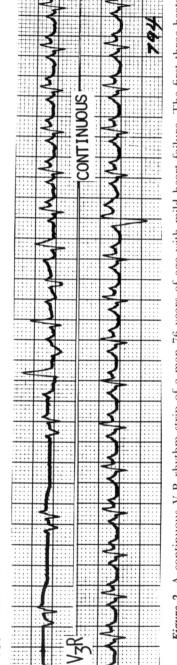

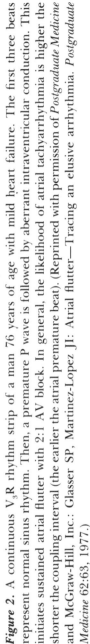

Figure 2. A continuous V₃R rhythm strip of a man 76 years of age with mild heart failure. The first three beats represent normal sinus rhythm. Then, a premature P wave is followed by aberrant intraventricular conduction. This initiates sustained atrial flutter with 2:1 AV block. In general, the likelihood of atrial tachyarrhythmia is higher the shorter the coupling interval (the earlier the atrial premature beat). (Reprinted with permission of *Postgraduate Medicine* and McGraw-Hill, Inc.: Glasser SP, Martinez-Lopez JI: Atrial flutter—Tracing an elusive arrhythmia. *Postgraduate Medicine* 62:63, 1977.)

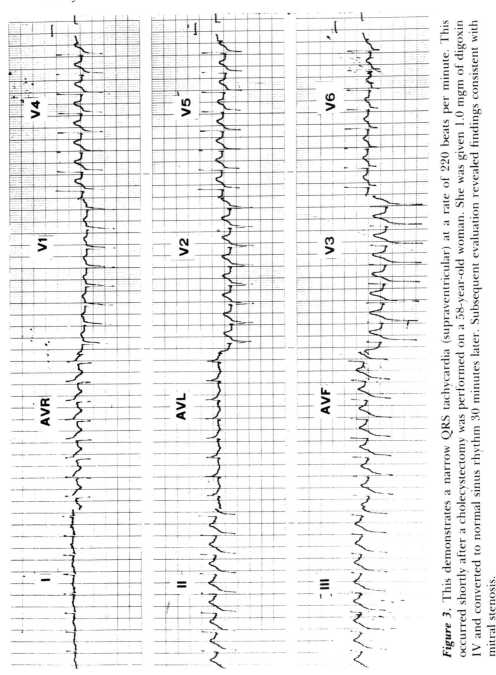

Figure 3. This demonstrates a narrow QRS tachycardia (supraventricular) at a rate of 220 beats per minute. This occurred shortly after a cholecystectomy was performed on a 58-year-old woman. She was given 1.0 mgm of digoxin IV and converted to normal sinus rhythm 30 minutes later. Subsequent evaluation revealed findings consistent with mitral stenosis.

Ventricular Extrasystoles

What should be done if ventricular premature beats occur de nova in the postoperative period? Rare or sporadic beats may be ignored. Treatment with lidocaine should be instituted until a cause is found, if the beats appear to be multifocal in origin, if pairs or runs occur, and if the extrasystole is close to the apex of the T wave of the sinus beat (R on T phenomenon). Procainamide, propranolol, disopyramide, quinidine, and diphenylhydantoin may also be used.

A search should be instituted for evidence of myocardial ischemia, digitalis toxicity, electrolyte imbalance, or pulmonary embolism (Figure 4). If these are absent, ventricular extrasystoles are unlikely to be malignant.

Ventricular tachycardia and ventricular fibrillation should be treated by immediate countershock. Recurrent fibrillation may require the use of bretylium or magnesium, or overdrive pacing.

Postoperative AV Block

The indications for pacing for block appearing after surgery are the same as for preoperative block. Note that sinus bradycardia, SA block and AV block, type I, are often transient, vagal, and benign.

A QRS axis shift may indicate hemiblock. This rarely progresses to complete AV block, but its appearance should occasion careful observation and monitoring.

Diagnosis of Aberration

The differential diagnosis between aberration and ectopy is often difficult and causes much heartache (or unwarranted pride) to cardiologists. It should be remembered that an aberrantly conducted beat is not physiologically abnormal and requires no treatment of itself. If an incorrect diagnosis of ventricular ectopy is made and the usual dose of lidocaine is given, very seldom will any harm be done (Figure 5).

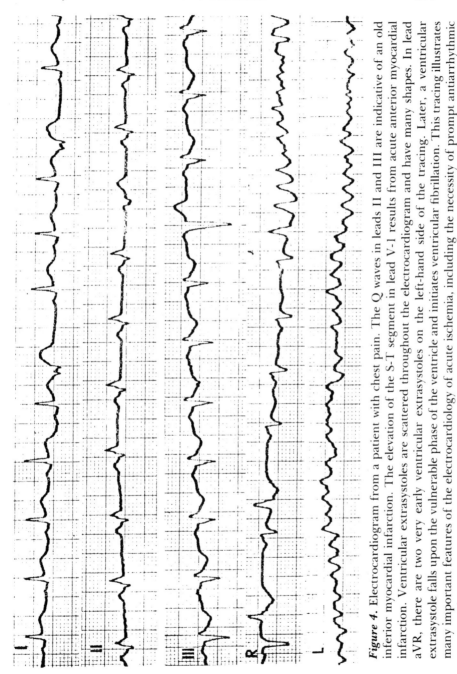

Figure 4. Electrocardiogram from a patient with chest pain. The Q waves in leads II and III are indicative of an old inferior myocardial infarction. The elevation of the S-T segment in lead V-1 results from acute anterior myocardial infarction. Ventricular extrasystoles are scattered throughout the electrocardiogram and have many shapes. In lead aVR, there are two very early ventricular extrasystoles on the left-hand side of the tracing. Later, a ventricular extrasystole falls upon the vulnerable phase of the ventricle and initiates ventricular fibrillation. This tracing illustrates many important features of the electrocardiology of acute ischemia, including the necessity of prompt antiarrhythmic treatment!

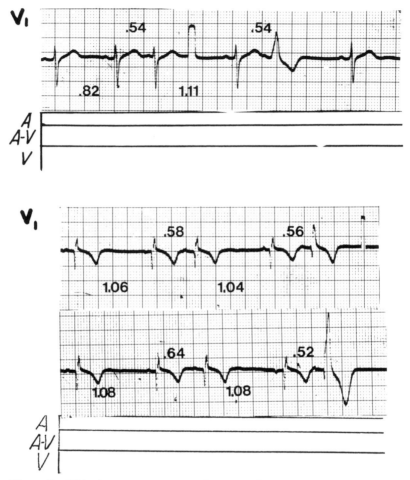

Figure 5. This demonstrates many features of the Ashman phenomenon. Note that the aberrantly conducted premature atrial beats occur after a shorter coupling interval or a longer preceding R-R interval.

Factors Favoring Aberration

Factors include: a small, deformed P wave preceding a broad QRS complex may produce a subtle change in the configuration of the preceding S-T segment and T wave; the phenomenon of a critical rate: the appearance of bundle branch block when the heart rate exceeds a certain figure is a form of aberration. Aberration may also occur with bradycardia; the second beat of a run of tachycardia is the one most likely to show aberration. This is related to the Ashman phenomenon; if definite preceding P waves are not available (because of lead selection, atrial fibrillation, or tachycardia) and considerations of timing do not help, a clue may be gained from the shape of the QRS complex. In favor of aberration are: typical right bundle branch block patterns, unchanged initial QRS vector, triphasic complex in lead VI, and qR, qRs, or QRS complexes in lead V6.

Factors Favoring Ventricular Origin

In lead VI, a monophasic QRS complex or qR, gR-R', or R'R with R taller than R', or atypical right bundle branch block patterns; in lead V6, a QS or rS complex; the deepest QS complex in lead V4; all precordial QRS complexes in the same direction; and a very unusual frontal plane QRS axis.

Tachycardia with Wide QRS Complexes

This may be: supraventricular tachycardia with pre-existing bundle branch block or intraventricular conduction defect; a supraventricular tachycardia with aberration; a supraventricular tachycardia with Wolff-Parkinson-White (WPW) syndrome; or ventricular tachycardia (Figure 6).

A tachycardia with wide QRS complexes must initially be presumed ventricular in origin: the clinical status of the patient is the overriding consideration. When one has time to analyze the arrhythmia fully, one should presume that it is ventricular in origin and attempt to disprove the presumption.

Digitalis Toxicity

An excess of digitalis in a heart perhaps sensitized by hypokalemia produces: *ventricular extrasystoles*, which may be multiform or multifocal, progressing to ventricular tachycardia and ventricular

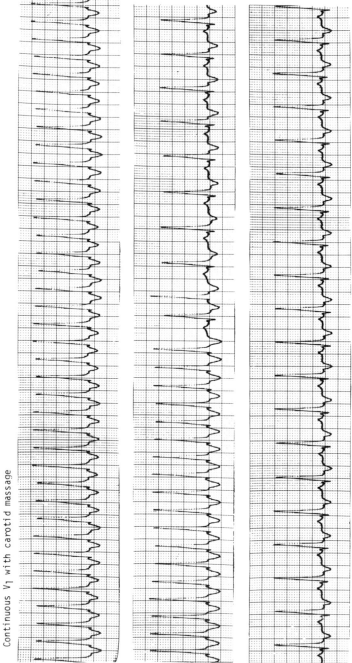

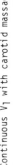

Continuous V₁ with carotid massage

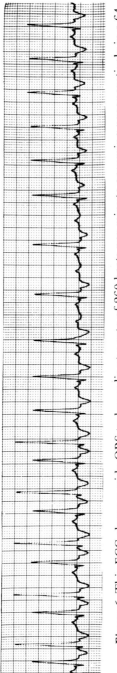

Figure 6. This ECG shows a wide QRS tachycardia at a rate of 260 beats per minute occurring preoperatively in a 64-year-old woman scheduled for gynecological surgery. Carotid sinus massage was applied midway through the second strip. This demonstrates that the rhythm was atrial flutter with 1 to 1 conduction. Carotid massage induced 2:1 and then 3:1 block, allowing for diagnosis. History revealed that she had been on digitalis, but that this had not been ordered upon hospital admission. Further, she had recently been placed on Dilantin for the treatment of "seizures" (probably dizzy spells due to paroxysmal atrial flutter). Apparently, the absence of digitalis in the presence of Dilantin (known to increase A-V conduction) allowed for the rapid atrial rate to conduct to the ventricles. The Dilantin was discontinued and the patient was redigitalized. (Reprinted with permission of *Postgraduate Medicine* and McGraw-Hill, Inc.: Glasser SP, Martinez-Lopez JI: Atrial flutter—Tracing an elusive arrhythmia. *Postgraduate Medicine* 62:63, 1977.)

fibrillation; an ectopic atrial rhythm *(idioatrial tachycardia)* with abnormal p' waves; the above arrhythmia may be complicated by the presence of varying AV block *(PAT with block).* The P waves are often small and may be seen only in lead VI. The atrial rate is usually 100 to 160; an *accelerated junctional rhythm* (nonparoxysmal junctional tachycardia, idiojunctional tachycardia). This may be associated with regular retrograde conduction to the atria. Often retrograde V-A block is present and the atria are under the control of a sinus mechanism. This results in AV dissociation. Both an idioatrial and an idiojunctional tachycardia may coexist—double tachycardia with dissociation; all degrees of AV block may occur with the exception of subnodal block and second-degree block, Type II, and trifascicular block: atrial fibrillation and atrial flutter are almost never the result of digitalis toxicity; digitalis, in general, depresses conductivity and enhances automaticity. It lowers the threshold for ventricular fibrillation, a point of some importance when myocardial ischemia is present; excessive sensitivity of the carotid sinus reflex and of the ocular cardiac reflex may occur.

References

1. Kirk JE, Kvorning SA: Sinus Bradycardia: A clinical study of 515 consecutive cases. *Acta Medica Scan* 142:625, 1952.
2. Agruss NS, Rosin EY, Adolph RJ, et al.: Significance of chronic sinus bradycardia in elderly people. *Circulation* XLVI:924, 1972.
3. Berg GR, Kotler MN: The significance of bilateral bundle branch block in the preoperative patient. *Chest* 59:62, 1971.
4. Kunstadt D, Punja M, Cagin N, et al.: Bifascicular Block: A clinical and electrophysiologic study. *Am Heart J* 86:173, 1973.
5. Venkataraman K, Madias JE, Hood WB Jr: Indications for prophylactic preoperative insertion of pacemakers in patients with right bundle branch block and left anterior hemiblock. *Chest* 68:501, 1975.
6. Pastore JO, Yurchak PM, Janis KM, et al.: The risk of advanced heart block in surgical patients with right bundle branch block and left axis deviation. *Circulation* 57:677, 1978.
7. Bellocci F, Santarelli P, DiGennaro M, et al.: The risk of cardiac complications in surgical patients with bifascicular block. *Chest* 77:343, 1980.
8. Rooney SM, Goldiner PL, Muss E: Relationship of right bundle-branch block and marked left axis deviation to complete heart block during general anesthesia. *Anesthesiology* 44:64, 1976.

9. Gertler MM, Finkle AL, Hudson PB, et al.: Cardiovascular evaluation in surgery. 1. Operative risk in cancer patients with bundle branch block. *Surgery, Gynecology and Obstetrics* 99:441, 1954.
10. Goldman L, Caldera DL, Southwick FS, et al.: Cardiac risk factors and complications in non-cardiac surgery. *Medicine* 57:357, 1978.

Suggested Reading

1. Schamroth L: *The Disorders of Cardiac Rhythm.* Oxford, Blackwell Scientific Publications, 1971.
2. Marriott HJL: *Workshop in Electrocardiography.* Oldsmar, Tampa Tracings, 1972.
3. Chung EK: *Principles of Cardiac Arrhythmias.* Baltimore, Williams & Wilkins Co., 1977.

CHAPTER XII

Coronary Artery Disease

*Jorge I. Martinez-Lopez, M.D.**

Coronary artery disease, per se, does not exclude noncardiac surgery. Often, in the preoperative period, the consultant is asked to determine the risk of noncardiac surgery and anesthesia in patients known to have coronary artery disease. While that judgment may be primarily intuitive, the consultant should make every effort to support his or her decision with objective data. The actual operative risk in any given patient is dependent upon multiple factors, the most important of which relate to the clinical manifestations and to the presence or absence of coronary artery disease complications. Therefore, the decision-making process begins with the pre-operative clinical evaluation, which includes a thorough history and physical examination, and the use of relevant noninvasive laboratory studies. Not infrequently, the evaluation cannot be completed without invasive studies.

At the outset, the consultant should not accept the given diagnosis of coronary artery disease until completeing his or her own evaluation, and reviewing the pertinent available data. Many patients have been told they have coronary artery disease that cannot be subsequently substantiated by a thorough cardiologic study. In one study, one-fourth to one-third of heart patients referred as "cardiacs" were found to have no recognizable heart disease.[1] The erroneous diagnosis was based on faulty interpretation of symptoms and/or signs present for some time. For this reason, questions of paramount importance which the consultant must raise at the time the patient is seen include: Is heart disease present? If it is,

---

*Due to overlapping in subject matter, a small portion of this chapter was contributed by Drs. Eric Harrison and Sheldon Sbar (see Chapter IX).

215

is it coronary artery disease, or is it some other form of heart disease? If it is coronary artery disease, what is the functional status of the heart? Is there any concomitant disease complicating coronary artery disease?

The consultant must also be knowledgeable about data pertaining to surgery and anesthesia in patients with coronary artery disease.

Basic Considerations

Is heart disease present? This question is relevant. Most of the symptoms due to heart disease are not specific for that organ and can be produced by a variety of noncardiac organic disorders, and by anxiety and other emotional disturbances. Among these symptoms are fatigue, weakness, and syncopal and near-syncopal episodes. Palpitations frequently are neither related to heart disease nor to cardiac arrhythmias. Dyspnea, at rest or on exertion, and orthopnea can be experienced not only by patients with cardiac dysfunction but also by patients with pulmonary parenchymal disease. On the other hand, paroxysmal nocturnal dyspnea is almost specific for left-sided cardiac failure. Acute pulmonary edema is most frequently due to cardiac failure, but it can also be noncardiac in origin. Swelling of both lower extremities is frequently noncardiac, particularly in women. In heart disease, pedal edema is a relatively late manifestation of cardiac failure. Unilateral swelling favors the presence of local vascular disease.

Patients frequently associate chest pain with underlying heart disease. While it is true that precordial pain can be a manifestation of coronary artery disease, pain itself can neither be measured nor graphically documented. And careful analysis of all its characteristics, as related by the patient, is essential. Noncoronary chest pain or chest discomfort may have its origin in any of the intrathoracic structures (pericardium, aorta, lungs, pleura, esophagus, and mediastinum). Noncoronary chest pain may also be of extra-thoracic origin (from the spine, chest wall, ribs and shoulders, of neurogenic origin, or from the gastrointestinal system).

Abnormal cardiac findings do not necessarily indicate the presence of heart disease. Arrhythmias can be found in normal healthy subjects with no recognizable heart disease. Murmurs, particularly systolic, may be transient and innocent, or may be related to noncardiac disorders which produce cardiocirculatory changes, e.g., anemia, febrile illnesses, etc. Loud heart sounds, third heart sounds, and fourth heart sounds can be normal findings. Whether these sounds are normal or abnormal has to be determined by "the company they keep."

Once it is established that the patient does have heart disease, the next step is to decide whether or not that disease is coronary atherosclerosis. It may be extremely difficult to make the diagnosis of coronary artery disease on the basis of history and physical examination alone. Mimics of coronary artery disease include the mitral valve prolapse syndrome, cervico-precordial angina, idiopathic hypertrophic subaortic stenosis, and other obstructive lesions of the left ventricular outflow tract, systemic arterial hypertension, and the so-called "syndrome X" in women. Not infrequently, the decision has to be made by correlating the noninvasive radionuclide imaging and treadmill tests with invasive coronary angiography and left ventriculography.

Atherosclerosis is the commonest cause of acquired coronary artery disease, and is associated with an extremely broad clinical spectrum (Table 1). That spectrum ranges from the totally asymptomatic to the patient with symptoms related to significant obstruc-

Table 1
Pre-Operative Patients with Coronary Disease

Clinical Subsets:

Asymptomatic
Symptomatic
    Prior infarction
      recent (< 6 months)
        uncomplicated
        complicated
      remote (> 6 months)
        uncomplicated
        complicated
    Angina pectoris
      stable
      unstable
      postinfarction
      variant
    Ischemic cardiomyopathy
    Arrhythmia
    Antecedent aorto-coronary bypass

tion of one or more major epicardial coronary arteries. Between these two extremes are patients with angina pectoris, cardiac failure, rhythm disturbances, and antecedent aorto-coronary bypass. All have varying risks of subsequent acute myocardial infarction or sudden cardiac death.

The prevalence of coronary artery disease in the asymptomatic adult population is estimated to be about four percent.[2] Although the preoperative likelihood of coronary artery disease in asymptomatic subjects can be estimated from the *Coronary Risk Handbook,*[3] there is probably no merit in doing so. Goldman and co-workers[4] found that established "risk factors" for long-term development of coronary artery disease (i.e., smoking, hyperlipidemia, left ventricular hypertrophy, and glucose intolerance) did not predict perioperative cardiac death. Also, it must be kept in mind that the absence of angina pectoris does not preclude the presence of multivessel coronary lesions.

Whenever possible, it is important for the consultant to identify the precise clinical diagnosis when coronary artery disease is present. It must be recalled that "ischemic heart disease is not one disease but rather an oversimplified term to represent a large group of patients with varied clinical presentations, physical findings, ECG changes, coronary anatomy and pathology, and ventricular function."[5] As a matter of fact, a completely satisfactory classification for coronary artery disease in which to place its various clinical expressions has yet to evolve.

The functional status of the heart in patients with coronary artery disease is determined by the consultant after the evaluation of the etiologic, anatomic, and physiologic data is completed. Also taken into consideration are the absence or presence of concomitant disease and its possible adverse role in the perioperative management of patients with coronary artery disease.

Specific Considerations

The discussion which follows touches on the cardiac risks for noncardiac surgery in patients with angina pectoris and myocardial infarction, and in patients in whom aortocoronary bypass surgery is contemplated or has been performed.

What is known about the risk of noncardiac surgery in patients with coronary artery disease? Our knowledge is imperfect because past studies which attempted to estimate morbidity and mortality all had inherent deficiencies. One of the main problems encountered in trying to answer the question of risk has been the lack of well-designed, controlled, prospective clinical studies. In the majority, reported over a decade ago, the data was analyzed retrospectively. In many reports, there was no preoperative cardiac evaluation, and postoperative follow-up was inadequate. Some had either no concurrent control group or used control groups which were not comparable either in age or type of operation. A systematic approach to the preoperative and postoperative cardiac diagnosis was not followed in others. Still in others, the group of patients studied was not always clearly defined, and/or was designated by a variety of diagnostic criteria now obsolete. Finally, virtually every study derived its conclusions from univariate analysis, rather than from analysis of multiple cardiac variables.

Notwithstanding the above limitations, the reports generally indicated that patients with coronary artery disease can undergo noncardiac surgery, but with a significantly higher morbidity and mortality than patients without.[6] The major and most serious complications which can develop during or after noncardiac surgery are myocardial infarction and death. Other complications include hypotension, cardiac failure, and cardiac arrhythmias which, though serious in nature, often can be reversed.

More recently, Goldman and co-workers[7] conducted the largest prospective study of cardiac risk in noncardiac surgery and based their conclusions on the results of multivariate analysis. That study consisted of 1,001 consecutive patients over the age of 40 who had surgical procedures; excluded were patients who had either transurethral prostatic resection or uncomplicated endoscopy. The majority of the operations were performed with general anesthesia, and the rest either under spinal or epidural anesthesia or under local or regional anesthesia.

Patients with Angina Pectoris

The risk of noncardiac surgery in patients with angina pectoris remains ill-defined. Most studies failed to comment on the type of angina pectoris present or its stability, and grouped all patients under a single major category. This is unfortunate because subsets of angina pectoris present entirely different prognoses and require different management. Perusal of the literature suggests a surgical mortality for patients with angina pectoris which may vary from a low of 0 to a high of almost 17 percent, with the overall mortality for combined series reported to be almost 9 percent.[8]

In the early 1960s, Mattingly[9] provided insight into this problem. He categorized patients with angina pectoris into three groups. Those *with stable angina pectoris* with no demonstrable cardiac abnormalities, and a normal ECG taken at rest, during, and after exercise presented about the same operative risk as patients of the same age without angina. In this group, postoperative infarction was unlikely to be fatal when it occurred unless a lethal arrhythmia supervened. By contrast, the second group, consisting of patients with *stable angina pectoris with ischemic findings on the ECG*, was more likely to develop troublesome arrhythmia and myocardial infarction, often fatal, in the intra- and post-operative period. The more serious prognosis in this group was attributed to the presence of more generalized and more severe coronary atherosclerosis. Patients with *angina decubitus* or *unstable angina pectoris* were in the third group. The presence of either one was noted to create a poor surgical risk.

The more recent data from Goldman and associates[4] suggested that stable angina, per se, was not a risk factor.

While *unstable angina* pectoris may indeed carry a significant operative risk, there is scant data from which to draw solid conclusions. Most reports do not mention unstable angina, as such. It is likely that a major contributing factor for this lack of information is the natural reluctance to operate on patients whose cardiovascular status is obviously unstable. Fear of provoking untoward complications and death would cause the treating physician to postpone noncardiac surgery until stabilization is accomplished. One study reported on 192 patients with angina pectoris.[10] Of these, there were 20 with unstable angina. They had a 10 percent total operative mortality. Six of the 20 patients had either intra-abdominal or intra-thoracic surgery, and two died postoperatively (33% mortality). However, the number of patients with unstable angina in this study was too small to be representative of the operative risk.

Two published reports included *postinfarction angina* as a subset of angina pectoris. In Skinner's series,[10] the overall total mortality was 16 percent, whereas a much higher mortality (27%) was observed when the operative procedure performed was either intra-thoracic or intra-abdominal. The study by Sapala et al.[11] suggested a two- to three-fold increase in the number of postoperative complications and death among patients with postinfarction angina in the preoperative period.

Finally, quantitative data does not exist regarding the risk of noncardiac surgery in patients with *vasospastic angina* (Prinzmetal or variant). It would appear logical to assume that the outcome following surgery would be determined, to a major extent, by the status of the coronary circulation between episodes of vasospastic angina, as well as by the degree of associated left ventricular dysfunction. In other words, the operative risk would likely be influenced by whether coronary vasospasm occurred in the presence of otherwise normal coronary vessels or in combination with single-, double-, or triple-vessel disease, and by the presence or absence of previous myocardial infarction.

It is clear, from the available observations, that patients with angina pectoris, as a whole, are at some risk of developing cardiac complications after noncardiac surgery, and that those with unstable angina patterns are at significant risk.

The Patient with Previous Myocardial Infarction

Whereas the operative risks in patients with angina pectoris remain undefined, there is less debate on risks in patients who are survivors of a previous myocardial infarction. Although there is a higher incidence of both fatal and nonfatal postoperative complications, the consensus is that not all patients with documented preoperative infarction share the same operative risk. Factors which play a major role in the outcome of noncardiac surgery include the temporal proximity of the infarction to surgery and the preoperative functional status of the heart. A major factor is the interval which has elapsed between the preoperative infarction and the time of operation. In other words, was the infarction *recent* or *remote*? In general, there is an inverse relationship between the two, so that the more recent the preoperative infarction, the greater the perioperative morbidity and mortality, and vice versa (Tables 2 and 3).[4,10,12-16]

There is no universal definition for *recent* infarction. It has been

Table 2
Recent Myocardial Infarction and Noncardiac Surgery
Mortality Rate

Author	Patient Number	Cardiac Mortality M.I. < 15 Days	Cardiac Mortality M.I. < 3 Months	Overall Mortality M.I. < 3 Months	Overall Mortality M.I. > 3 Months
Fraser[15]	50	12%	14%	—	—
Arkins[14]	27	—	—	40%	22.6%
Goldman[4]	12	—	23%	—	—
Skinner[10]	10	—	40%	—	—
TOTAL	99	12%	19% Mean	40%	22.6%

Table 3
Recent Myocardial Infarction and Noncardiac Surgery
Incidence of New Postoperative Myocardial Infarction

Author	Patient Number	New M.I. Incidence M.I. 3 Months	Patient Number	New M.I. Incidence M.I. 4–6 months	Patient Number	New M.I. Incidence M.I. 0–6 Months
Steen[16]	15	27%	18	11%	—	—
Tarhan[12]	8	37%	19	16%	22	54%
Topkins[13]	—	—	—	—	—	—

Patient Number	New M.I. Incidence M.I. 6 mos.–1 yr.	Patient Number	New M.I. Incidence M.I. 1–2 yrs.
36	25%	49	22.4%

variously defined as one occurring less than three months or less than six months before the contemplated surgical procedure. There are some areas of agreement regarding recency of infarction and noncardiac surgery, however. So great is the risk of major surgery performed during an acute myocardial infarction—with a mortality near ninety percent—that any form of elective surgery is totally unjustified. Great risk also is encountered when lifesaving emergency surgical procedures are carried out. Under such adverse circumstances, the decision *is best made* after weighing the increased risk of surgery against the risk if the operation is either postponed or not performed. Surgical procedures of less urgency or those elective in nature are best postponed until the infarction is well healed and associated complications controlled.

In the series reported by Tarhan et al.,[12] 37% of patients operated on within three months of myocardial infarction had postoperative infarction. The incidence decreased to 16% when the operation was performed between three and six months of the infarction, and remained at 4% to 5% in patients operated on more than six months after previous infarction.

Topkins and Artusio[13] found a 55% incidence of reinfarction when the interval between the previous infarction and subsequent operation was less than six months, whereas between six months and two years, the recurrence rate was almost the same, between 20% and 25%. A dramatic drop in the rate of postoperative reinfarction, to 6%, was observed between the second and third year after previous infarction. Thereafter, the rate declined further to 1%. They concluded that the risk of recurrent infarction in the perioperative period was high within the first two years after an acute infarction, with the greatest danger during the first six months.

According to Arkins and his co-workers,[14] subendocardial infarction had a better prognostic significance than previous transmural infarction. In their report, 10 of 13 patients (77%) with recent transmural infarction died postoperatively, whereas only 1 of 14 patients (7%) with subendocardial infarction died. Differences in risk between the two groups were not confirmed in Goldman's series.[4] In view of Goldman's recent study, and of the weight of evidence which shows that both transmural and subendocardial infarction have similar long-term prognosis,[17–19] it would be advisable to manage both groups in the same manner until further data become available.

The operative risk associated with *remote* infarction, i.e., infarction occurring more than six months before noncardiac surgery, gradually declines and eventually levels off at about 4% or 5%. Goldman's series[4] reported cardiac death in 5 of 22 patients (22.7%) with preoperative infarction six months or less before surgery, but only in 2 of 79 patients (2.5%) whose infarction was remote. These workers could not establish any statistical correlation, however, between the recency of the preoperative infarction and occurrence of a nonfatal reinfarction. Among patients with remote infarction, they found that the risk of cardiac death was no higher than in those who never had an infarction (12 of 894 patients, 1.3%).

The preoperative functional status of the heart in patients with remote infarction also plays a prominent role in determining the operative risk. In general, as procedures become more extensive, the functional status assumes more importance.[4] Among patients with poor cardiac status, mortality is highest during emergency surgical procedures. Sapala and co-workers[11] subdivided patients with remote infarction into three groups: uncomplicated; postinfarction angina; and complicated by cardiac failure, bundle branch or AV block, arrhythmia, or ECG changes compatible with myocardial ischemia or injury. Patients with *uncomplicated* infarction tolerated anesthesia and operative procedures very well, and had the lowest incidence of cardiorespiratory complications (6%), whereas patients with *postinfarction angina* had an incidence of 14%, and those with *complicated* infarction had the greatest chance of postoperative complications (40%). Mortality in these three groups was 2.8%, 11%, and 10%, respectively. Cardiac complications were three times more frequently the cause of death than were pulmonary complications.

The Patient with Aortocoronary Bypass

The presence of coronary artery disease in patients who are also in need of noncardiac surgery poses another dilemma in management. If the patient is a candidate for aorto-coronary bypass surgery, should this procedure be performed before, concomitantly with, or after noncardiac surgery? The selection of the proper sequence for the contemplated surgical procedures appears to be critical for patient survival. The question becomes even more critical when there is disease of the aortic, cerebral, renal, or peripheral vasculature.

Bernhard and his co-workers[20] were first to address this question. Thirty-one patients with documented coronary artery disease, candidates for aorto-coronary bypass surgery, had coexisting extracranial cerebrovascular disease. Their patients were categorized into three groups, depending upon the sequence of the operations. In one group, carotid artery repair was done first. In the second group, aorto-coronary bypass was done first and carotid endarterectomy four months later. The third group was subjected to simultaneous aorto-coronary bypass and carotid artery repair. Although the number of patients in this series was small, the authors recommended the combined approach (aorto-coronary bypass and carotid artery repair) as the safest course to follow to avoid myocardial damage and cerebral injury. Okies et al.[21] suggested basing the decision for combined vascular surgery on the severity of the lesions in both vasculatures, rather than on symptoms alone. Hence, when symptoms related to carotid artery and coronary artery disease are severe, and the associated stenoses critical—as determined by angiography—the combined approach should be used. Otherwise, the sequence of operations must be planned to fit the circumstances.

Others have reported similar experiences. Seventy-one noncardiac procedures were performed concomitantly with aorto-coronary bypass surgery in 68 patients reported by Dalton et al.[22] The operations were for associated vascular disease, for surgical diseases of the gastrointestinal tract, for associated neoplasia, and for hernia. There were two operative deaths among the 68 patients, for an operative mortality of 2.9%. Both deaths occurred in patients with moderately compromised left ventricular function. Korompai and Hayward[23] concluded that the combined approach allowed a smoother and less complicated recovery.

Of the patients who have had direct myocardial revascularization, 10% to 20% will develop problems requiring a noncardiac operation. In 1976, Scher and Tice[24] reviewed the records of patients with antecedent aorto-coronary bypass surgery, who were then free of symptoms of coronary artery disease. Of the 141 patients, 20 underwent 24 subsequent noncardiac operations. Of those 20 patients, 16 had a total of 19 *elective* procedures with no mortality. Major complications, observed in only five patients, included transient arrhythmias, cardiac failure, atelectasis, and ECG evidence of ischemia without cardiac enzyme changes. Five *emergency* procedures were required in four patients with previous revascularization of the heart; only one patient died postoperatively, with sepsis and hypertension refractory to all measures. Data presented on 60 patients with previous aorto-coronary bypass surgery, by McCollum and co-workers,[25] showed no mortality. Eight episodes of postoperative cardiac complications were recorded in the 77 operative procedures, but all of these complications were easily controlled medically.

Crawford and associates[26] reported data on 358 patients with prior aorto-coronary bypass surgery, who underwent noncardiac surgery from 10 days to 89 months after bypass. The majority (74%) had only one subsequent operation; the remainder had two or more surgical procedures. There were four deaths (1.1%), but none were cardiac deaths. Three of the four deaths occurred in patients subjected to subsequent operation within 30 days of aorto-coronary bypass.

In summary, the above studies suggest that *successful* revascularization of the myocardium before subsequent surgery may have a "protective" effect on the myocardium, reducing operative morbidity and mortality. But, the risk of the bypass procedure should be included in the overall mortality and morbidity. However, once patients have undergone successful revascularization, they are acceptable risks for subsequent emergency or elective noncardiac operations.

Percutaneous Transluminal Coronary Angioplasty

At the present time, there are no data available showing how patients with coronary artery disease treated by percutaneous transluminal coronary angioplasty fare during or after noncardiac surgery.

Other Considerations

The consultant must also be aware of other factors which may increase the operative risk in patients with coronary artery disease.

It is extremely important to know which medication(s) the patient is taking before the operation. Of particular interest are digitalis, antiarrhythmic agents, salt-depleting and potassium-depleting agents, beta-blockers, antihypertensives, anticoagulants, steroids, and central nervous system antidepressants. In some instances, it may be desirable to discontinue the administration of one or more drugs before surgery. In others, continuation of the drug(s) may be necessary. Additionally, the possibility of drug interaction with other agents given postoperatively must be kept in mind (see Chapter 3).

To be taken into consideration also are the expertise and skills of the surgical and the anesthesia teams. It is obvious that a lower morbidity and mortality should be expected with the more experienced teams.

Finally, other factors which can have adverse effects on the outcome of noncardiac surgery in patients with coronary disease include age beyond 70 years, certain associated diseases, and the general status of the patient.

References

1. Goldwater LJ, Bernstein LH, Kresky B: Study of one hundred seventy-five "cardiacs" without heart disease. *JAMA* 148:89, 1952.
2. Diamond GA, Forrester JS: Analysis of probability as an aid in the clinical diagnosis of coronary-artery disease. *N Engl J Med* 300:1350, 1979.
3. American Heart Association: New York, *Coronary Risk Handbook*, 1973.
4. Goldman L, Caldera DL, Southwick FS, et al.: Cardiac risk factors and complications in noncardiac surgery. *Medicine* 57:357, 1978.
5. Conti CR, Christie LG Jr: Coronary artery bypass surgery. *Cardiov Rev and Rep* 2:127, 1981.
6. Nachlas MM, Abrams SJ, Goldberg MM: The influence of arteriosclerotic heart disease on surgical risk. *Am J Surg* 101:447, 1961.
7. Goldman L, Caldera DL, Nussbaum SR, et al.: Multifactorial index of cardiac risk in noncardiac surgical procedures. *N Engl J Med* 297:845, 1977.
8. Salene DN, Homans DC, Isner JM: Management of cardiac disease in the general surgical patient. *Current Problems in Cardiology* 5(2):22, 1980.
9. Mattingly TW: Patients with coronary artery disease as a surgical risk. *Am J Cardiol* 12:279, 1963.
10. Skinner JF, Pearce MI: Surgical risk in the cardiac patient. *J Chron Dis* 17:57, 1964.

11. Sapala JA, Ponka JL, Duvernoy WF: Operative and nonoperative risks in the cardiac patient. *J Am Geriatr Soc* 23:529, 1975.
12. Tarhan S, Moffit EA, Taylor WF, et al.: Myocardial infarction after general anesthesia. *JAMA* 220:1451, 1972.
13. Topkins MJ, Artusio JF: Myocardial infarction and surgery: A five-year study. *Anesth Analg* 43:715, 1964.
14. Arkins R, Smessaert AA, Hicks RG: Mortality and morbidity in surgical patients with coronary artery disease. *JAMA* 190:485, 1964.
15. Fraser JG, Ramachandra PR, Davis HS: Anesthesia and recent myocardial infarction. *JAMA* 199:96, 1967.
16. Steen PA, Tinker JH, Tarhan S: Myocardial reinfarction after anesthesia and surgery. *JAMA* 239:2566, 1978.
17. Scheinman MM, Abbot JA: Clinical significance of transmural versus nontransmural electrocardiographic changes in patients with acute myocardial infarction. *Am J Med* 55:502, 1973.
18. Madias JE, Chahine RA, Gorlin R, et al.: A comparison of transmural and non-transmural acute myocardial infarction. *Circulation* 49:498, 1974.
19. Rigo P, Murray M, Taylor DR, et al.: Hemodynamic and prognostic findings in patients with transmural and non-transmural infarction. *Circulation* 51:1064, 1975.
20. Bernhard VM, Johnson WD, Peterson JJ: Carotid artery stenosis. Association with surgery for coronary artery disease. *Arch Surg* 105:837, 1972.
21. Okies JE, MacManus Q, Starr A: Myocardial revascularization and carotid endarterectomy: A combined approach. *Ann Thorac Surg* 23:569, 1977.
22. Dalton ML Jr, Parker TM, et al.: Concomitant coronary artery bypass surgery and major noncardiac surgery. *J Thorac Cardiovasc Surg* 75:621, 1978.
23. Korompai FL, Hayward RH: Noncoronary surgery combined with coronary artery bypass. *Cardiovasc Dis, Bull Texas Heart Inst* 5:265, 1978.
24. Scher K, Tice DA: Operative risk in patients with previous coronary bypass. *Arch Surg* 111:807, 1976.
25. McCollum CH, Garcia-Rinaldi R, Graham JM, et al.: Myocardial revascularization prior to subsequent major surgery in patients with coronary artery disease. *Surgery* 81:302, 1977.
26. Crawford ES, Morris GS, Howell JF, et al.: Operative risk in patients with previous coronary artery bypass. *Ann Thorac Surg* 26:215, 1978.

CHAPTER XIII

Peripheral and Cerebrovascular Disease

James W. Williams, M.D.

The evaluation of patients with vascular disease who have known or occult cardiac disease is a common problem. The high incidence of coronary artery disease in the individuals with peripheral vascular disease has been recognized for many years.[1-5] Singer and Rob,[5] for instance, have reported that the incidence of coronary artery disease in patients with lower extremity claudication is approximately 33%. Routine coronary arteriography in a series of patients with aortoiliac occlusive disease or abdominal aortic aneurysm has shown that 30% to 40% have significant coronary artery disease.[4] Studies of the natural history of patients with intermittent claudication also reveal the effect of coronary artery disease, since the mortality of patients with vascular disease approaches 20% at five years to approximately 50% at ten years[3] (Table 1), and the major causes of death are coronary artery disease and cerebrovascular disease.[2]

Peripheral Arterial Disease

In spite of the unfavorable statistics mentioned above, the physician must deal with the patient whose life is seriously limited by claudication or who is in imminent danger of limb loss, since the risk of amputation during a five to ten-year follow-up is about 10% (Table 1). In the patient with overt cardiac disease, it is imperative that the physician carefully weigh the benefits of palliation or limb

229

Table 1

Natural History of Patients with Intermittent Claudication

Author	N	% Requiring Amputation	Mortality
Bloor[2]	1,476	at 9% (10 years)	at 46% (10 years)
Singer and Rob[5]	359	at 7% (3 years)	at 21% (3 years)
Eastcott[3]	3,735	at 10% (5 years)	at 20% (5 years)

N = Number

salvage against the risks of surgery. Often, however, an accurate assessment of the extent of coronary artery disease is not available in patients with peripheral vascular disease, since the symptoms of even severe cardiac disease may be masked by activity restriction. This makes the assessment of risk subject to error. Since the specter or coronary artery disease must be considered, only patients with far-advanced arterial insufficiency should be considered for operation. Cooperman et al.[6] noted an overall 8.5% mortality in 566 patients with peripheral vascular operations. Cardiovascular complications were responsible for 62% of these deaths (23 of 37). Overall, 71 patients experienced a cardiovascular complication and one in three of those patients died. The postoperative cardiovascular complications included congestive heart failure (31%), cardiac arrhythmia (31%), myocardial infarction (25%), peripheral embolus (7%), and cerebrovascular accident (6%). Five preoperative risk factors showed a statistically significant individual association with postoperative cardiovascular complications. The incidence of postoperative cardiovascular complications was 20% in patients with a previous myocardial infarction (compared to 7% in patients without prior myocardial infarctions). Table 2 reviews the other risk factors. When all risk factors were considered and patients at the two extremes of risk were evaluated, the incidence of cardiovascular complications was 23% for high risk, and 1–2% for low risk patients.

It should be realized that the management of many patients who present with claudication and superficial femoral or iliac occlusive

Table 2
Preoperative Cardiac Risk Factors Compared to Outcome*

Risk Factor	% Complication With Risk Factor	% Complication Without Risk Factor
MI	20%	7%
CHF	33%	8%
Arrhythmias	33%	9%
Abnormal ECG	13%	3%
CVA	24%	9%
Angina**	16%	9%

*From Cooperman et al.[6]
**Not statistically significant
MI = myocardial infarction

CHF = congestive heart failure
CVA = cerebrovascular accident

disease does not have to include surgery. Studies of the natural history of patients with claudication have demonstrated that most have improved exercise tolerance after six to twelve months of conservative medical management.[7] Although the etiology of peripheral arterial disease is unclear, cigarette smoking is probably one of the most pertinent related factors in our culture. Physicians are in a unique position to counsel patients on the effects of this habit and, if not require, at least strongly urge them to stop smoking. This approach has not been emphasized often enough. Of course, nonoperative therapy might be more successful if the etiology of arterial disease were known, but a program of weight loss, cessation of smoking, and graded exercise should be proposed, when applicable. (Even if surgery is performed, cessation of smoking is mandatory. Myers et al.[8] noted a three-fold increase in occlusions in the grafted limb in patients who continued to smoke more than five cigarettes daily.) Adherence to a program of this type can cause significant improvement in exercise tolerance in over one-half of patients. Contrast arteriography is not necessary at this stage, but the patient should be followed with serial noninvasive pressure and flow studies at two to four month intervals. (See Chapter 7) In addition, there is indirect evidence that occlusion of a major artery may delay or diminish the appearance of atheromatous changes in the arterial tree distal to the occlusion.[9]

Since the risk of limb loss is low and many patients improve with nonoperative therapy, we recommend arterial surgery for occlusive disease only in certain situations. One such situation is when the patient cannot support himself financially because of severe limitation of activity, and a program of conservative management has failed to improve his symptoms. Another situation is when existing ischemia is associated with gangrene, impending gangrene, an ulcer which will not heal, or pain which is present at rest. When the patient has cardiac disease which imposes significant functional limitations, he is clearly not a candidate for an operation aimed solely at relieving claudication. But, for the patient with impending limb loss, a bypass procedure is indicated and may be as easily tolerated as an amputation. Increasing experience with extra-anatomic bypass (axillo-femoral) suggests that limb salvage may be obtained and sustained without the stress of entering the peritoneal cavity and with the acceptable penalty of only slightly diminished long-term patency. It is, thus, apparent that multiple factors including cardiac impairment, generalized medical diseases, and the extent and location of arterial disease affect the decision to perform a surgical procedure in these patients. When the decision for surgery is made, studies suggest a reasonable outcome (Table 3).[10]

Abdominal Aortic Aneurysm

The situation with regard to the abdominal aortic aneurysm is relatively more clear cut. The indication for surgery is to lengthen life. DeBakey et al.[11] and Szilagyi et al.[12] have shown that elective resection of such aneurysms significantly prolongs the life expectancy of these patients. O'Donnell et al.[13] have suggested that even in the very elderly, elective resection of an aortic aneurysm can be safe (overall operative mortality under 5%) and can restore survival to that expected in the general population. Emphasis on physiologic considerations, rather than chronologic age, holds true for this as for most surgical procedures.

One must always be aware that the natural history of the aneurysm is ultimate rupture,[14] but the timing and indications for surgery must be considered. The mean rupture rate of aneurysms smaller than 5 cm is 5%, while aneurysms of 6 cm have a mean rupture rate of 16%, and aneurysms 7 cm or greater may have a rupture rate greater than 75%.[10] Thus, there is little disagreement that a healthy patient, less than 70 years of age, with an aneurysm

Table 3

Results of Femoropopliteal Bypass Grafts with Autologous Saphenous Vein

Study	Number of Limbs	Indication for Operation	Patency Rate in Survivors (%)	Limb Preservation (%)	Mortality, Long-Term (%)	Duration of Follow-up* (yr)
DeWeese and Rob	67	Salvage	45	64	62	5
Naji et al.	100	Salvage	47	70	40	5
DeWeese and Rob	67	Salvage	14	63	88.5	10
DeWeese and Rob	46	Claudication	74	100	26	5
Naji et al.	100	Claudication	70	97	26	5
DeWeese and Rob	46	Claudication	45	100	48	10

*All patients were followed for five or ten years.
(Reprinted with permission of the New England Journal of Medicine: Thompson JE, Garrett WV: New England Journal of Medicine 302:497, 1980.)

greater than 5 cm, should have aneurysmectomy. Likewise, the patient with a symptomatic aneurysm should be operated immediately, since his life expectancy is diminished to less than a few months. However, there is less consensus regarding the patient who is more than 75 years of age or who has significant systemic disease with limited reserve in a vital organ, and who has an aneurysm of 5–6 cm. The problem of operability in these poor risk patients requires a slightly different approach. If the aneurysm is 7–8 cm or more in the greatest diameter, the risk of rupture within two years is 50% or greater,[15,16] and the mortality of rupture is at least 75%. This estimate is based on reports from Szilagyi et al.[16] and is consistent with our experience. Thus, the risk of death with elective surgery must be judged to be quite high or the likelihood of death over the following two years from other causes, very great, before surgery is withheld. Other patients can be followed carefully and only if the aneurysm begins to enlarge suddenly, (thereby increasing the likelihood of rupture), is surgery, in general, indicated.[17]

The use of ultrasound to calibrate and follow the progression of the aneurysm has added significantly to our understanding of the cause of this disease[18] and in our ability to follow patients for aneurysmal enlargement. It should be remembered that ultrasound yields a more accurate estimate of the size of an aneurysm compared to physical examination or abdominal x-ray, both of which magnify or overestimate the aneurysm's size. This is important to realize, since most of the published mortality figures were based upon x-ray evaluation or physical examination of aneurysmal size (e.g., an aneurysm of 6 cm on x-ray may be only 4–5 cm on ultrasound). Thus, a smaller-sized aneurysm is considered surgical when ultrasound is used to assess aneurysmal size in the evaluation for need of surgery. Although the degrees of risk mentioned above are estimates, there are certain other principles to observe. For instance, lung disease or heart disease severe enough to produce marked dyspnea when walking up a single flight of stairs (15 steps), is a manifestation of limited reserve, and significantly increases the risk of surgery and complicates convalescence. In some cases, careful attention to reversible medical problems and the cessation of cigarette smoking may improve a patient's risk of operation and permit him to have the aneurysm safely resected.

Since repair of these aneurysms generally requires a dacron and teflon prosthesis, a number of complications can be seen in the postoperative period. These include graft infections (which may occur in 1–3%), aortoenteric fistulae, anastomatic aneurysms, ureteral obstruction, and others.[10] Discussion of each is beyond the scope of this chapter, but points out the need for careful postoperative follow-up.

Peripheral Aneurysms

Peripheral aneurysms do not present a significant threat to the life of the patient, since rupture can be controlled more readily than rupture of the abdominal aortic aneurysm. They do, however, present a sizeable risk of embolization and thrombosis. Since the physiologic challenge of operation is not particularly great, these aneurysms should be resected and grafted unless the concurrent medical conditions are extremely grave, such as recent myocardial infarction, chronic intractable heart failure, severe angina, coexisting malignancy, or debilitating neurologic or metabolic disease. The mortality of above-the-knee amputation, a common result of a neglected popliteal artery aneurysm, is approximately 10% and probably higher than that of elective popliteal artery surgery.

Cerebrovascular Disease

Extracranial carotid arterial disease produces cerebrovascular symptoms in two ways. The internal carotid may become severely stenotic, producing diminished cerebral blood flow and eventual occlusion; or, an atheromatous plaque can cavitate or ulcerate, producing a source for thromboembolism to the vessels supplied by the internal carotid. This second mechanism provides the more common manifestations of carotid disease. The development of transient ischemic attacks (TIA) portends a serious threat of permanent neurologic deficit. Over five years, up to 35% of such episodes are followed by permanent neurologic deficit.[19–22] Carotid endarterectomy is an effective method of diminishing this risk of neurologic deficit, and operative mortality is now 1–2% if patients are carefully and properly selected. Neurologic deficits related to operation should be no more than 2–4%, compared to a 30–35% incidence of permanent stroke in untreated patients with TIAs (Table 4).[10] It must be noted, however, that overall long-term mortality is not as greatly affected by endarterectomy, since these patients generally have diffuse vascular disease and the ravages of coronary artery disease are not controlled.

Interest in the use of drugs affecting platelet activity for treatment of patients with TIAs is bolstered by reports of protection against stroke in men by use of aspirin.[23] Hopefully, other data will support these findings. Until support is forthcoming, one must not precipitously abandon carotid endarterectomy, which is a proven method of stroke prevention. Additionally, in the symptomatic patient with a very high degree of carotid stenosis, whose symptoms are due to a reduction in cerebral blood flow, it is not logical to expect any currently available drug to be effective.

A bothersome patient is the one with no cerebrovascular symptoms, who is scheduled for a major surgical procedure, and a carotid bruit is found on physical examination. Several studies have suggested that patients with asymptomatic carotid bruits may have a subsequent incidence of TIAs as high as 27% and of stroke in 17% within three to five years.[10] Prophylactic endarterectomy may reduce this incidence six-fold.[10] The use of newly developed noninvasive methods to evaluate the extent of stenosis will, hopefully, eliminate an unnecessary carotid arteriogram in these individuals. Blackshear et al.[24] have shown that ultrasonic imaging of the internal carotid and pulsed doppler spectrum analysis correlates very closely with arteriography. When hemodynamically significant stenosis is detected by noninvasive methods and visualized by arteriography, we have recommended surgery for the asymptomatic patient if the obstruction is 75% or greater.

If a major operative procedure is planned for the patient with carotid artery disease, we strongly recommend considering carotid endarterectomy prior to the proposed operation. The patient with high grade carotid stenosis (greater than 85%), who has an urgent indication for cardiac surgery, may have both procedures performed simultaneously. The carotid endarterectomy can be performed with little increase in anesthesia time, while the saphenous veins are harvested. This, hopefully, protects the patient from thrombosis of a stenotic carotid in the event of an episode of low

Table 4

Results of Carotid Endarterectomy for Transient Cerebral Ischemia

Study	Operative Mortality (%)	Normal or Improved, Long-Term (%)	Strokes, Long-Term (%)	Length of Follow-up (yr)
Fields et al. Joint Study 1970	3.6	47	4	3.5*
Thompson et al. 1970	1.1	93	5.4	1–13
Wylie and Ehrenfeld 1970	—	94	5.7	1–10
DeWeese et al. 1973	1	88	10.6	5†
Toole et al. 1975	6.1	71	7	3.8*

*Mean
†All patients
(Reprinted with permission of New England Journal of Medicine: Thompson JE, Garrett WV: New England Journal of Medicine 302:494, 1980.)

flow in the postoperative setting. Bernhard et al.[25] first discussed this approach in 1972, after noting that a group of patients approached with a carotid endarterectomy as a first procedure suffered a 20% mortality due to cardiac complications. Since then, several studies have demonstrated the feasibility of such a combined approach, but no studies exist with a satisfactory control group.[26,27] The fact that the combined procedure is feasible is probably so because carotid endarterectomy is usually not a long operation, and the postoperative physiologic derangements mentioned in Chapter III are not as great as in those operations in which a body cavity is entered, unless the patient has very severe or unstable heart disease. Pulmonary and renal diseases are not severely jeopardized by the procedure and, therefore, usually do not preclude its performance.

Peripheral Arterial Embolism

Another peripheral vascular problem which arises in cardiac patients is that of peripheral arterial embolism, which continues to be a common problem. Arterial embolism usually presents as a sudden dramatic change in perfusion, with pain, pallor, and parasthesia in the involved extremity. Unless an overriding contraindication to anticoagulation exists, the patient should be heparinized immediately. The success of embolectomy depends on the extent of thrombosis in the small vessels peripheral to the occluded artery; therefore, anticoagulation can improve the likelihood of successful embolectomy. Embolectomy should be done under local anesthesia as soon as possible. Because of an obligatory blood loss of approximately 300 ml, type specific and cross-matched blood should be available. Ony the moribund individual or one with established infection near the operation site should be denied consideration for embolectomy if the condition is diagnosed early. If the ischemia is severe and prolonged, however, embolectomy may prove fatal. When the limb is anesthetic, diffusely cyanotic, and muscles are paralyzed, revascularization may flush potassium, myoglobin, and aggregates of platelets, white blood cells, and fibrin into the systemic circulation producing hyperkalemia, arrhythmias, renal failure, and pulmonary insufficiency. The patient with limited cardiac reserve tolerates these complications very poorly and mortality is high, varying from 15–30% with the usual cause of death related to the underlying cardiac disease. Amputation rates have declined and overall limb salvageability among operative survivors is 80–90%.

Venous Diseases

Patients with cardiac disease have long been recognized as being at increased risk of pulmonary embolism, as venous disease is common. Other important risk factors include age, obesity, previous history of deep venous thrombosis or pulmonary embolism, estrogen use and major surgery, especially orthopedic, abdominal, and pelvic surgery. These predisposing effects are cumulative, so that patients with multiple risk factors are in much greater jeopardy. In the perioperative patient, measures which should be routine include the avoidance of dehydration, leg exercises, and early ambulation. These measures have decreased the incidence of thromboembolism to some degree. However, the number of cases of deep venous thrombosis and pulmonary embolism remains high.

There is little evidence that "anti-embolism" stockings are useful. Elevation of the foot of the bed 10–15 degrees is probably more helpful in promoting venous drainage.

Two measures recently introduced to prevent postoperative thromboembolism appear to be highly effective. They consist of low doses of heparin and certain mechanical measures to increase venous drainage. "Low dose" heparin (5,000 units given subcutaneously every eight to twelve hours) has been shown to be extremely effective in preventing thromboembolism in patients undergoing general surgical procedures (See Chapter 3 for further discussion).

Intravenous dextran has also been employed for thrombosis prophylaxis and may be as effective as low dose heparin. However, since dextran expands the blood volume, it has limited use in most cardiac patients. Finally, aspirin and other antiplatelet agents have been demonstrated to have some prophylactic effects.

The mechanical measures consist of calf muscle contraction during surgery, using a mechanical pedal to flex and extend the ankle, electrical stimulation of leg muscles, and intermittent pneumatic compression of the leg. A number of studies[28–30] have shown that these prophylactic measures can reduce the incidence of thromboembolism from 30–50% in nontreated patients to 6–10% in patients treated with this measure.

In general, surgery for venous disease is not recommended for the patient with severe heart disease. The benefits are questionable, and gratifying results can be obtained by other means. Venous thrombectomy should be considered only when vigorous heparin administration has failed and venous gangrene appears imminent (phlegmasia cerulea dolens). Surgery for pulmonary embolism, for all practical purposes, is limited to interruption of the vena cava to prevent further pulmonary embolism. Indications for this surgery include recurrent pulmonary embolism in spite of adequate anticoagulation, pulmonary embolism occurring in a patient for whom anticoagulation is excessively dangerous (esophageal varices, active duodenal ulcer, intracranial aneurysm, etc.), and septic thromboembolism. The preferred method of interruption of the vena cava for nonseptic embolism has been application of a clip which compresses the vena cava producing channels of blood flow small enough to trap a large embolus, yet preserve patency of the vena cava. Several of these devices have been designed and used with overall good results. For the patient who is very ill and unable to safely undergo general anesthesia, transvenous insertion of an intraluminal filter device has been proposed. Unfortunately, migration of the filter and improper placement occasionally occur with this method of vena cava interruption. More recent modifications of this type of device may diminish some of these problems and provide acceptable protection against embolization,[31] but it should be remembered that one must continue anticoagulation after insertion of the device to prevent excessive venous thrombosis in the legs.

The successful management of patients with peripheral vascular disease and cardiac disease demands close attention to the details of surgical technique and medical care, and close cooperation and communication between the surgeon and the medical physician. In few other areas of surgery are the results of casual or sloppy surgical technique or patient care more apparent or damaging. Preoperative evaluation is the same as for all surgical patients, e.g., careful assessment of the presence and degree of associated diseases and optimization of therapy. Because of the high incidence of coronary artery and cerebrovascular disease, as well as hypertension and diabetes, special emphasis should be placed on these disorders. These same problems require attention postoperatively.

References

1. Mitchell JRA, Schwartz CJ: Relationship between arterial disease in different sites. *Brit Med J* May, 1293, 1962.
2. Bloor K: Natural history of arteriosclerosis of the lower extremities. *Ann Roy Coll Surg Eng* 28:36, 1961.
3. Eastcott HHG: *Arterial Surgery* Pitman, London, p. 56, 1969.
4. Hertzer NR, Young JR, et al.: Routine coronary angiography prior to elective aortic reconstruction. *Arch Surg* 114:1336, 1979.
5. Singer A, Rob C: Fate of the claudicator. *Brit Med J* Aug, 633, 1960.
6. Cooperman M, Pflug B, Martin EW, Jr, et al.: Cardiovascular risk factors in patients with peripheral vascular disease. *Surg*:84:505, 1978.
7. Ekroth R, Dahloff A, Grundevall B: Physical training of patients with intermittent claudication: Indications, methods and results. *Surgery* 84:640, 1978.
8. Myers KA, King RB, Scott DF, et al.: The effect of smoking on the late patency of arterial reconstructions in the legs. *Brit J Surg* 65:267 1978.

9. Mozersky DJ, Sumner DS, Strandness DE: Disease progression after femoropopliteal surgical procedure. *SGO* 135:700, 1972.
10. Thompson JE, Garrett WV: Peripheral arterial surgery. *NEJM* 302:491, 1980.
11. DeBakey ME, Crawford ES, Cooley DH, et al.: Aneurysm of abdominal aorta: Analysis of results of graft replacement therapy one to eleven years after operation. *Ann Surg* 160:622, 1964.
12. Szilagyi DE, Smith RF, DeRusso FJ, et al.: Contribution of aortic aneurysmectomy to prolongation of life: 12 year review of 480 cases. *Ann Surg* 164:678, 1966.
13. O'Donnell TF, Jr, Darling RC, Linton RR: Is 80 years too old for aneurysmectomy? *Arch Surg* III:1250, 1976.
14. Klippel AP, Butcher HR: The unoperated abdominal aortic aneurysm. *Am Jour Surg* 111:629, 1966.
15. Schatz IJ, Fairbairn JF, Juergens JL: Abdominal aortic anuerysms: A reappraisal. *Circulation* XXVI:200, 1962.
16. Szilagyi DE, Elliott JP: Clinical fate of the patient with asymptomatic abdominal aortic aneurysm unfit for surgical treatment. *Arch Surg* 104:600, 1978.
17. Bernstein E, et al.: Growth rate of small aortic aneurysms. *Surg* 80 (6):765, 1976.
18. Wheeler WE: Ultrasonic evaluation of abdominal masses. *JAMA* 239 (5):419, 1978.
19. Whisnant JP: A population study of stroke and TIA: Rochester, Minn. In FJ Gillingham, C Mawdsley, Eds. *Stroke*: Williams, New York, Churchill Livingstone pp 21–39, A.E. 1976.
20. Ziegler DK, Hazzaneiu RS: Prognosis in patients with transient ischemic attacks. *Stroke* 4:666, 1973.
21. DeWeese JA, Rob CG, Satran R, et al.: Results of carotid endarterectomies for transient ischemic attack: Five years later. *Ann Surg* 178:258, 1973.
22. Fields WS, Maslenikov V, Meyer JS, et al.: Joint study of extracranial arterial occlusion. V. Progress report of prognosis following surgical or non-surgical treatment for transient ischemia attacks and cervical carotid artery lesions. *JAMA* 211:1993, 1970.
23. Fields WS, Lemak NA, Frankowski RF, et al.: Controlled trial of aspirin in cerebral ischemic stroke. *JAMA* 211:1997, 1970.
24. Blackshear WM, Phillips DJ, Thiele BL, Hirsch JH, Chikos PM, Marinelli MR, Ward KJ, Strandness DE: Detection of carotid occlusive disease by ultrasonic imaging and pulsed Doppler spectrum analysis. *Surgery* 86 No. 5:698, 1979.
25. Bernhard VM, Johnson WD, Peterson JJ: Carotid artery stenosis: Association with surgery for coronary artery disease. *Arch Surg* 105:837, 1972.
26. Oakies JE, MacManus Q, Starr A: Myocardial revascularization and carotid endarterectomy: A combined approach. *Ann Thorac Surg* 23:560, 1977.

27. Eckstein PF, Vijayanagar R, Bognolo DA, et al.: Management of combined coronary and peripheral vascular disease. *J Florida MA* 66:1051, 1979.
28. Cotton LT, Roberts VC: The prevention of deep vein thrombosis, with particular reference to mechanical methods of prevention. *Surgery* 81:228, 1977.
29. Hills KH, Pflug JJ, Jeyasingh K, Boardmann L, Calnan JS: Prevention of deep vein thrombosis by intermittent compression of the calf. *Brit Med Journal* 1:131, 1972.
30. Rosenberg IL, Evans M, Pollock AV: Prophylaxis of postoperative leg vein thrombosis by low dose subcutaneous heparin or preoperative calf muscle stimulation: A controlled clinical trial. *Brit Med Journal* 1:649, 1975.
31. Greenfield LJ, Zocco J, et al.: Experience with the Kim-Ray Greenfield vena cava filter. *Annals of Surgery* 185:692, 1977.

CHAPTER XIV

Valvular Heart Disease

Thomas J. Linnemeier, M.D., R. Joe Noble, M.D.,
and Edward F. Steinmetz, M.D.

The clinical assessment of the patient with valvular heart disease will be dichotomized into two phases: the preoperative evaluation and intraoperative assessment and management.

Preoperative Evaluation

Preoperatively, the evaluation evolves around several points: the lesion involved, and the hemodynamic significance of the lesion; the cardiac rhythm; prophylaxis against infectious endocarditis; and anticoagulation (in some patients).

The Hemodynamic Significance of Valvular Lesions

Of utmost importance is the determination of the hemodynamic significance of the valvular abnormality. If the lesion is not of sufficient severity to embarrass the circulation under usual circumstances, then it is highly unlikely to embarrass the circulation during the operative procedure.

With the important exception of left ventricular outflow tract obstruction (i.e., aortic stenosis and subaortic stenosis) *symptoms* are the principle clue to the hemodynamic significance of the lesion. The patient who is *symptomatic* from his valvular lesion is the patient who requires meticulous care and attention during the surgical procedure.

243

The hemodynamic significance of the valvular lesion is determined by eliciting a careful history; performing a meticulous physical examination; and by analyzing the electrocardiogram, the chest radiogram, and often an echocardiogram. Rarely is cardiac catheterization essential to this assessment.

Five of the more common valvular lesions will be considered.

Mitral Stenosis

As an example of the clinical assessment required of the patient with valvular disease, consider first the patient with mitral stenosis. One inquires as to dyspnea, reflecting an elevation in left atrial and hence pulmonary capillary pressure; as to fatigue, resulting from a decrease in cardiac output; and palpitations, which may suggest atrial fibrillation.

The physical examination is extremely helpful. If the patient has severe mitral stenosis, the examination should reveal right ventricular hypertrophy, an accentuation in the first heart sound, a long diastolic rumble, and an early opening snap with less than 0.08 seconds separating the opening snap from the aortic component of the second heart sound.

If severe, mitral stenosis should be manifested electrocardiographically as atrial fibrillation with a "squatty" QRS in V_1, due to a relative predominance of right ventricular over left ventricular electrical forces, right axis deviation is often seen. Indeed, a tracing such as illustrated in Figure 1 demonstrating atrial fibrillation with

MITRAL STENOSIS

HISTORY
  Dyspnea
  Fatigue
  Palpitations
PHYSICAL EXAMINATION
  Right ventricular hypertrophy
  ↑ S_1
  Opening snap (OS); A_2-OS interval
  Diastolic rumble
ELECTROCARDIOGRAM
  Atrial fibrillation
  Right ventricular predominance

RADIOGRAM
  ↑ Left atrium
  Pulmonary venous
    hypertension
ECHOCARDIOGRAM
  ↑ Left atrium
  Mitral valve thickening
  ↓ E to F slope
  Paradoxical diastolic septal
    motion

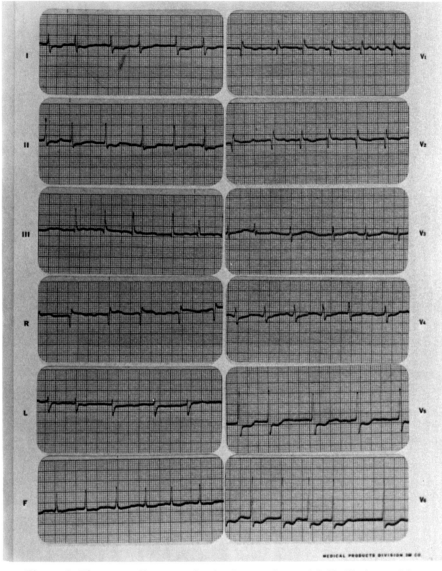

Figure 1. Electrocardiogram of mitral stenosis. Atrial fibrillation, with a vertical axis and diminutive QRS in V_1 are all features of mitral stenosis. The qr complex in V_1 is often associated with right atrial dilatation, thereby indicating clinical tricuspid regurgitation. The explanation for the q wave is uncertain; it may result from the enlarged right atrium presenting as an "intra-atrial" complex in V_1; alternately, the convexity of the interventricular septum toward the left ventricle may alter septal forces in this direction.

right axis deviation and a qr complex in lead V_1, suggests not only mitral stenosis, but also right atrial dilatation secondary to severe pulmonary hypertension.

The chest radiogram would be expected to demonstrate an enlarged left atrium and pulmonary arterial and venous hypertension.

Finally, the echocardiogram would demonstrate thickening of the mitral valve with a reduced E to F slope, restricted motion of both leaflets, and early diastolic motion of the septum toward the left ventricle (Figure 2).

Considering the above techniques of assessment of the hemodynamic significance of mitral stenosis, particular attention should be paid to:

The *symptoms*. If the patient is completely asymptomatic, it is quite unlikely that he has significant, severe mitral stenosis. But, symptoms must be diligently sought before concluding that the patient is asymptomatic. This is so because, in slowly progressing disease, patients may learn to "live within" their cardiac limitation without their being aware of it.

The *physical examination*. If the opening snap is quite late and the rumble quite short in duration and there is no evidence of right ventricular hypertrophy, it is quite unlikely that the mitral stenosis is severe.

The *electrocardiogram* is not so helpful. The electrocardiogram may actually be normal, even in the presence of moderately severe stenosis.

The *radiogram* is helpful. Particular attention should be directed to the degree of pulmonary venous hypertension.

The *echocardiogram*, of course, is quite helpful. The cross-sectional echocardiogram provides an approximation of mitral valve area.[1] Such a noninvasive assessment of the mitral valve correlates closely with data collected at catheterization and surgery, and may provide additional assurance, when needed.

Mitral Regurgitation

Mitral regurgitation is of importance not only from the standpoint of the hemodynamic overload it imposes, but also from the standpoint of the anatomic lesion responsible for valvular leakage. Regurgitation may result from disease in any of the six components

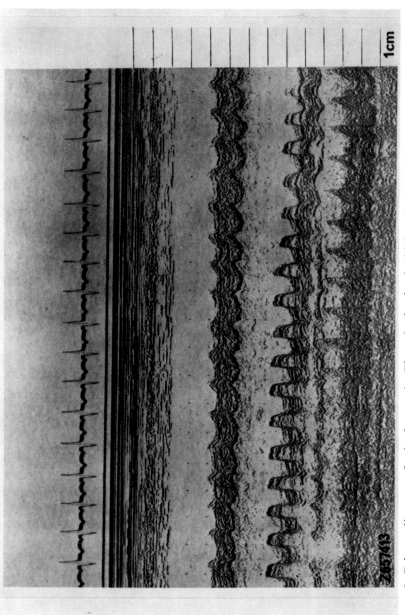

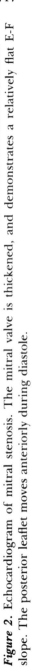

Figure 2. Echocardiogram of mitral stenosis. The mitral valve is thickened, and demonstrates a relatively flat E-F slope. The posterior leaflet moves anteriorly during diastole.

MITRAL REGURGITATION

HISTORY
   Rheumatic fever history
   History of myocardial infarction, angina
   Dyspnea
   Palpitations
PHYSICAL EXAMINATION
   Right ventricular heave
   Apical systolic murmur
   S_3G
ELECTROCARDIOGRAM
   Evidence of previous myocardial infarction
   Left atrial abnormality
   Left ventricular hypertrophy
Radiogram
   Left ventricular and left atrial dilatation
ECHOCARDIOGRAM
   Left ventricular and left atrial dilatation
   Mitral valve thickening and/or calcification if rheumatic
   Possible left ventricular aneurysm and/or ↓ left ventricular wall motion
      if coronary artery disease

of the mitral apparatus: the left atrium, the annulus, the valve, the chordae tendineae, the papillary muscles, or the left ventricular wall.[2] The length of time mitral regurgitation has been present is also important. In this discussion, we will consider only chronic mitral regurgitation since acute mitral regurgitation imposes such severe hemodynamic impairment that elective, noncardiac surgery is precluded by its mere presence.

Left atrial dilatation, though it may beget further mitral regurgitation, is not a primary cause of mitral insufficiency. Mitral annular fibrosis and calcification may result in significant, chronic mitral regurgitation—this particular lesion is most frequent in elderly females. Valvular lesions such as those resulting from rheumatic carditis or bacterial endocarditis, may produce severe mitral regurgitation. Rupture of the chordae tendineae results in acute mitral regurgitation or, if chronic, the regurgitation is severe. Papillary muscle dysfunction and left ventricular wall disease are generally due to coronary artery disease with its resultant myocardial ischemia and/or infarction.[2]

The symptoms of chronic mitral regurgitation are those of heart failure with or without palpitations due to atrial tachyarrhythmias. Interestingly, the degree of mitral regurgitation may be quite severe without marked symptomatology. The left atrium simply enlarges in response to the regurgitant volume so that the increased capacity accepts the increased volume without an elevation in left atrial, and hence pulmonary capillary wedge pressure. Similarly, the left ventricle may dilate appreciably, yet continue to eject a reasonable stroke volume with even lesser contractile motion.

If severe, chronic mitral regurgitation will nearly always be associated with atrial fibrillation. Even if sinus rhythm is maintained, an S_4 gallop is unlikely, because the left atrium is dilated, and presumably contracts weakly. Left ventricular enlargement, an S_3 gallop, and a prominent, long systolic apical murmur are all expected.

The electrocardiogram will demonstrate either atrial fibrillation or evidence of left atrial abnormalities; left ventricular hypertrophy is also expected.

The chest radiogram will confirm dilatation of both the left atrium and the left ventricle; pulmonary venous distention and pulmonary congestion are likely.

The echocardiogram will confirm dilatation of both left-sided chambers; mitral valve thickening and doming of the anterior leaflets will be seen if rheumatic fever is the etiology of the regurgitation. On the other hand, prolapse of the mitral valve on the echocardiogram confirms this to be the etiology. Mitral annular calcification can be demonstrated as a dense mass beneath the mitral leaflets in other cases. Hence, the echocardiogram confirms not only the hemodynamics of mitral regurgitation but also suggests the specific anatomic structure responsible for the insufficiency.[3]

The simple diagnosis of mitral insufficiency does not adequately determine the patient's surgical risk. Not only must the physician carefully assess the hemodynamic significance of the regurgitation, but he must also be aware of the specific etiology; for example, coronary artery disease with myocardial ischemia would add an additional surgical risk factor over and above the degree of mitral insufficiency.

Aortic Stenosis

Contrast a patient with mitral stenosis to a patient with aortic stenosis. Though relatively asymptomatic, the patient may harbor

AORTIC STENOSIS

HISTORY
    Angina
    Syncope
    Exertional dyspnea

PHYSICAL EXAMINATION
    Systolic ejection murmur
    Absent A2 (paradoxical split)
    Left ventricular hypertrophy
    Weak, delayed carotid pulses

ELECTROCARDIOGRAM
    Left ventricular hypertrophy

RADIOGRAM
    Left ventricular hypertrophy
    Ca^{++}
    Post-stenotic dilatation

ECHOCARDIOGRAM
    Two dimensional: restricted
    opening of thickened leaflets

critical stenosis. Though the physician anticipates eliciting a history of angina, syncope, or exertional dyspnea from his patient with significant aortic stenosis, the patient may be asymptomatic, particularly when elderly and relatively inactive. Incidentally, this is the same patient who commonly presents a systolic ejection murmur at the base of the heart during preoperative evaluation.

Careful analysis of this murmur generally suffices to determine its significance. If it is long, peaks late in systole, and radiates into the carotids, then it is likely to represent significant aortic stenosis. Other findings are of critical importance; principally, the delay in upstroke of the carotid pulse distal to the obstruction, and the evidence of left ventricular hypertrophy proximal to the obstruction. Indeed, the careful palpation of the carotid pulse is *the* most important part of the preoperative clinical assessment of the *asymptomatic* patient—for the physician cannot afford to overlook critical aortic stenosis.

The electrocardiogram demonstrates left ventricular hypertrophy, though the voltage may not be impressive. The chest radiogram generally shows evidence of left ventricular hypertrophy and, in addition, poststenotic dilatation of the ascending aorta and calcium in the aortic valve may also be evident.

Finally, when it is difficult to be certain of the degree of stenosis, the two-dimensional echocardiogram is quite helpful.[4] Figure 3A illustrates the record of a young patient with a systolic ejection murmur in whom the leaflets of the aortic valve can be seen to open widely during systole, thus excluding significant aortic stenosis. In contrast, the two-dimensional echocardiogram recorded from an elderly patient with a similar murmur is shown in Figure 3B. In this recording, the aortic leaflets do not separate widely, but are markedly restricted in their opening dimensions, indicating quite significant aortic stenosis, and thereby providing a good reason not to proceed with purely elective surgery without better characterization of the degree of stenosis.

In summary, when a murmur of aortic stenosis is heard by physical examination, careful palpation of the carotid pulse is extraordinarily important in determining the significance of the lesion. The electrocardiogram is quite helpful as a noninvasive test, since the absence of left ventricular hypertrophy almost excludes significant aortic stenosis. Also, in the elderly patient, the absence of calcification in the vicinity of the aortic valve, and the absence of post-stenotic dilatation on the chest radiogram argue strongly against significant obstruction. In this case, the two-dimensional echocardiogram might be diagnostic.

The reason for concern is that the patient with critical aortic stenosis is at a very high risk for the development of a potentially lethal ventricular arrhythmia when subjected to general anesthesia or sudden changes in blood volume. Should such an arrhythmia develop, it is notoriously difficult to convert or to control. Resuscitation also is quite difficult in a patient with critical aortic stenosis. Consequently, if critical aortic stenosis is suspected, cardiac catheterization is probably indicated, and elective surgery should be deferred for this more definitive evaluation.

Idiopathic Hypertrophic Subaortic Stenosis

The same sort of considerations that apply to the patient with valvular aortic stenosis also apply to the patient with idiopathic hypertrophic subaortic stenosis, i.e., IHSS.

Again, one can generally determine the degree of obstruction noninvasively, though not by history, since the patient may de-

IDIOPATHIC HYPERTROPHIC SUBAORTIC STENOSIS

HISTORY	ELECTROCARDIOGRAM
Angina	Q waves
Syncope or presyncope	Left ventricular hypertrophy
Exertional dyspnea	ECHOCARDIOGRAM
PHYSICAL EXAMINATION	Asymmetric septal hypertrophy
Paradoxical split of S2	Systolic anterior motion
Thrill	Early closure of aortic valve
Bisferiens pulse	

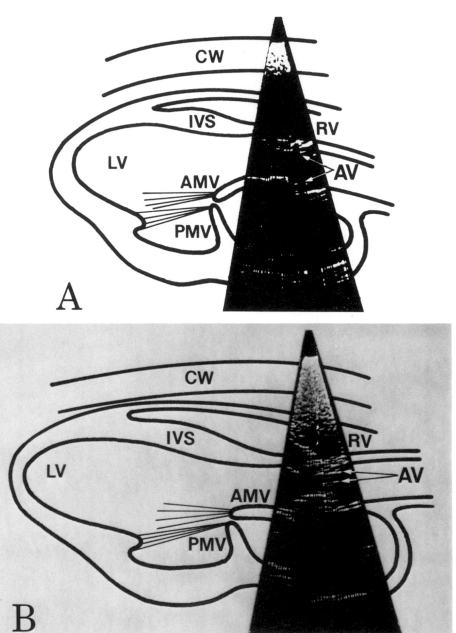

Figure 3. Cross-sectional echocardiogram of patients with systolic ejection murmurs. (A) The aortic leaflets are seen to separate widely in systole, excluding significant aortic stenosis. (B) The maximal separation of the aortic leaflets is markedly reduced, suggesting severe aortic stenosis.

scribe the same symptoms as with aortic stenosis, or he may be asymptomatic despite tight obstruction. In IHSS, the physical findings are important: a paradoxical split of the second heart sound, a palpable thrill, or a bisferiens pulse each indicates significant obstruction, with a gradient across the outflow tract generally exceeding 70 mmHg. The electrocardiogram may show pathological Q waves, and will virtually always be abnormal, with evidence of left ventricular hypertrophy when the obstruction is significant. If the electrocardiogram is quite normal, significant obstruction can virtually be eliminated from consideration. The radiogram is not so helpful in IHSS. The echocardiogram is helpful in that the M-mode record may show asymmetrical septal hypertrophy (ASH), systolic anterior motion (SAM) of the mitral valve, or early closure of the aortic valve (Figure 4). Each of these findings indicate obstruction.

The patient with IHSS represents a significant risk at surgery. Principally, the risks are three-fold: stimulation of the sympathetic nervous system by the anesthetic agent; reduction in blood volume which, by reducing the size of the left ventricle, accentuates the obstruction and virtually pulls the mitral valve into the aortic outflow tract by the Venturi effect; and tachycardia which, presumably, by augmenting the contractile state and reducing left ventricular volume, accomplishes the same as a reduction in blood volume.

With either valvular aortic stenosis or subvalvular obstruction, elective surgery should be avoided if possible. The valvular lesion can be corrected preoperatively if it is determined to be significant. The obstruction of IHSS may be controlled with high dose beta blockade or calcium antagonists preoperatively and during the operative intervention.

Aortic Regurgitation

The operative risk of a patient with aortic regurgitation is not substantially increased, as long as he is asymptomatic. On the other hand, if the individual describes symptoms of left ventricular failure, the risk is appreciable. Angina pectoris may occur, even in the absence of coronary artery disease, but almost always is associated with left ventricular failure.

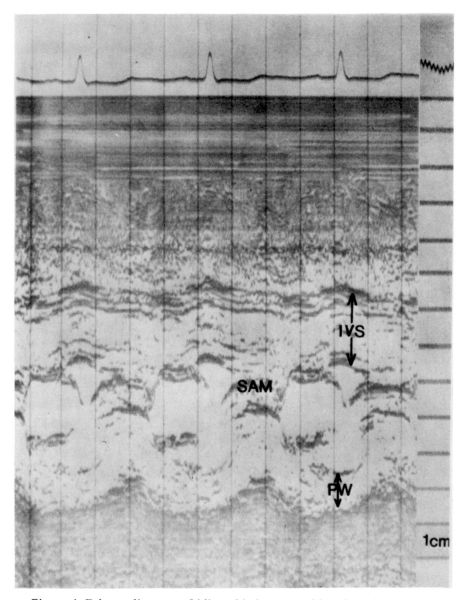

Figure 4. Echocardiogram of idiopathic hypertrophic subaortic stenosis. The interventricular septum (IVS) is asymmetrically hypertrophied with respect to the posterior wall (PW). The mitral valve demonstrates systolic anterior motion (SAM).

AORTIC REGURGITATION

HISTORY
    Dyspnea, edema
    Angina
PHYSICAL EXAMINATION
    High frequency diastolic
      decrescendo murmur of long
      duration
    Third heart sound
    Hyperdynamic peripheral pulses

ELECTROCARDIOGRAM
    Left ventricular hypertrophy
RADIOGRAM
    Cardiomegaly
    Pulmonary congestion
ECHOCARDIOGRAM
    Fluttering anterior mitral
      valve leaflet
    Left ventricle
    Dynamic wall motion

Physical examination is helpful in determining the severity of the lesion. Peripheral pulse pressure is one of the best ways of determining the hemodynamic significance of aortic regurgitation, though pulse pressure may diminish as heart failure intervenes. A high frequency, diastolic, decrescendo murmur, generally of maximum intensity along the left sternal border, is characteristic. When the murmur is best heard along the right sternal border, disease of the aortic root rather than valvular disease is to be expected. The duration of the murmur correlates better with the severity of the regurgitation than its intensity. The longer the murmur, the more significant the lesion. A third heart sound gallop is to be expected with severe aortic regurgitation.

With severe, chronic aortic regurgitation, the electrocardiogram will virtually always show evidence of left ventricular hypertrophy, with increased QRS voltage, ST segment depression, and T wave inversion in the leads reflecting the electrical activity over the anterolateral left ventricle. Atrial fibrillation is a poor prognostic sign in the absence of mitral valve involvement.

The chest radiogram will almost always show substantial cardiomegaly if the aortic regurgitation is severe. Similarly, the echocardiogram will demonstrate dilatation of the left ventricle and dynamic contractile motion, each as the result of a volume overload of the left ventricle. Fine fluttering of the anterior leaflet of the mitral valve or even the interventricular septum are other echocardiographic findings in significant aortic regurgitation.

Thus, as with most other valvular lesions, the symptoms of aortic regurgitation determine the significance of the lesion at the time of noncardiac surgery. An asymptomatic patient is unlikely to decompensate hemodynamically, and hence is at a relatively low risk for surgery. The symptomatic patient with evidence of left ventricular enlargement, heart failure, a long diastolic murmur, an S_3 gallop, or echocardiographic evidence of left ventricular dilatation presents a significant risk.

Cardiac Arrhythmias

A documented or potential rhythm disturbance requires careful evaluation if it: compromises hemodynamics; or increases the risk of sudden cardiac death. Any rhythm disturbance—supraventricular or ventricular—may compromise hemodynamics by reducing the cardiac output, elevating left ventricular filling pressure, or increasing the myocardial requirements for oxygen, thereby eliciting the symptoms of weakness or syncope, dyspnea or angina. On the other hand, only rhythm disturbances of ventricular origin are likely to produce sudden electrical death—either ventricular fibrillation or asystole. Hence, a supraventricular rhythm disturbance is of particular interest when it elicits symptoms; a complex ventricular rhythm disturbance, on the other hand, requires evaluation not only as a result of symptoms, but also because of the threat of sudden death. (Also see Chapter XI).

Let us consider the four basic types of cardiac arrhythmias: the bradycardias and tachycardias, of both supraventricular and ventricular origin. Bradycardia of supraventricular origin, i.e., sinus bradycardia, sinus exit block, sinus arrest, and Type I AV block, are unusual in patients with valvular heart disease. When present, they generally denote a concomitant disease process, such as the "sick sinus syndrome." Slow ventricular responses to atrial fibrillation due to inappropriate AV block may be the result of the administration of excessive digitalis in the patient with mitral valve disease. Simple observation of the ventricular response by discontinuing digitalis, or with moderate exercise will generally suffice to assure adequate AV conduction. If bradycardia is sufficient to elicit symptoms, and does not readily resolve with alterations in pharmacologic management, then at least temporary transvenous pacing is required during the operative precedure.

Infra-His (ventricular) Type II block requires more careful evaluation and possible therapy. If the PR interval is normal, and the patient is asymptomatic, no further evaluation is required. Asymptomatic patients with bifascicular block, such as the combination of right bundle branch block and left anterior hemiblock illustrated in Figure 5 do not require additional evaluation or temporary pacing. On the other end of the spectrum are patients with second or third degree, Mobitz II, Type II, infra-His block (Figure 6). Pacing is clearly mandatory in these patients, not only during the operative procedure, but permanently. Intermediate between these two extremes are patients with: bifascicular block with normal PR interval, but with a history of syncope; or patients with trifascicular block. In such patients, the options would appear to be three-fold:

Exercise the patient on a treadmill. As the heart rate accelerates in response to stress, higher grade block may develop.

Perform an invasive His-bundle electrogram. If the HV interval is abnormally prolonged, or if higher grade block develops in response to atrial pacing, then at least temporary pacing is clearly indicated.

Temporary pacing. Other physicians would recommend temporary pacing during the operative procedure, regardless of a neg-

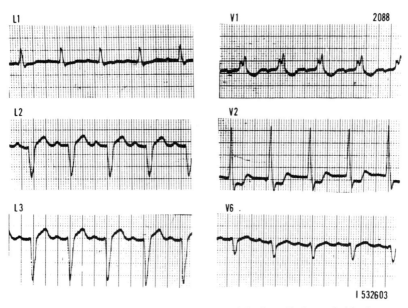

Figure 5. Bilateral bundle branch block. Right bundle branch block, confirmed by the rsr' complex in V_1, with prolonged QRS duration; and left anterior hemiblock, indicated by the marked left axis deviation in leads II and III, indicate bifascicular block.

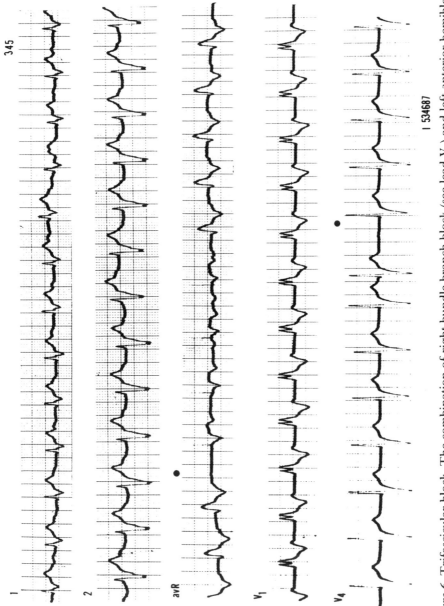

Figure 6. Trifascicular block. The combination of right bundle branch block (see lead V_1) and left anterior hemiblock (see lead II) indicate bifascicular block. In addition, the marked prolongation in the PR interval would suggest either a coexistent conduction defect in the AV node or the remaining, left posterior hemifascicle. In lead aVR, beneath the dot, the p wave fails to conduct. Preceding PR intervals were constant, indicating Mobitz II, infra-His conduction delay. The subsequent four complexes are paced, before conduction resumes. The evidence of bifascicular block plus Mobitz II block indicates trifascicular conduction delay.

ative response to either of the above tests, thus obviating the necessity for these tests.

In the patient with aortic valve disease with bifascicular block and syncope, it is mandatory to determine the cause of syncope—whether exertional (related to the severity of the aortic stenosis) or, instead, transient heart block, due to transient trifascicular block.

All varieties of supraventricular tachyarrhythmias may occur in patients with mitral valve disease, the most common being atrial fibrillation. The control of the ventricular response to atrial fibrillation is most important. Recall that digitalis exerts a vagal and an extra-vagal effect to slow AV conduction. If the patient is inadequately digitalized, the heart rate may be controlled at rest, yet with any moderate exertion, the ventricular rate reaches unacceptable levels as the vagal effects are superseded by the adrenergic effect of exercise. The same consideration applies to the preoperative administration of atropine. By blocking the vagal effect of digitalis, the ventricle may accelerate to reduce diastolic filling time, elevate left atrial pressure, and elicit pulmonary edema. Hence, the degree of digitalization should be carefully assessed preoperatively by demonstrating the extent of vagal effect with an analysis of the ventricular response to moderate exercise.

Ventricular rhythm disturbances are unusual in patients with valvular heart disease. Ventricular arrhythmias may accompany aortic valve disease, but in such instances the lesion is quite severe from a hemodynamic point of view; such patients require careful hemodynamic assessment preoperatively.

In our experience, premature ventricular complexes are usually transiently suppressed by anesthesia, and hence do not pose much of a problem. However, one must consider the specific valvular disease which is associated with the ventricular ectopy to determine its significance. In patients with IHSS, for example, ventricular arrhythmias are probably the cause of sudden cardiac death, independent of the component of obstruction.[5] Full beta blockade preoperatively and intraoperatively seems essential. When patients with mitral valve prolapse present complex ventricular arrhythmias, such as symptomatic, sustained ventricular tachycardia, then therapeutic blood levels of their proven effective antiarrhythmic agent should be maintained throughout the operative precedure.

Antibiotic Prophylaxis of Infective Endocarditis

Another consideration in the preoperative assessment of patients with valvular heart disease is prophylaxis against infective endocarditis. Every patient with suspected valvular heart disease undergoing a procedure which is expected to introduce an organism into the blood stream should receive antibiotic prophylaxis. This includes patients with valvular heart disease of all etiologies, including rheumatic heart disease, degenerative disease such as aortic stenosis, and congenital heart disease, such as IHSS and mitral valve prolapse. An exception is uncomplicated atrial septal defect, secundum variety, which probably does not require prophylaxis.

Even though a lesion may be hemodynamically insignificant, prophylaxis is still indicated. Indeed, there may be an inverse relationship between the anatomic severity of the valvular lesion and the likelihood of developing infective endocarditis. A densely fibrotic, calcified, and stenotic mitral valve is less likely to become infected than the less scarred, more pliable prolapsed valve. In addition, regurgitant lesions seem more susceptible to endocarditis than stenotic lesions. Although there are no conclusive studies to prove that prophylactic antibiotics prevent endocarditis, it is acceptable medical practice to attempt to do so in patients with valvular heart disease who are likely to become bacteremic during a surgical procedure.

The American Heart Association (AHA) has divided its recommendations for the prophylaxis for bacterial endocarditis into two categories:[6] dental procedures and upper respiratory tract surgery and instrumentation; and gastrointestinal and genitourinary tract surgery and instrumentation. *Streptococcus viridans* (an alpha hemolytic species of streptococcus) is the organism most commonly implicated in bacterial endocarditis following dental procedures. Other bacteria recovered from the blood stream following surgical procedures of the upper respiratory tract, such as tonsillectomy and adenoidectomy or bronchoscopy (especially with a rigid bronchoscope), have similar antibiotic sensitivities to those recovered from dental procedures. The AHA suggests two possible antibiotic regimens for prophylaxis of patients undergoing these procedures, including a more aggressive approach to patients felt to be at extremely high risk (namely those with prosthetic heart valves). Alternative antibiotics are listed for those who are allergic to penicillin (Table 1).

Prophylactic therapy for genitourinary tract or gastrointestinal tract surgery or instrumentation is directed against *Streptococcus fecalis* (the enterococcus). Situations not requiring prophylaxis, as recommended by the AHA, include uncomplicated vaginal delivery, upper G.I. panendoscopy, percutaneous liver biopsy, proctoscopy, sigmoidoscopy, barium enema, pelvic exam, D & C of the uterus, and insertion and removal of pelvic devices. Although sometimes associated with bacteremia, these procedures rarely if ever, have been associated with endocarditis; however, some authors believe that patients with cardiac valve prosthesis should receive prophylaxis even with these procedures. These recommendations are empiric, and are based more upon concern than definitive data (Table 1).

Different recommendations have been offered by Petersdorf,[7] who argues for a briefer duration of treatment (Table 1). Petersdorf cites experimental animal studies in which endocarditis is prevented by a single dose of antibiotics. Consequently, he recommends only three doses following the initial dose rather than the usual eight. Such a regimen may be equally efficacious while reducing cost and increasing patient compliance. In addition, Petersdorf also recommends a combination of penicillin (or ampicillin) plus gentamicin as the regimen of choice for gastrointestinal or genitourinary tract surgery and manipulation, since 40 percent of enterococci are not inhibited *in vitro* by a combination of penicillin and streptomycin.

Anticoagulation

The final step in the preoperative analysis of the patient with valvular heart disease is to question whether or not he is anticoagulated. At this point, we are not interested in the indications for anticoagulation, but rather one's assessment of the patient with mitral stenosis and atrial fibrillation, or the patient with a prosthetic heart valve, for instance, who has required anticoagulation. Anticoagulated patients are obviously at increased risk for excessive

Table 1

Current Recommendations for Prophylaxis of Bacterial Endocarditis

Indications	American Heart Association's Recommendations—1977	Petersdorf's Recommendations—1978
Oral regimen for dental and upper respiratory tract manipulation in *low* risk patients	Penicillin V 2g p.o. followed by penicillin V 500 mg p.o. 1.6.h. for 8 doses postoperatively	Penicillin V 2g p.o. followed by penicillin V 500 mg p.o. 1.6.h. for 3 doses postoperatively Parenteral regimens need not be used in low risk patients
Parenteral regimen for dental and upper respiratory tract manipulation in *low* risk patients	Aqueous penicillin 1,000,000 units with procaine penicillin 600,000 units IM followed by penicillin V 500 mg p.o. 1.6.h. for 8 doses postoperatively	
Parenteral regimen for dental and upper respiratory tract manipulation in *high* risk patients (i.e., prosthetic heart valves)	Aqueous penicillin 1,000,000 units with procaine penicillin 600,000 units, *plus* streptomycin 1 g IM followed by penicillin V 500 mg p.o. q.6.h. for 8 doses postoperatively	Single administration of 1.2 million units of aqueous procaine penicillin *plus* 1 g streptomycin IM
Regimen for surgery or instrumentation of G.I. or G.U. tracts	Aqueous penicillin 2,000,000 units IM or IV or ampicillin 1 g IM or IV *plus* gentamicin 1.5 mg/kg (not to exceed 50 mg) IM or IV or streptomycin 1g IM, followed by gentamicin 1.5 mg/kg (not to exceed 80 mg) IM q.8.h. for 2 additional doses *or* streptomycin 1g IM q.12.h. for 2 additional doses postoperatively	Aqueous penicillin 2,000,000 units IM or IV or ampicillin 1g IM or *plus* gentamicin 1.5 mg/kg IM followed by gentamicin 1.5 mg/kg IM q.8.h. for 2 doses (however, prophylaxis could be completed on same day for single day procedures such as cystoscopy)
Regimen for dental and upper respiratory tract manipulation in patients allergic to penicillin	Erythromycin 1g p.o. followed by erythromycin 500 mg p.o. q.6.h. for 8 doses postoperatively	Erythromycin 1g p.o. followed by erythromycin 500 mg p.o. q.6.h. for 3 doses postoperatively Does not specifically recommend, however, does not argue with AHA's recommendations
Regimen for surgery or instrumentation of G.I. or G.U. tracts in patients allergic to penicillin	Vancomycin 1g IV *plus* Streptomycin 1g IM followed by same dose of each 12 hours	

blood loss at the time of surgery; conversely, an invitation for a thromboembolic episode by discontinuation of the anticoagulant unnecessarily is also undesirable.

Several factors are important in the decision to continue or discontinue anticoagulation—first, the type of surgery to be performed. Procedures such as cardiac catheterization, for example, do not require discontinuation of anticoagulation unless the transseptal technique is employed. In contrast, intra-abdominal surgery, neurologic surgery, and genitourinary surgery do require a reversal of the state of anticoagulation. In such an instance, anticoagulants can generally be discontinued during the perioperative period with minimal risk. With high risk patients, such as those with caged-disc prostheses, reversal of coumadin-like anticoagulation with vitamin K preoperatively may be accompanied by transient anticoagulation with intravenous heparin until the actual operative procedure.[8] As a general rule, coumadin-like agents should be discontinued about 5 days preoperatively in order to reduce the prothrombin time to less than 15 seconds. If necessary, vitamin K may be administered to hasten reversal of the anticoagulation. Aspirin should be discontinued about five to seven days preoperatively so that its antiplatelet aggregating effect is reversed by the time of surgery. A bleeding time (not a platelet count) is the test needed for measuring this function.

Postoperatively, there is no reason to provide large, loading doses of coumadin anticoagulation. These agents act by depressing the hepatic synthesis of clotting factors II, VII, IX, and X. A finite period of time is required for these factors to decrement, depending upon their half-life. A loading dose does not accelerate this depression, but may lead to a bleeding diathesis without the desired intravascular anticoagulated state.

Intraoperative Assessment and Management

Again, the intraoperative assessment of patients with valvular heart disease includes an analysis of hemodynamics and rhythm, but the physician is now also concerned with the agents and techniques of anesthesia.

Hemodynamics

The necessity for monitoring parallels the preoperative assessment of the hemodynamic severity of the lesion. If the lesion is merely of auscultatory interest, no special hemodynamic monitoring is required. If, however, the lesion is assessed to be severe, or heart failure or hypotension are a problem, then monitoring should include at least:

An intra-arterial pressure line for the purpose of continuously measuring blood pressure, and also providing periodic samples for blood gas and other laboratory analysis.

Either central venous pressure, or preferably, a Swan-Ganz catheter positioned in the pulmonary artery to reflect left heart filling pressure.

Optimally, when the Swan-Ganz is provided with a thermister probe, cardiac output can be followed by the thermodilution technique.

Urinary output, by an indwelling catheter.

The status of the patient can then be followed meticulously (Table 2). Hypotension, accompanied by a fall in pulmonary capillary wedge pressure, generally indicates inadequate volume which should respond to volume replacement. Hypoventilation can be recognized by hypercarbia, hopefully prior to the development of hypotension and a depression of cardiac output. Hypoxemia and an elevation in pulmonary capillary wedge pressure reflect heart failure, and require careful management. Depending upon the precise valve lesion present, impedance reduction may provide the key alteration necessary–perhaps supplementing digitalization and diuresis. For instance, if the valve lesion is mitral regurgitation, the

Table 2
Intraoperative Hemodynamics

	BP	pcw	pO_2	pCO_2	Cardiac Output
Hypovolemia	↓	↓	↓	—	↓
Hypoventilation	↓	—	↓	↑	↓
Heart failure	—	↑	↓	—	↓

actual regurgitant fraction can be substantially reduced by reducing afterload or impedance to forward ejection with nitroprusside, as illustrated in Figure 7.

Nitroglycerin, administered as a continuous intravenous infusion, is an ideal agent to reduce pulmonary capillary wedge pressure, and hence, reverse pulmonary edema in almost every situation, both because it dilates the systemic veins to reduce preload, and because it dilates the pulmonary vascularity. This applies to mitral stenosis as well, where even a single sublingual nitroglycerin reduces mean left atrial pressure substantially.

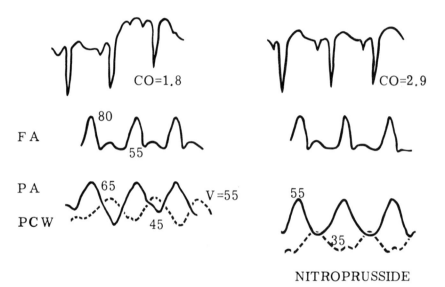

NITROPRUSSIDE

Figure 7. Effect of nitroprusside on mitral regurgitation. In the control (left panel) the elevation in mean pulmonary capillary wedge (PCW) and V wave pressure confirms mitral regurgitation. Pulmonary arterial (PA, continuous line) pressure is also elevated; the femoral arterial (FA) pressure is diminished. With nitroprusside (right panel) the V wave diminishes from 55 to 35 mmHg; but systemic pressure remains unaltered due to the simultaneous increase in cardiac output from 1.8 to 2.9 liters per minute.

Arrhythmias

Of course, the cardiac rhythm must be monitored continuously, and the anesthesiologist should have a monitor which can provide a written recording of the rhythm. Ideally, lead II and a precordial lead, such as V_1, should be recorded, though this is rarely available. V_5 is particularly helpful in assessing ST-T changes as a result of ischemia.

In this discussion, we will be concerned only with the emergency management of the bradycardias and tachycardias, stressing some newer ideas rather than the standard, usually successful approaches. It is of paramount importance to recall the axiom: do not treat a rhythm disturbance unless sustained, recurrent and resulting in hemodynamic deterioration; otherwise, the therapy is probably worse than the disease. Assuming this to be the case, if a bradycardia is manifested by a narrow QRS complex, it is of supraventricular (supra-His) origin, and hence susceptible to atropine. Conversely, if the bradycardia is accompanied by a broad QRS complex, then it may arise in the ventricle (infra-His), and therefore be unresponsive to atropine. In this case, a catecholamine or a pacemaker may be required. (Also see Chapter II)

A supraventricular tachycardia, manifested by a narrow QRS complex, such as an accelerated ventricular response to atrial fibrillation, is common, and difficult to manage. Assuming adequate digitalis has already been provided, the vagal effects of digitalis can be augmented with an agent like edrophonium.[9] By blocking acetylcholinesterase, and hence increasing the concentration of the vagal mediator, acetylcholine, edrophonium can supplement the digitalis effect and at least transiently slow the ventricular response. In Figure 8, the ventricular response to atrial flutter is decelerated from 150 to 75 with this technique.

Postoperatively, recurrent supraventricular tachycardia can best be managed by intra-atrial cardioversion,[10] to obviate the need for repetitive external cardioversion, the latter probably contraindicated by recent surgery. A pacemaker in the right atrium captures the right atrial activity, as seen in panel C, Figure 9, and then converts it to sinus rhythm (panel D).

Should ventricular tachycardia repetitively recur during or immediately following an operation in a patient with aortic valve or other valvular heart disease, the first step is to assure optimal ventilation and volume management; subsequently, lidocaine or procainamide are generally administered. However, should the rhythm prove refractory to these usual maneuvers, then the newer agent, Bretylol, is often quite efficacious.[11] It seems to be particularly valuable when the blood pressure is elevated or quite labile,

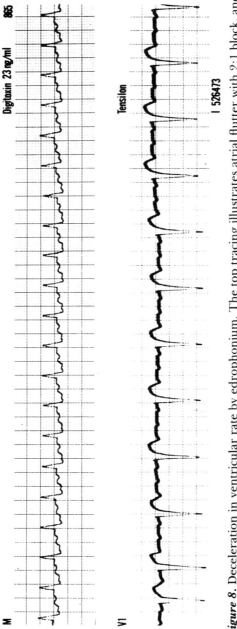
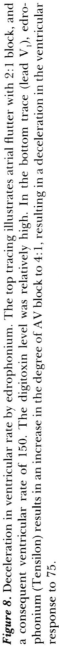

Figure 8. Deceleration in ventricular rate by edrophonium. The top tracing illustrates atrial flutter with 2:1 block, and a consequent ventricular rate of 150. The digitoxin level was relatively high. In the bottom trace (lead V_1), edrophonium (Tensilon) results in an increase in the degree of AV block to 4:1, resulting in a deceleration in the ventricular response to 75.

demonstrating wide swings between hyper- and hypotension. Perhaps these alterations in pressure are a result of fluctuation in sympathetic tone. Figure 10 provides an example of repetitive ventricular tachycardia refractory to a combination of lidocaine and procainamide, yet partially suppressed with the first, and subsequently totally suppressed with the second loading dose of Bretylol. Simultaneously, the fluctuation in systolic blood pressure between 80 and 200 mmHg was also reversed.

Anesthesia

When considering anesthetic agents and techniques, the best advice which the authors can provide is to employ an accomplished anesthesiologist. However, the consulting physician must clearly outline the patient's specific valvular lesion so that the anesthesiologist can properly select his anesthesia. (Also see Chapter II)

Nearly all inhalation anesthetic agents depress the myocardium. Ethrane is probably preferable to Halothane for most patients with valvular heart disease since, in contrast to Halothane, Ethrane does not sensitize the myocardium to catecholamines; hence, it is less likely to induce ventricular tachyarrhythmias. In addition, because of its relatively potent negative inotropic effect, Halothane is contraindicated in patients with significant left ventricular failure.

A new agent, soon to be released—isoflurane (Forane)—is probably even better. This new agent is less negatively inotropic than most other inhalation agents; in addition, by reducing afterload, cardiac output is often maintained.[12]

Nitrous oxide is a good inhalation agent for patients with valvular heart disease. However, a small but significant depression in contractility results from the inhalation of as little as 40 percent nitrous oxide.[13] With higher inspired concentrations, significant myocardial depression and hypotension result.

Morphine may be used effectively as a primary anesthetic agent and is excellent for patients with mitral valve disease, in whom essentially no change in hemodynamics is recorded. In one study of patients with aortic valve disease undergoing aortic valve replacement, primary anesthesia with morphine actually resulted in an increase in cardiac output and no evidence of significant myo-

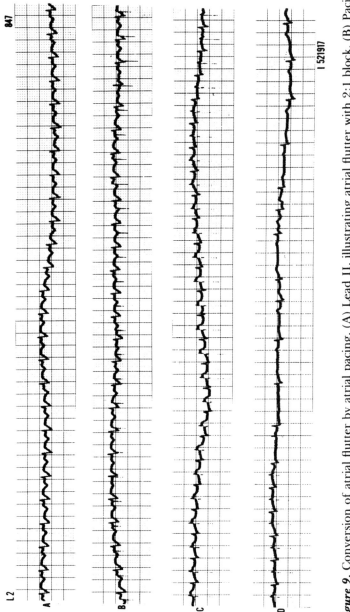

Figure 9. Conversion of atrial flutter by atrial pacing. (A) Lead II, illustrating atrial flutter with 2:1 block. (B) Pacing artifacts are identified, yet do not capture the atrium. (C) The pacing artifacts now capture the atrium, with a p wave following each pacing artifact, and the heart rate is thus controlled by the pacemaker. (D) As the pacemaker is decelerated and discontinued, sinus rhythm resumes.

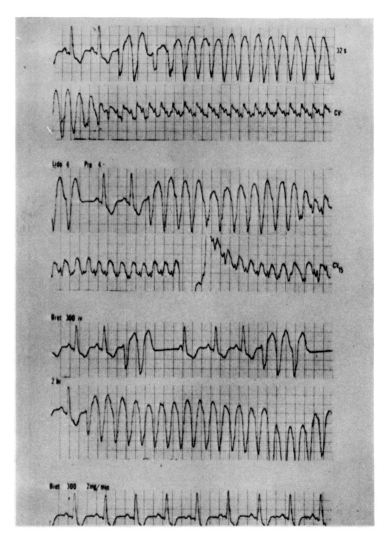

Figure 10. Bretylium Therapy. Ventricular tachycardia recurs repetitively, requiring 35 countershocks over several hours. In the top two tracings (from which 32 seconds is excluded), ventricular tachycardia requires cardioversion. In the second two tracings, ventricular tachycardia recurs despite an appropriate loading dose of both Lidocaine and Procainamide, with a continuous infusion of each at 4 mg/min. In the 5th trace, pairs and triplets of premature ventricular complexes follow the first loading dose of Bretylium, but at 2 hours, ventricular tachycardia recurs. In the final tracing, normal sinus rhythm is maintained after a second loading dose of Bretylium with a continuous infusion of 2 mg/min.

cardial depression. In doses of 1.0 mg/kg, morphine has been demonstrated to increase cardiac index and stroke index, and to diminish total peripheral resistance and myocardial oxygen consumption.[14]

Ketamine is a nonbarbiturate, analeptic, intravenous agent which stimulates the cardiovascular system—i.e., it induces moderate tachycardia and hypertension, and hence increases the myocardial consumption of oxygen.[15] Though this agent may be undesirable for patients with coronary artery disease, it is an excellent agent for the induction of anesthesia in patients with significant left ventricular dysfunction or hypertension consequent to valvular heart disease.

Scopolamine is an excellent preoperative agent for induction, inducing less tachycardia than atropine. It is also an excellent agent to provide amnesia during the operative procedure.

The combination of droperidol and fentanyl (Innovar) probably has little effect on cardiac contractility and has been increasingly employed for patients with impaired myocardial function[16]; the inability to lighten the degree of anesthesia quickly is a potential disadvantage of this combination.

Actually, the sole use of an intravenous agent is unusual in clinical anesthesia practice today. Rather, these agents are often used in combination with other drugs, such as the inhalation agents or neuromuscular blockers.

Metubine may be preferable to Pavulon as a muscle relaxant in patients with valvular heart disease since it has little if any cardiovascular effect. Either of these agents, however, are of considerable utility in patients with valvular heart disease.

Regional anesthesia is a possibility for patients being considered for operations. The use of local or nerve block anesthesia is satisfactory, provided exceedingly large doses of the anesthetic agent are not used. Remember that local anesthetics are absorbed systemically, and as such, may depress myocardial contractility. Epidural anesthesia requires more time than spinal anesthesia for effect; this added time may actually be an advantage to the anesthesiologist for correcting or preventing any hypotension that could result from either technique as a result of sympathetic blockade.

To repeat, the well trained, expert anesthesiologist must be aware of the precise anatomy and hemodynamic effects of the valvular lesions.[17] An agent which is desirable for one patient could be disastrous for a patient with a different valvular lesion. Several ideas must be kept in mind. For instance, in patients with aortic stenosis, significant hypotension must be avoided at all costs. Sustained tachycardias are poorly tolerated and require urgent therapy. In patients with mitral stenosis, the ventricular response to atrial fibrillation may be greatly accelerated with atropine, but also with Ketamine or Pavulon, both of which increase the rate of conduction through the AV node. Finally, the regurgitant lesions, either aortic or mitral, seem to tolerate the insult of surgery and anesthesia much better than stenotic lesions.

It is the role of the consulting physician to inform the anesthesiologist of the specific pathology, so that the anesthesiologist can more intelligently select the ideal anesthetic agent from his armamentarium.

Conclusion

In summary, the preoperative assessment of the patient with valvular heart disease requires nothing more than a careful clinical analysis of the hemodynamics, the cardiac rhythm, infectious endocarditis prophylaxis, and a consideration of the state of anticoagulation. The cardiologist is particularly interested in excluding valvular or subvalvular aortic stenosis.

During the operation, one must be prepared to follow the hemodynamics and rhythm. Remember the potential benefits of preload and afterload reduction, for instance, in the form of nitroprusside or nitroglycerin in patients with valvular heart disease. In addition, the usual therapy for cardiac rhythms may require some supplementation during or immediately following the operative procedure (such as with edrophonium or intra-atrial pacing, as discussed).

Though this assessment and management often proves challenging, it is exactly the sort of challenge that makes clinical cardiology interesting, and hopefully beneficial to our patients.

References

1. Martin RP, Rakowski H, Kleiman JH, et al.: Reliability and reproducibility of two dimensional echocardiographic measurement of the stenotic mitral valve orifice area. *Am J Cardiol* 43:560, 1979.

2. Perloff JK, Roberts WC: The mitral apparatus: Functional anatomy of mitral regurgitation. *Circulation* 46:227, 1972.
3. Mintz GS, Kotler MN, Segal BL, et al.: Two dimensional echocardiographic evaluation of patients with mitral insufficiency. *Am J Cardiol* 44:670, 1979.
4. Weyman AE, Feigenbaum H, Hurwitz RA, et al.: Cross-sectional echocardiographic assessment of the severity of aortic stenosis in children. *Circulation* 55:773, 1977.
5. Frank MJ, Abdulla AM, Canedo MI, et al.: Long-term medical management of hypertrophic obstructive cardiomyopathy. *Am J Cardiol* 42:993, 1978.
6. American Heart Association Committee Report: Prevention of bacterial endocarditis. *Circulation* 56:139, 1977.
7. Petersdorf RG: Antimicrobial prophylaxis of bacterial endocarditis. Prudent caution or bacterial overkill? *Am J Med* 65:220, 1978.
8. Katholi RE, Nolan SP, McQuire LB: The management of anticoagulation during noncardiac operations in patients with prosthetic heart valves. A prospective study. *Am Heart J* 96:26, 1978.
9. Frieden J, Cooper JA, Grossman JI: Continuous infusion of edrophonium (Tensilon) in treating supraventricular arrhythmias. *Am J Cardiol* 27:294, 1971.
10. Zipes DP: The contribution of artificial pacemaking to understanding the pathogenesis of arrhythmias. *Am J Cardiol* 28:211, 1971.
11. Koch-Weser J: Bretylium. *N Engl J Med* 300:473, 1979.
12. Stevens WC, Cromwell TH, Halsey MH, et al.: Cardiovascular effects of a new inhalation anesthetic, Forane, in human volunteers at constant arterial carbon dioxide tension. *Anesthesiology* 35:8, 1971.
13. Eisele JH, Smith NT: Cardiovascular effects of 40 percent nitrous oxide in man. *Anesth Analg* 51:956, 1972.
14. Lowenstein E, Hallowell P, Levine FL, et al.: Cardiovascular responses to large doses of intravenous morphine in man. *N Engl J Med* 281:1389, 1969.
15. Tweed WA, Minauck M, Mymin D: Circulatory responses to Ketamine anesthesia. *Anesthesiology* 37:613, 1972.
16. Graves CL, Downs NH, Browne AB: Cardiovascular effects of minimal analgesic quantities of Innovar, fentanyl and droperidol, in man. *Anesth Analg* 54:15, 1975.
17. Kaplan JA (Ed.): *Cardiac Anesthesia.* New York, Grune & Stratton, 1979.

CHAPTER XV

Hypertension*

Ronald L. Katz, M.D.
and Leah E. Katz, C.R.N.A., M.A.

This review will interpret the title in a broad sense; that is, discuss drugs which are given for their cardiovascular effects and, also, discuss drugs which may produce untoward cardiovascular effects in patients undergoing elective surgery even though the primary purpose for receiving the drug may have been for other than its cardiovascular effects. One of the most important points to be made in this review is that not only should the cardiovascular effects of the drugs discussed be considered, but equally important, if not more important, is the underlying disease which is responsible for the patient receiving the drug. Proper appreciation of this point might have prevented many of the misconceptions and erroneous conclusions drawn in the past. Therefore, we will review the historical background of the problem in order to provide better understanding of how misconceptions developed and how proper appreciation of the importance of the patient's condition can lead to rational management of patients without denying them necessary drugs. In order to make the review meaningful, common drugs which patients may be receiving when presenting for operation will be discussed briefly. A review of their pharmacology will be necessarily brief. Although pertinent literature will be cited, much of the information to be presented is based on clinical experience. Our own clinical experience is based on interest in this area over the past twenty years. This personal experience is sup-

*This chapter was modified and adapted with permission from an article published in *Cardiovascular Medicine,* November, 1978.

plemented by discussions with other clinicians who have done a great deal of thinking about these problems and have had much clinical experience.

We will first discuss how common hypertension is in order to put the problem in perspective. Estimates of the frequency of hypertension vary between 10–15% of the population. A commonly quoted figure is that 23,000,000 Americans suffer from hypertension.[1] It is well established that the untreated hypertensive has a 10% greater death rate in the male and an eight-fold greater death rate in the female.[2] Furthermore, the frequency of myocardial infarction and angina is twice as great in the hypertensive as in the normotensive.[3] Congestive heart failure is more frequent in the untreated hypertensive and the mortality is higher.[4] It has also been estimated that: half of these hypertensives are not aware of their high blood pressure; only half of those aware of their high blood pressure are under medical care; and half of those under care are not adequately treated and remain hypertensive.[5,6] Although there have been improvements in the numbers of patients under adequate control, there are still large numbers of patients who are inadequately controlled. Finally, of the estimated 23 million Americans with hypertension, up to 10% in any given year will undergo a surgical procedure requiring anesthesia. A discussion of the risks of anesthesia and operation in the uncontrolled hypertensive will also be presented.

Antihypertensive Medications

Reserpine

Reserpine, although initially one of the mainstays of the treatment of hypertension, is no longer used as much as formerly. Its mode of action is by depletion of central and peripheral stores of norepinephrine.[7] Its actions are complex and include inhibition of norepinephrine uptake by the postganglionic adrenergic nerve terminal. The major effect of reserpine appears to be through depletion of norepinephrine from adrenergic nerve endings. This depletion probably results from an action of reserpine on neuronal vessicles where norepinephrine is stored. As a result, long-term administration of reserpine is associated with a decrease in sym-

Table 1
Antihypertensives and Side Effects

Drug	Adverse Effects
Reserpine	depression, lethargy, nasal congestion, bradycardia, parkinsonian rigidity, diarrhea, increasing weight
Propranolol	bronchoconstriction, cardiac failure, bradycardia, depression, lassitude, insomnia, Raynaud's phenomenon, nausea, vomiting, myocardial ischemia, angina, infarction on abrupt withdrawal
Clonidine	bradycardia, cardiac failure, hypertensive crisis on abrupt withdrawal, drowsiness, depression
Hydralazine	reflex tachycardia, angina, lupus erythematosis-like reaction, headache, palpitations, fluid retention
Diuretics	hypokalemia, hypovolemia, hyperglycemia, hyperuracemia, hypercalcemia, anemia, necrotizing vasculitis
Methyldopa	somnolence, depression, hemolytic anemia, drug fever, positive Coombs test leading to blood crossmatching difficulty, liver damage, postural hypotension
Guanethidine	morning hypotension, exercise hypotension, bradycardia, weakness, diarrhea, nasal congestion

pathetic activity leading to a reduction of cardiac output and peripheral resistance. Whether this effect is primarily central, peripheral, or a combination of the two is still a subject of debate. Some of the adverse side effects are central nervous system sedation and depressive reactions. Nasal congestion, flushing, and gastrointestinal side effects are also common. Rarely, seizure activity and extrapyramidal disturbances have been observed following the use of large doses.

Historically, the problem of patients on cardiovascular drugs was most prominently discussed in the middle 1950s. It was suggested in 1955 that patients receiving reserpine or Rauwolfia alkaloids tolerated anesthesia and operation poorly and that these patients should not be operated upon except in emergencies.[8] The main problem was said to have been hypotension during anesthesia which responded poorly or not at all to the intravenous injection of vasopressors. While the initial paper in 1955 dealt with patients receiving Rauwolfia alkaloids and undergoing electroconvulsive therapy, it was suggested in 1956 that the problem extended to all patients undergoing anesthesia, who were on Rauwolfia therapy, and that in all patients on reserpine, elective surgery should not be undertaken, and that the reserpine should be discontinued for two weeks prior to surgery.[9,10] These views were widely accepted and taught as gospel in the late 1950s. Interestingly, this two-week period, which is reasonable for reserpine, based on its pharmacology, seems to have assumed magical properties so that even today this two-week figure is recommended for stopping other antihypertensive medication and is commonly recommended in spite of pharmacological evidence to the contrary. In fact, distinguished professors at distinguished universities still perpetuate this misconception.[11,12] It is clear that with most other antihypertensive drugs the half life of the drug and its duration of action is such that the drug effects are dissipated within a matter of hours to a few days, depending upon which drug one is considering, and that the two-week abstinence period is irrational. This continuing use of the two-week period will be discussed later in the paper.

Although aware of the reported difficulties, from 1955 through 1961, one of us (RLK) did not observe unusual problems in the management of patients on Rauwolfia alkaloids and gradually came to believe that treatment of these patients with these agents was not a contraindication to elective anesthesia and operation. In 1961, an article was published[13] which, based on an experience with 48 reserpine patients reported that: small amounts of anesthetic agent were sufficient to maintain anesthesia throughout the entire procedure; in 70% of the patients, it was necessary to use a vasopressor at least during part of the operation; it was necessary to omit opiates as premedicant drugs; the use of spinal anesthesia was not recommended, except for specific indications; ether and halothane were not recommended; succinylcholine chloride was adequate for relaxation; however, the use of long-acting curarizing agents was not advised; anesthesia and operation should not be performed on patients taking Rauwolfia medications, except in emergencies. This paper was widely publicized. As a result, many of our colleagues who had been sending us surgical patients on Rauwolfia alkaloids now, instead, began to hospitalize the patients, withdraw the reserpine, and present the patients for operation two weeks after the reserpine was discontinued. In some cases, the patient remained at home during the two-week withdrawal period.

Frequently, the realization that the patient was on reserpine did not occur until after the patient had been admitted to the hospital and it was then necessary to delay the operation and decide whether the patient should remain at home or in the hospital for the two-week period. This delay played havoc with the operating schedule as well as with the use of hospital beds, and was expensive for the patient or his hospital insurance carrier. In addition, it was our clinical impression that we were encountering more, rather than fewer, clinical difficulties in these patients. As a result, we decided to carefully review our past experience with patients on Rauwolfia therapy with special attention directed to the seven points listed above. Our results differed from those of others[8–13] and were at variance with all of the conclusion listed above. We, therefore, undertook a prospective study in late 1961 and continued it through December, 1962. We studied 100 patients on Rauwolfia therapy for hypertension. The duration of therapy varied from six months to six years. These patients received for preanesthetic medication a barbiturate and/or a narcotic and a belladonna alkaloid. The anesthetic agents were selected on the basis of clinical indications and included a wide variety of agents: halothane, cyclopropane, methoxyflurane, diethyl ether, trichlorethylene, halopropane, ethylene and nitrous oxide supplemented by other agents. Long-acting nondepolarizing agents were employed and regional anesthesia was employed where indicated. These 100 patients on reserpine therapy were compared to a randomly selected group of known hypertensive patients operated on during the same time period. However, these latter patients were either not treated or, in eleven patients, were treated with drugs other than Rauwolfia, i.e., barbiturates in seven patients, and chlorothiazide in four. We observed that the patients on Rauwolfia presented no special problems and that, in fact, the hypertensives treated with Rauwolfia had fewer hypotensive episodes than hypertensive patients not treated with Rauwolfia. We, therefore, concluded that patients on Rauwolfia tolerated anesthesia and operation satisfactorily and at least as well as hypertensive patients not treated with Rauwolfia. We also concluded that elective surgery could be safely undertaken without discontinuing Rauwolfia therapy. The most reasonable explanation for these results was that the treated hypertensive patient presented a better risk than the untreated hypertensive patient. Although there was difficulty in publishing the paper because it was contrary to current opinion, the paper was ultimately published.[14] Since then, other investigators reported results similar to ours.[15,16] It is fair to say that in the anesthetic community today it is commonly accepted that patients on Rauwolfia need not have their therapy discontinued prior to operation. Although the problem rarely comes up, in part because of the decreased use of reserpine in the treatment of hypertension, we still periodically receive comments from internists or surgeons that a patient was on reserpine and that the reserpine was discontinued two weeks prior to the date of proposed operation.

Propranolol

Propranolol[17-19] is a beta adrenergic blocking drug which is commonly used in the treatment of angina pectoris, sinus tachycardia, cardiac arrhythmias, and obstructive cardiomyopathy. It is also used in the treatment of hypertension. While there is some debate on the issue, it appears that the major mechanism of action of this drug is its ability to block beta adrenergic receptors. The one exception to this general statement involves its use in the treatment of hypertension, where its antirenin effect seems to be the mechanism responsible for its effectiveness.

Propranolol antagonizes the beta adrenergic effects of catecholamines, whether released by sympathetic nerve stimulation, released from the adrenal, or from exogenous sources. It produces a negative chronotropic effect (decrease in heart rate), and a negative inotropic effect (decrease in myocardial contractility); effects which may explain its value in the treatment of sinus tachycardia, arrhythmias, and obstructive cardiomyopathy. The decrease in work of the heart due to the negative chronotropic and inotropic effects appears to account for its effectiveness in the treatment of angina pectoris by improving the supply/demand ratio for oxygen in the heart. Some of the beta adrenergic blocking effects can be deleterious, however. These include bronchoconstriction which occurs in normal subjects and which may in asthmatic patients result in an asthmatic attack. Propranolol may also induce cardiac failure in patients with borderline myocardial function. It has also been suggested that propranolol adds to the myocardial depressant effects of anesthetics and may precipitate failure in these patients.

Propranolol may produce hypoglycemia, which may produce problems in insulin dependent diabetic patients. This hypoglycemia may be masked by propranolol, since many of the warning signs of impending hypoglycemia are due to sympathetic activation. It is important to point out that doses of propranolol may vary markedly, depending upon the condition being treated. For arrhythmias and angina control, doses ranging from 160–320 mg/day usually suffice. The same is true in patients with hypertension who have high plasma renin levels. However, in hypertensive patients in whom plasma renin levels are low, doses of propranolol of 1,000–2,000 mg/day have been used.

Because propranolol is so effective in the treatment of angina, large numbers of patients receive the drug for this condition. In 1972, Viljoen et al.[20] reported difficulty in resuscitating patients who had been treated with propranolol and who developed cardiac failure immediately after coronary bypass operations. These five patients with advanced coronary artery disease received 100–320 mg/day of propranolol to within 24 hours of surgery. Four of the patients died and one had a stormy postoperative course. It was felt that the propranolol was a major factor responsible for the deaths of these patients, and it was recommended that propranolol be discontinued for two weeks in patients scheduled for coronary bypass procedures. When this work was published, the cardiac anesthesia group at Columbia University (which is now the cardiac anesthesia group at UCLA) reviewed its data and could not find similar difficulties in patients receiving propranolol up to the time of coronary bypass surgery. In order to properly review this controversy, two factors should be considered. The first is the pharmacology of propranolol, particularly in terms of its duration of action and second, is what the course of patients continuing on propranolol to the time of surgery is likely to be.

The duration of action of propranolol suggests that discontinuing propranolol for two weeks is inappropriate. It was reported by Shand and Rangno in 1972[21] that the serum half life of this drug was only three to six hours. In an elegant set of studies by Coltart et al.[22,23,24] it was observed that there was no difference in plasma or atrial tissue levels of propranolol in patients on chronic therapy, in whom the drug had been discontinued 24 to 72 hours before surgery compared to control patients who had never received propranolol. Furthermore, the isoproterenol dose-contrac-

Table 2

Evidence in Favor of Continuing Propranolol up to Time of Operation

- Little or no biochemical or pharmacological evidence of lingering effect 24–74 hours after propranolol discontinued[21–26]
- Patients receiving propranolol up to time of operation did not have greater problems than patients in whom it was discontinued prior to operation[24,26–30]
- Problems associated with discontinuing propranolol prior to surgery angiography or for other reasons
    - 2 of 57 had acute myocardial infarction after abrupt cessation of propranolol[31]
    - 3 acute myocardial infarctions and 2 deaths in 8 patients in whom propranolol withdrawn[32]
    - myocardial infarction following propranolol withdrawal[30,33,34,36,37]
    - 4 of 6 patients developed progressive anginal symptoms following withdrawal[35]
    - 6 of 20 patients either died or suffered life-threatening complications after cessation of propranolol. 4 other patients had increasing angina on withdrawal[38]
    - 15 acute coronary events (death, myocardial infarction, acute coronary insufficiency) in 14 patients on cessation of propranolol[39]

tile response curve from atria in patients whose propranolol had been discontinued 24 to 72 hours earlier was similar to that of control atria. In other studies carried out by this group, it was clear that there was neither biochemical nor pharmacological evidence of a lingering effect of propranolol following its discontinuation for 24 to 72 hours. Other studies by Evans and Shand[25] reported a serum half life of propranolol of three to six hours after discontinuation of chronic administration in normal man. Faulkner et al.[26] also showed that propranolol disappears from the plasma and atrium (at a similar rate) within 24–48 hours after discontinuing the propranolol and that the chronotropic and inotropic responses returned to normal within 24 to 48 hours after discontinuing propranolol. Thus, it is clear that, pharmacologically, the effect of propranolol, measured by a variety of techniques, is dissipated within 24 to 48 hours at most.

As to the course of patients receiving propranolol up to the time of surgery, Moran et al.[27] in 1973, and Jones et al.[28] in 1974, reported that with appropriate selection, there was no greater risk when compared with patients who had not received propranolol. Coltart et al.[24] also observed no significant differences in patients who were on propranolol close to the time of surgery as compared with those in whom it was discontinued. Similar results were also reported by Faulkner et al.[26] in 1973. In addition, Caralps et al.[29] reported on a group of patients on propranolol to within 24 hours of operation, and did not observe an increased mortality. Kaplan et al.[30] also reported that patients whose propranolol was discontinued less than 24 hours prior to operation did not have a higher mortality or complication rate than patients in whom propranolol was not received. From all of the above, it is clear that patients on propranolol can successfully be carried through coronary bypass operation without increased mortality.

These data apply to patients undergoing coronary bypass procedures. Does the same hold true for patients on propranolol undergoing other kinds of surgery, in whom coronary blood flow will not be increased postoperatively? In a review of our data on patients maintained on propranolol up to the time of surgery, whose surgery did not involve the heart or coronary blood vessels, (most of whom were on propranolol because of angina), we found that with careful anesthetic management, patients tolerated anesthesia and operation without untoward difficulty. There were no unexplained intraoperative or postoperative problems. As a result of these observations, as well as the observations reported above in patients undergoing bypass surgery, our current recommendation is to review the indications for propranolol in patients scheduled for surgery and, if the propranolol is clearly necessary for the patient, it is continued up until the time of surgery. This policy has been in effect for over six years and we have had no cause to consider modifying it.

Having demonstrated that pharmacologically there is no basis for discontinuing propranolol two weeks prior to surgery and that continuing propranolol up until the time of surgery has not had any deleterious effects, we must now consider the results of discontinuing propranolol. There have been a number of reports that such a course is not only unnecessary, but may in fact be dangerous. In 1972, Mizgala and Meldrum[31] reported that two of fifty-seven patients had an acute myocardial infarction shortly after abrupt cessation of propranolol. At the time, the authors concluded that this was a chance occurrence. However, Mizgala et al.[32] subsequently noted three acute myocardial infarctions with two deaths when propranolol was discontinued in eight patients.

Slome[33] and Nellin[34] independently reported myocardial infarctions following propranolol withdrawal. Alderman et al.[35] reported that four of six patients had progressive anginal symptoms for 2 to 21 days preceding myocardial infarction. Diaz et al.[36,37] also reported myocardial infarction following withdrawal of propranolol.

Miller et al.,[38] in a series of 20 patients, reported six who died or experienced life-threatening complications within 14 days of abrupt cessation of propranolol. Anterior wall myocardial infarction with shock and death occurred in one patient, sudden death in another, ventricular tachycardia requiring DC cardioversion in another, and intermediate coronary syndrome manifested by angina at rest persisting for more than 15 minutes (with incomplete relief with nitroglycerin) in three others. Four other patients in the group of 20 suffered an increase of more than 50% in the number of anginal attacks as well as increased nitroglycerin consumption in the two-week period after abrupt withdrawal of propranolol, as compared with the two-week period prior to its withdrawal. Thus, 50% of the 20 patients suffered serious adverse effects following withdrawal of propranolol. Mizgala and Counsell[39] similarly reported disastrous results following abrupt cessation of propranolol therapy. Fifteen acute coronary events occurred in 14 patients who had been receiving 80–400 mg of propranolol for seven days to six years. The propranolol had been stopped anywhere from one to fourteen days before the acute event. Cessation of propranolol was followed by rapid progression of symptoms in 11 of the 15 acute events. There were six acute transmural myocardial infarctions resulting in death in three patients, three intramural myocardial infarctions, and six episodes of acute coronary insufficiency. The mean dose of propranolol was 220 mg, (range of 80–400 mg), and the mean duration of therapy was 11 months (range of seven days to three years). In seven of the patients, the propranolol was stopped because of angiographic studies and in one because of elective surgery. Kaplan et al.[30] also reported complications in patients in whom propranolol was discontinued while awaiting operation. Five such patients developed preoperative myocardial infarctions within 48 hours of discontinuing the drug. Two of these patients died.

The mechanism of occurrence of the acute coronary syndromes following acute propranolol withdrawal is not known. It has been speculated that propranolol favorably affects the balance between myocardial oxygen supply and demand, and that its sudden withdrawal may result in myocardial ischemia and necrosis. Miller et al.[38] speculated on the mechanism of exacerbation of symptoms. They felt that because propranolol improved angina-limited exercise in patients with coronary artery disease, the continued increased exercise after discontinuing the propranolol might precipitate or further aggravate imbalances between myocardial oxygen supply and demand. They also suggested as another possibility that, in patients receiving large doses of propranolol, an increase in sympathetic tone becomes unmasked upon cessation of beta adrenergic blockade resulting in an increase in cardiac contractility and heart rate which produces an increased myocardial oxygen requirement, even at rest. Another possible factor is a shift of the oxyhemoglobin dissociation curve. Propranolol produces a favorable displacement of the curve to the right, and sudden withdrawal could produce adverse changes in oxygen affinity for hemoglobin. Another possibility is that propranolol may diminish platelet aggregation and suppress renin secretion, thus producing adverse changes in platelet adhesiveness and activation of the renin angiotensin system upon propranolol withdrawal. Other possible explanations include a denervation hypersensitivity to circulating catecholamines and alterations in ventricular volumes and wall stress which might lead to an increase in myocardial metabolic needs.[40]

Clonidine

Clonidine[42-44] is a relatively new antihypertensive agent which is effective in the treatment of moderate to severe hypertension. The magnitude of response varies markedly among patients, and doses ranging from 0.2 to 2.4 mg/day are required, although the most common range of dose is 0.2 to 0.8 mg/day. Clonidine produces a fall in blood pressure in both the supine and standing position. Its side effects include drowsiness, lethargy, and dryness of the oral mucosa. In general, because of the sedation it produces, it is wise to administer a major portion of the dose at bedtime. The mechanism of action of clonidine is by a central nervous system alpha adrenergic blockage, which results in decreased sympathetic neuronal stimulation of the heart, kidneys, and peripheral vasculature. In addition, clonidine may stimulate presynaptic alpha receptors in the neuron, which can reduce the release of neurotransmitters from the peripheral sympathetic nerves. There is usually a decrease in heart rate and cardiac output; however, the patient's response to exercise is normal. Peripheral vascular resistance usually decreases. The onset of activity usually occurs within 30 to 60 minutes after oral administration, with a maximum effect in 2 to 4 hours. The half life of clonidine is 16 to 40 hours. When the drug is discontinued, the antihypertensive action usually is gone within 24 to 36 hours, but may diminish markedly after 4 to 6 hours in some patients. Clonidine diminishes renin release either by a central nervous system action or an effect on the kidney involving alpha adrenergic receptor inhibition.

The normal course of therapy is to begin the patient on a dose of 0.1 to 0.2 mg/day and increase this dose at weekly intervals by 0.1 to 0.2 mg/day. The agent can be used in combination with other agents, such as vasodilators or beta blockers. When clonidine is used with other drugs, its antihypertensive action is usually additive. If toxicity due to overdose of clonidine occurs, the alpha adrenergic blocking agent tolazoline can be used to reverse the toxicity, since this agent passes the blood–brain barrier and can inhibit the central nervous system effects of clonidine. Because clonidine can potentiate insulin induced hypoglycemia in man, diabetic patients on hypoglycemic agents should be carefully watched for excessive hypoglycemia.

Clonidine in animal studies initially increases and then decreases blood pressure when given intravenously. This may be due to initial stimulation of central nervous system alpha receptors followed by alpha block. Thus, clonidine is a partial agonist as well as antagonist. In addition to the central alpha adrenergic block, clonidine inhibits the release of norepinephrine as well as the cardiac response to postganglionic adrenergic stimulation. However, these peripheral effects cannot account for the acute hypotension clonidine produces. Clonidine also produces a reduction in salivary flow, which results in a dry mouth.

Clonidine abruptly discontinued may produce a dangerous withdrawal syndrome in which blood pressure may sharply increase to levels seen prior to therapy or to greater than pretherapy levels.[45–49] During the withdrawal syndrome, anxiety and nervousness, headache, abdominal pain, nausea, and vomiting may all be present. Elevated blood and urine catecholamine levels are associated with this syndrome and, therefore, indicate increased sympathetic nervous system activity. In a few cases, deaths have been reported. The withdrawal syndrome can be prevented by gradually reducing the clonidine over a period of two to four days. It can also be treated by reinstituting clonidine. The hypertensive crisis usually occurs within 12 to 24 hours. It should be pointed out that although there have been several case reports, we are once again left with a numerator without a denominator in that the case reports of the withdrawal syndrome do not provide information on the number of patients in whom withdrawal did not produce difficulty. The study by Whitsett et al.[50] of 12 patients on clonidine who were abruptly withdrawn suggests that the phenomenon does not occur routinely, since in none of the 12 patients that they studied was the rebound phenomenon seen. However, the patients they studied had only mild to moderate hypertension, rather than severe hypertension, and therapy in their patients was not chronic. Since I have already observed one patient in whom abrupt withdrawal of clonidine led to a severe rebound phenomenon and, since it is still common for some physicians to withdraw antihypertensive medication prior to operation, it is important to be aware of this potential complication, even though its true incidence is not known. Faced with a patient on clonidine presenting for operation, it would be reasonable to either continue the clonidine preoperatively and postoperatively or, if preferred, to substitute other antihypertensive drugs a week or more prior to the operative procedure. Once again, as with reserpine and propranolol, the well controlled hypertensive would appear to be a better operative risk than the patient in whom therapy has been withdrawn.

Hydralazine

Hydralazine[44,51] has been used since the 1950s. It has a direct relaxing action on arterial smooth muscle and produces vasodilation and a decrease in peripheral resistance. Blood flow in skeletal muscle and skin is unaffected, but splanchnic, coronary, cerebral, and renal blood flow increase due to a decrease in vascular resistance. Hydralazine has no direct effects on the heart. Blood pressure is reduced in both the horizontal and standing position. Hydralazine is administered orally and reaches a peak effect in one hour with its half life being approximately four hours, although there is variation among patients. Hydralazine has a predominant effect on arterial smooth muscle with little or no effect on venous smooth muscle. As a result, the venous return to the heart is enhanced secondary to reflex vasoconstriction and an increased preload may be imposed on the heart. When used in doses of less than 300 mg/day hydralazine is an effective drug with minimal risk of side effects. Associated with the fall in blood pressure is a reflex increase in heart rate and cardiac output. The reflex tachycardia may result in angina in patients with underlying coronary disease. Therefore, hydralazine is often combined with propranolol in order to block the reflex increase in heart rate and cardiac output. The decrease in arterial pressure in hypertensive patients during hydralazine therapy is associated with an increase in peripheral plasma renin activity. This effect can be minimized by the simultaneous administration of propranolol. Many experts feel that hydralazine is a useful drug when added to diuretics and propranolol.

Some of the side effects of hydralazine are related either to its direct or reflex mediated hemodynamic effects and include flushing, nasal congestion, dizziness, headache, palpitations, anginal attacks, and myocardial ischemia. The reflexly induced increase in heart rate and cardiac output raises cardiac work and oxygen consumption, but these problems can be prevented or diminished when the patient is treated with a beta adrenergic blocker. When doses of hydralazine greater than 300 mg/day are administered, a lupus erythematosis-like syndrome may be seen. In our experience with hydralazine, this drug has not caused any problems in patients undergoing anesthesia and operation.

Diuretics

Since one-third of hypertensive patients can be controlled by diuretics alone,[52] these agents are often the first ones tried in patients with mild to moderate hypertension. Even if other drugs are necessary, diuretics still are the first line of defense in antihypertensive therapy. The most commonly used diuretics are the thiazides.[44,53] They decrease blood pressure by reducing blood volume and/or through a peripheral vascular effect.

According to Mundy and Raisz,[54] the action of diuretics is largely by direct vasodilation of the arterial bed with a subsequent fall in peripheral vascular resistance. Another factor is a decrease in vascular volume due to sodium diuresis. Thiazides have been shown to cause a decrease in both venous reactivity and arterial resistance. Diuretics are valuable not only in and of themselves, but also because they are able to counteract the sodium retaining effect of other more potent antihypertensive agents. Thus, thiazides are valuable to augment the effects of other antihypertensives.

One of the problems of the diuretics is that they are prone to produce hypokalemia. It is well known that hypokalemia frequently is responsible for cardiac arrhythmias in both anesthetized as well as unanesthetized patients. This problem can be prevented by the addition of potassium supplements to the diet. The major problem we have experienced in patients on diuretics is the hypovolemia often seen in these patients. Their diminished blood volume, which is little or no problem in the awake state, does sometimes present problems in maintenance of blood pressure during anesthesia. The hypotension can usually be treated by the rapid administration of fluid. An alternate approach is to discontinue the diuretics three to seven days prior to operation. This usually does not result in a loss of control of blood pressure, but does appear to result in recovery of blood volume to satisfactory levels.

Methyldopa (Aldomet)

Methyldopa or alpha methyldopa is an extremely effective antihypertensive agent.[18,44,53] Its mode of action has been the subject of much confusion. Originally, it was thought that methyldopa worked by interfering with norepinephrine synthesis through the inhibition of the decarboxylation of dopamine. While this effect occurs, it is probably not the major mechanism of action. It was also thought that methyldopa worked by the production of a false transmitter, alpha methylnorepinephrine, which competed with norepinephrine for adrenergic receptors. While alpha methylnorepinephrine undoubtedly is produced, the false transmitter does not seem to be the major mechanism of action of methyldopa. The current theory is that methyldopa has an effect on autonomic nervous system function in the central nervous system similar to that of clonidine. Possibly as a result of the accumulation of alpha methylated amines, the sympathetic outflow from the central nervous system is diminished, leading to a decrease in blood pressure due to a fall in pulse rate, cardiac output, and peripheral resistance. The decrease in vascular resistance appears to be the most important effect. The effects of methyldopa are potentiated by thiazide diuretics.

Some of the side effects of methyldopa include lassitude, somnolence, and postural hypotension. Other major toxic effects include hepatitis, which is rare, drug fever (which is seen in approximately 1% of patients), and the development of a positive Coombs' test in approximately 10–30% of the patients. This makes crossmatching of blood difficult. However, an autoimmune hemolytic anemia is rarely seen in patients who develop a positive Coombs' test.

There have been no special problems observed intraoperatively or postoperatively in patients on methyldopa.

Guanethidine

Guanethidine[18,53] is a potent antihypertensive agent which acts at the postganglionic adrenergic neuron. By inhibiting depolarization of the terminal end of the neuron, norepinephrine is not released. This results in a decreased peripheral sympathetic outflow. Furthermore, norepinephrine in the intraneuronal storage granule is partially released by guanethidine and the reuptake of the neurotransmitter, norepinephrine, is blocked. As a result, guanethidine produces a diminished tissue level of norepinephrine.

It has been observed that inhibition of responses to adrenergic nerve activity develops rapidly and prior to detectable changes in tissue catecholamine stores which subsequently decline slowly. Therefore, the adrenergic neuron block appears to be more important than depletion of catecholamine stores although the latter may also be a factor in the action of this drug. Guanethidine is taken up and stored in adrenergic nerves. The uptake involves the same mechanism responsible for the nerve membrane transport of norepinephrine and can be inhibited by tricyclic antidepressants and cocaine. Guanethidine accumulates in and displaces norepinephrine from intraneuronal storage granules and is itself released by nerve stimulation. Thus, it could be described as a false transmitter, but this mechanism appears not to be responsible for its major effects. Supersensitivity is also seen with chronic administration of guanethidine. If one understands these mechanisms and the peripheral adrenergic neuronal block produced by guanethidine, it is possible to predict the effects of this agent as well as its side effects which include orthostatic hypotension, diarrhea, and failure of ejaculation.

Oral absorption of guanethidine is unpredictable and varies from 3–40% of the orally administered dose. However, it is relatively constant in a given patient. The dose of guanethidine varies from 35 mg/day to 300 mg/day. The maximum effect occurs in four to five days. The half life of this drug is two to five days. Thus, it is necessary to wait one to two weeks in order to evaluate the effect of changes in dosage. It can, therefore, be seen that this agent is difficult to work with and side effects are annoying. Because the effects of guanethidine are cumulative, adverse effects may persist for days or even weeks after cessation of its administration. Although guanethidine is an effective agent, the problems of its use have led to its being used mainly in patients who do not adequately respond to diuretics, hydralazine, methyldopa, propranolol, or combinations thereof.

There is an important interaction between guanethidine and tricyclic antidepressants which one should be aware of. Tricyclic antidepressants inhibit the neuronal pump for norepinephrine, and since guanethidine gains access to the neuron by means of this pump, the tricyclic antidepressants inhibit the action of guanethidine. If one is unaware of this drug interaction and attempts to overcome it by giving large amounts of guanethidine, and the tricyclic antidepressant is discontinued, a suddenly increased action of guanethidine will occur and may produce severe hypotension. The action of guanethidine is also blocked by amphetamines, which inhibit the uptake of guanethidine at postganglionic nerve endings. In general, it is wise to avoid the concomitant use of tricyclic antidepressants, amphetamines, and guanethidine.

Our experience with patients on guanethidine is such that we continue the patients on therapy up to the time of operation.

Anesthetic Drug Interactions

L-Dopa (Levo-dopa)

Levo-dopa[18,19,55,58] is commonly used in the treatment of Parkinsonism. Its cardiovascular and other actions may produce problems during anesthesia and operation. Levo-dopa produces cardiovascular effects primarily through the production of dopamine since levo-dopa is the precursor of dopamine. Cardiac stimulation is produced by dopamine by direct action on adrenergic receptors and by the release of norepinephrine. Dopamine also produces vasodilation in the renal and mesentery bed by an action on dopaminergic receptors. It also produces vasoconstriction in most other vascular beds by an action on alpha adrenergic receptors. The normal use of levo-dopa in a dose of 1–2 gms usually has little effect on heart rate and blood pressure. However, in the two-hour period following its ingestion, cardiac contractility is increased due to stimulation of beta adrenergic receptors. There is a theoretical danger in that a patient receiving anesthetic agents such as halothane or cyclopropane, which sensitize the myocardium to the arrhythmic effects of catecholamine, might develop ventricular arrhythmias if a dose of levo-dopa had been given within the two hours prior to surgery. A more likely problem with levo-dopa is hypotension, which is frequently seen in patients receiving this agent. Hypotension appears to be due to decreased sympathetic nerve activity, with both central and peripheral mechanisms being proposed. Levo-dopa reduces renin release, which results in a decreased stimulus to the renin-aldosterone system and a decrease in intravascular volume. Another possible cause of hypotension is the replacement of norepinephrine by dopamine at adrenergic storage sites. Dopamine is a weaker pressor agent than norepinephrine. Patients on levo-dopa who have been operated on have been reported to have, on the one hand, hypotension associated with operation and, on the other hand, hypertension associated with operation. We have observed several patients in whom discontinuing the levo-dopa prior to operation resulted in hypotension. The postulated mechanism is that the cardiac stores of dopamine were diminished because of the discontinuation of the levo-dopa. Another potential problem is the recurrence of the patient's symptoms of Parkinsonism if levo-dopa is discontinued,

Table 3
Drug Interactions and Adverse Cardiovascular Effects of Mao
Inhibitors, Tricyclic Anti-depressants and L-dopa

Drug	Interactions
MAO inhibitors	severe hypertension and cardiac arrhythmias when consuming foods containing large amounts of tyramine (wine, beer, some cheeses, herring) cardiovascular depression when using meperidine; also tachycardia and convulsions, hyperpyrexia and coma when used in combination with tricyclic anti-depressants
Tricyclic Antidepressants	profound hypertension, tachycardia, cardiac arrhythmias in the presence of increased levels of endogenous or exogenous catecholamines anticholinergic effects causing tachycardia, dry mouth, urinary retention, constipation hypotension and arrhythmias when using halothane or neostigmine
L-DOPA	antagonism of L-dopa effects by droperidol and chlorpromazine hypotension in association with cardiovascular depressant anesthetics recurrence of parkinsonism on discontinuation with possible aspiration of saliva or gastric contents cardiac arrhythmias if recent dose given and patient anesthetized with cyclopropane or halothane (theoretical risk)

since peak plasma concentrations of levo-dopa occur one to three hours after oral administration and the drug has a half life of about half an hour. The danger associated with recurrence of symptoms is that in the absence of adequate therapy, the patient with Parkinsonism suffers from drooling and dysphagia and, therefore, aspiration may be a problem. We, therefore, believe that patients on levo-dopa should continue on this agent up until the time of surgery, and that the levo-dopa should be restarted as soon as the patient is able to take medication by mouth. It is important to remember that agents such as chlorpromazine and droperidol antagonize the effects of dopamine and may precipitate a Parkinson-like syndrome by inhibiting the action of dopamine.

Monoamine Oxidase (MAO) Inhibitors

Monoamine oxidase inhibitors[18,19,44] have been used in the treatment of hypertension and depression. In 1951, isoniazid and its relative, iproniazid, were developed for the treatment of tuberculosis. It was soon discovered that these agents had mood elevating effects and that iproniazid was capable of inhibiting the enzyme monoamine oxidase. The monoamine oxidase inhibitors were then introduced into psychiatry for the treatment of depression. Some monoamine oxidase inhibitors are still used for the treatment of depression. One of the most common ones is tranylcypromine. Another monoamine oxidase inhibitor used is pargyline, which is used as an antihypertensive agent. Monoamine oxidase is an enzyme located mainly in the mitochondrial fraction of the cell in sympathetic nerves, the brain, liver, and kidney. It is believed that monoamine oxidase plays a major role in the degradation of intracellular biogenic amines including epinephrine, norepinephrine, dopamine, and five hydroxytryptomine. In addition to pargyline, which has an antihypertensive action and is the most commonly used monoamine oxidase inhibitor in the treatment of hypertension, other monoamine oxidase inhibitors have an antihypertensive action. There is much speculation as to the mechanism by which monoamine oxidase inhibitors produce their antihypertensive effect. The monoamine oxidase inhibitors modify the synthesis of catecholamines such that there is an accumulation of dopamine and octopamine, which may function as false transmitters and have lesser physiologic activity than epinephrine and norepinephrine. Whether this accounts for the antihypertensive action is not known. Recent studies of compounds structurally similar to monoamine oxidase inhibitors, which lower blood pressure but do not inhibit monoamine oxidase, suggest that inhibition of monoamine oxidase may not be responsible for the fall in blood pressure.

The decrease in blood pressure induced by monoamine oxidase inhibitors develops slowly, usually requiring three or more weeks. The fall in blood pressure appears to be due mainly to a decrease in peripheral resistance and in cardiac output.

Patients on MAO inhibitors present special problems for the anesthesiologist. Agents such as tryamine, which are found in wine, cheese, pickled herring, and other delicacies, cause the release of catecholamines. Normally, the action of tyramine is limited by its breakdown by monoamine oxidase. However, if the patient has received a monoamine oxidase inhibitor, ingestion of these foods will result in the tyramine contained in these foods releasing large amounts of catecholamines since the tyramine is not broken down by monoamine oxidase. Marked hypertension may occur. Another problem is the interaction between monoamine oxidase inhibitors and analgesics, particularly meperidine. There have been reports of hypertensive crisis in some patients, or hypotension in others. Tachycardia, convulsions, respiratory depression, and hyperpyrexia have also occurred. The mechanism responsible for this is not well established.

The monoamine oxidase inhibitors are not commonly used in the treatment of hypertension, and their use in treating depression is also diminishing. If anesthesia is required in a patient receiving a monoamine oxidase inhibitor, the usual recommendation is to discontinue the monoamine oxidase inhibitor for at least two weeks with the substitution of another antihypertensive agent. Although we have a small number of patients[22] who were anesthetized while receiving monoamine oxidase inhibitors and did not experience difficulty, it would appear reasonable to follow the course of discontinuing monoamine oxidase inhibitors since other excellent drugs are available for the management of the hypertension and because a large number of potential problems do exist in patients on monoamine oxidase inhibitors.

Tricyclic Antidepressants[19,59,60]

As the popularity of the monoamine oxidase inhibitors for the treatment of psychiatric problems decreased, there has been an increase in the use of tricyclic antidepressants. Among the common agents are imipramine, desmethylimipramine, amytriptaline, and doxepine. The action of the tricyclic antidepressants comes on slowly and wears off slowly. Therefore, it is customary to wait two to three weeks before increasing the dose or otherwise changing the therapy. The mechanism by which depression is relieved is not clear, but is probably related to effects on biogenic amines.

The tricyclic antidepressants block the re-uptake of norepinephrine by adrenergic nerve terminals. Since re-uptake of catecholamines is a major mechanism for termination of the action of catecholamines, this inhibition of uptake by tricyclic antidepressants may lead to an enhanced effect of catecholamines, resulting in severe hypertension or cardiac arrhythmias. Disastrous results have been observed in patients on tricyclic antidepressants who received sympathomimetic agents. Severe hypertension, stroke, and cardiac arrhythmias have been seen due to the tricyclic antidepressants inhibiting the re-uptake of the sympathomimetics which, as noted above, is the major mechanism for termination of the action of catecholamines. Thus, both endogenous and exogenous catecholamines may have their actions amplified by tricyclic antidepressants. Another side effect of tricyclic antidepressants is their anticholinergic action which results in dry mouth, constipation, urinary retention, and tachycardia. This anticholinergic action plus the blocking of re-uptake and termination of action of catecholamines both result in sympathetic predominance. Cardiac arrhythmias may be seen following the use of tricyclic antidepressants, particularly if large doses are used. The concurrent administration of tricyclic antidepressants and monoamine oxidase inhibitors has resulted in severe reactions characterized by hyperpyrexia, convulsions, and coma. It is recommended that two weeks or more elapse between discontinuation of monoamine oxidase inhibitors and initiation of tricyclic antidepressant therapy.

Tricyclic antidepressants, by blocking re-uptake of catecholamines from the extracellular synaptic cleft to the intracellular storage area, also produce depletion of catecholamine stores. Tricyclic antidepressants also have a direct action on the heart. Catecholamine levels in the myocardium are reduced and their action on myocardial tissue is blocked. As a result, congestive heart failure, profound hypotension, myocardial infarction, and cardiac arrest have been reported. Arrhythmias resulting in sudden death have also been reported.

Cardiovascular Disease and Hypertension

Up to this point, we have focused on drugs. However, as pointed out earlier in reviewing our 1963 reserpine study, just as important, if not more important than the drugs the patient is receiving, is the basic disease responsible for the patient being on therapy. We will, therefore, now discuss the role of hypertension, per se, and compare the response to anesthesia and operation of untreated hypertensive patients with treated hypertensive patients. In the previous section on reserpine, we suggested that, in terms of intraoperative blood pressure control, hypertensive patients under treatment did better than hypertensive patients not treated. Over the last few years, Prys-Roberts and his associates[61-66] at Oxford, have carried out a number of excellent studies which have clarified the role of hypertension as well as hypertensive therapy. In one study,[61] there were seven normotensive patients, seven untreated hypertensive patients, and fifteen treated hypertensive patients whose cardiovascular responses were compared during anesthesia. In five of the seven untreated patients, there was a marked fall in blood pressure as well as changes in the ST segment and T wave depression, indicative of myocardial ischemia. The fall in mean arterial pressure in these patients was to levels less than 50% of the awake values. In the fifteen treated patients, three were inadequately treated and, therefore, still hypertensive. In these three patients, there were marked decreases in blood pressure and electrocardiographic changes suggestive of myocardial ischemia. Thus, these inadequately treated patients behaved like untreated patients. It is important to point out that the situation may be even worse than indicated by these data since none of these patients were really undergoing major surgery. The surgery was brief in duration, lasting only 25 to 95 minutes, and none of the reported operations involved massive blood loss or fluid shifts. In any event, it was concluded that the response to anesthesia depends on the pre-existing level of arterial pressure more than, or whether or not, the patient is treated. Therefore, the inadequately treated patient appears to be just as great a risk as the untreated patient. In discussing the question as to whether one should recommend that symptom-free patients with hypertension be treated prior to surgery, Prys-Roberts et al. felt that this was desirable.

In a subsequent paper,[62] this group demonstrated that not only was hypotension a problem in the hypertensive patient, but that hypertension during induction and intubation could also be a problem. Again, studying untreated as well as treated hypertensives, it was observed that arrhythmias occurred in six of thirteen

untreated patients and five of sixteen treated patients. The arrhythmias were associated with sharp increases in blood pressure
and heart rate occurring during intubation, and evidence of myocardial ischemia was seen. Thus, it is obvious that in the hypertensive patient, one must be concerned with hypotension occurring
during anesthesia as well as with hypertension occurring during
induction of anesthesia.

Goldman et al.,[67] however, did not find preoperative hypertension to be an independent predictor of cardiac death, postoperative
myocardial infarction, heart failure, or arrhythmias. Patients with
preoperative hypertension, though, were more likely to develop
intra- or post-operative blood pressure elevation, and this was true
if they were on treatment and even if treatment had normalized
their blood pressure. Specifically, in their study, patients who had
persistent hypertension with diastolic pressures of 110 mmHg or
less, (on therapy or not) fared no worse than did patients in whom
hypertension was tightly controlled. Because mild to moderate hypertension did not seem to effect morbidity or mortality, it is not
recommended that surgery be cancelled in patients found to be
mildly hypertensive during the preoperative evaluation.

Prys-Roberts and associates[63] also reported that the mode of ventilation was an important determinant of blood pressure. Hypo-
capnia to a mean arterial PCO_2 of 23 patients anesthetized with
halothane produced severe falls in mean arterial pressure as well
as EKG evidence of ischemia. These changes occurred in four of
eight treated patients and in all of six untreated patients.

It is now clear that the hypertensive patient is a special problem
for anesthesia and operation and that the better the control of the
blood pressure prior to operation, the less the danger for the patient. Other authors have also concluded that stabilization of the
hypertensive should be achieved before elective surgery.[68,69] We
strongly support this point of view.

A key to the preoperative evaluation of the patient with hypertension is the cardiovascular assessment, for in the long run, it is
the effect of hypertension on the target organs that influence operative and postoperative mortality and morbidity. Thus, special
attention should be given the neurologic, cardiovascular, and renal
systems. For instance, fluctuations in blood pressure during anesthesia can be particularly poorly tolerated in the patient with cerebrovascular disease. It should also be realized that mild eleva-

tions of the blood urea nitrogen and creatinine indicates that there is a reduction of 50–70% in total renal function.

Another situation common to patients with hypertension relates to the serum potassium (K^+) level, since many of these patients are taking diuretics (see discussion in Chapter III). In addition, hyperventilation, common during the administration of anesthesia, causes further lowering of serum K^+ concentration. Arrhythmias occur more frequently when serum K^+ levels are low and, in patients with hypertensive heart disease, may be particularly dangerous. Although minimum acceptable K^+ levels generally used for patients undergoing surgery are 3.0 MEQ/L, if not concomitantly taking digitalis, and 3.5 MEQ/L, if they are (see Chapter III for a discussion of the potentiation of digitalis toxicity in patients with hypokalemia), these levels should serve only as a guide.

Recommendations

It has clearly been demonstrated above that the problems of the hypertensive patient include periods of excessive hypotension and periods of excessive hypertension. Therefore, in general, one should attempt to maintain as smooth a control of blood pressure as possible preoperatively as well as perioperatively. It should also be remembered that the treated hypertensive is a better risk than the untreated or inadequately treated hypertensive.

Concerning premedication and its value in allaying the apprehension of the hypertensive patient, there is no unanimity of opinion. There are those who feel that a well conducted preoperative visit prior to operation is sufficient to allay the apprehension of most patients, and that additional medication is not needed. In general, this is our usual practice. However, we recognize that others may prefer to use large doses of premedication. If appropriately done, this can be effective.

An important question in dealing with the hypertensive patient is monitoring. The electrocardiogram is essential, and a lead which allows the ST segment and T wave to be carefully monitored and which permits one to observe ST segment deviations is important. One way of accomplishing this is to place one lead on the manubrium sterni and the other in the V-5 position and connect to lead 1. Intra-arterial pressure monitoring is also of great value and,

often, indicated. Central venous pressure monitoring, particularly
the use of a Swan-Ganz catheter, is being increasingly used in our
department as well as in others. The induction of anesthesia must
be smooth and hypotension and hypertension avoided. If one waits
until the patient is anesthetized before giving the muscle relaxant
and intubating the patient, marked elevations in blood pressure
can often be avoided. Finally, anesthetic agents must be chosen
which maintain the blood pressure at a reasonable level for the
patient. Since it is known that extreme hyperventilation with reduction of PCO_2 to the low 20s can markedly lower blood pressure,
we prefer to maintain ventilation such that arterial PCO_2 is in the
middle 30s range. We attempt to avoid hypotension by avoiding
sudden changes in anesthetic concentrations and by careful attention to detail. If hypertension occurs, we usually have a sodium
nitroprusside drip available to lower the blood pressure.

Choice of anesthetic agents and techniques for hypertensive patients is not easy to determine. If one were to solicit opinions from
a number of experts, there would be those who felt that general
anesthesia was best, since it can be used regardless of the site of
surgery, is quickly reversible, and allows easy control of blood pressure. The fact that the patient is asleep also may eliminate anxiety.
There are, however, advocates and enthusiasts for regional anesthesia, spinal, or epidural. There are many excellent points both
for and against regional anesthesia. There are also advocates for
local anesthesia and, once again, this choice has its advocates as
well as detractors. While the use of drugs is minimized with local
anesthesia, one should be concerned about the emotional effect on
the patient. It is interesting that in a recent study of arrhythmias
during urologic procedures[70] the highest incidence occurred in
patients under local anesthesia. It may be that the anxiety associated with undergoing an operative procedure under local, and
without sedation, results in elevated levels of catecholamines, which
could have accounted for the higher incidence of arrhythmias. It
is, of course, possible to sedate the patient appropriately, so that
the operation can then satisfactorily be carried out under local
anesthesia.

It is not possible to reconcile in the abstract the three different
approaches to the patient: general versus regional versus local.
Much depends upon the patient and the physician. Every technique has advantages and disadvantages. The only logical common

sense way to handle the situation is to evaluate each patient individually, weigh the risks and benefits of a given form of anesthesia for a given patient and, then, choose the technique that appears best. Much less important than the choice of agent or technique is the presence of a physician well grounded in physiology, pharmacology, the pathophysiology of the patient's disease, and knowledge of the potential complications.

References

1. Vital and Health Statistics: Heart disease in adults: United States—1960–62. Series 11, No. 6, Washington DC, US Department of Health, Education and Welfare, 1964.
2. Mathisen H, Lohen H, Rean U: Complications in treated arterial hypertension. *Clin Soc Mol Med* 45:205, 1973.
3. Kannel WB, Schwartz MJ, McNamara PM: Blood pressure and risk of coronary heart disease: The Framingham study. *Dis Chest* 56:43, 1969.
4. McKee PA, Castelli WP, McNamara PM, Kannel WB: The natural history of congestive heart failure: The Framingham study. *N Engl J Med* 285:1443, 1971.
5. Wilber JA, Barrow JG: Reducing elevated blood pressure; experience found in a community. *Minn Med* 52:1303, 1969.
6. Wilber JA, Barrow JG: Hypertension—a community problem. *Am J Med* 52:653, 1972.
7. Nickerson M, Collier B: Drugs inhibiting adrenergic nerves and structure innervated by them. In: Goodman LS, Gilman A: *The Pharmacologic Basis of Therapeutics* Vol. 5, p. 533, N.Y.: MacMillan, 1975.
8. Foster MW Jr, Gayle RF: Dangers in combining reserpine (Serpasil) with electroconvulsive therapy. *JAMA* 159:1520, 1955.
9. Bracha S, Hes JP: Death occurring during combined reserpine-electroshock therapy. *Amer J Psychiat* 113:257, 1956.
10. Coakley CS, Alpert S, Boling JS: Circulatory responses during anesthesia of patients on rauwolfia therapy. *JAMA* 161:1143, 1956.
11. Perlroth MG, Hultgren HN: The cardiac patient and general surgery. *JAMA* 232:1279, 1975.
12. Logue RB. Surgery in patients with heart disease. In: Hurst JW, Logue RB, Schlant RC, et al. (Eds.): *The Heart, Arteries and Veins*, ed. 3, New York: McGraw-Hill Book Co., Inc., 1974, p. 1446.
13. Smessaert AA, Hicks RG: Problems caused by rauwolfia drugs during anesthesia and surgery. *N Y State J Med* 61:2399, 1961.
14. Katz RL, Weintraub HD, Papper EM: Anesthesia, surgery and rauwolfia. *Anesthesiology* 25:142, 1964.
15. Alper MH, Flacke W, Krayer O: Pharmacology of reserpine and its implications for anesthesia. *Anesthesiology* 24:524, 1963.

16. Ominsky AJ, Wollman H: Hazards of general anesthesia in the reserpinized patient. *Anesthesiology* 30:443, 1969.
17. Shand DG: Drug Therapy: Propranolol. *NEJM* 293:280, 1975.
18. Goldberg LI: Anesthetic management of patients treated with antihypertensive agents or levo-dopa. *Anesth Analg* 51:625, 1972.
19. Schwartz AJ, Wollman H: Anesthetic considerations for patients on chronic drug therapy: L-dopa, monoamine oxidase inhibitors, tricyclic antidepressants and propranolol. Refresher course in *Anesthesiology* 4:99, 1976.
20. Viljoen JF, Estafanous FG, Kellner GA: Propranolol and cardiac surgery. *J Thorac Cardiovasc Surg* 64:826, 1972.
21. Shand DG, Ragno RE: The disposition of propranolol. *Pharmacology* 7:159, 1972.
22. Coltart DJ, Gibson DG, Shand DG: Plasma propranolol levels associated with suppression of ventricular ectopic beats. *Br Med J* 1:490, 1971.
23. Coltart DJ, Cayen MN, Stinson EB, et al.: Determination of the safe period for withdrawal of propranolol therapy. *Circulation* 47 & 48 (Suppl. IV) 4–7, 1973.
24. Coltart DJ, Cayen MN, Stinson EB, et al.: Investigation of the safe withdrawal period for propranolol in patients scheduled for open heart surgery. *Brit Hrt J* 37:1228, 1975.
25. Evans GH, Shand DG: The disposition of propranolol VI. Independent variation in steady state circulatory drug concentration and half life as a result of plasma binding in man. *Clin Pharmacol Therap* 14:494, 1973.
26. Faulkner SL, Hopkins JT, Boerth RC, et al.: Time required for complete recovery from chronic propranolol therapy. *N England J of Med* 289:607, 1973.
27. Moran JM, Mulet J, Caralps JM, Pifarre R: Coronary revascularization in patients receiving propranolol. *Circulation* 49 & 50 (Suppl II) 2–116, 1974.
28. Jones EL, Dorney ER, King SB, et al.: Propranolol therapy in patients undergoing myocardial revascularization. *Circulation* 50, Suppl. III, 3, 1974.
29. Caralps JM, Mulet J, Wienke HR, et al.: Results of coronary artery surgery in patients receiving propranolol. *J Thorac Cardiovasc Surg* 67:526, 1974.
30. Kaplan JA, Dunbar RW, Bland JW, et al.: Propranolol and cardiac surgery: A problem for the anesthesiologist? *Anesth Analg Curr Resch* 54, No. 5:571, 1975.
31. Mizgala HF, Meldrum DAN: Propranolol prophylaxis of high risk unstable coronary artery disease: A preliminary report (abstr.). *Ann R Coll Phys Surg Can* 5:14, 1972.
32. Mizgala HF, Tinmouth AL, Waters DD, et al.: Prospective controlled trial of long-term propranolol on acute coronary events in patients with unstable coronary artery disease. *Circulation* 50 (Suppl. 3): 235: 1974.

33. Slome R: Withdrawal of propranolol and myocardial infarction. *Lancet* 1:156, 1973.
34. Nellen M: Withdrawal of propranolol and myocardial infarction. *Lancet* 1:558, 1973.
35. Alderman EL, Coltart DJ, Wettach GE, Harrison DC: Coronary artery syndromes after sudden propranolol withdrawal. *Ann Intern Med* 81:625, 1974.
36. Diaz RG, Somberg J, Freeman E, et al.: Withdrawal of propranolol and myocardial infarction. *Lancet* 1:1068, 1973.
37. Diaz RG, Somberg J, Freeman E, et al.: Myocardial infarction after propranolol withdrawal. *Am Heart J* 88:257, 1974.
38. Miller RR, Olson HG, Amsterdam EA, Mason DT: Propranolol withdrawal rebound phenomenon. *N Engl J Med* 293:416, 1975.
39. Mizgala HF, Counsell J: Acute coronary syndromes following abrupt cessation of oral propranolol therapy. *CMA Journal* 114:1123, 1976.
40. Bennett KR: Cessation of propranolol therapy and rebound angina pectoris. *Chest* 70: 2:314, 1976.
41. Viljoen JF: *Guest Discussion Anesth & Analg* 54:577, 1975.
42. Pettinger WA: Clonidine, a new antihypertensive drug. *NEJM* 298, No. 23:1179, 1975.
43. Dollery CT, Davies DS, Draffan GH, et al.: Clinical pharmacology and pharmacokinetics of clonidine. *Clin Pharmacol Ther* 19:11, 1976.
44. Nickerson M, Ruedy J: Antihypertensive agents and the drug therapy of hypertension. In: Goodman LS, Gilman A (Eds.) *The Pharmacol. Basis of Therapeutics*, Vol. 5, p. 705, N.Y.: MacMillan, 1975.
45. Hokfelt B, Hedeland H, Dymling JF: Studies on catecholamines, renin and aldosterone following catapresan (2-(2,6-dichlor-phenylamine)-1-imidazoline hydrochloride) in hypertensive patients. *Eur J Pharmacol* 10:389, 1970.
46. Hansson LM, Hunyor SN: Blood pressure over-shoot due to acute clonidine (Catapres) withdrawal: Studies on arterial and urinary catecholamines and suggestions for management of the crisis. *Clin Sci Mol Med* 45:181, 1973.
47. Hansson L, Hunyor SN, Julius S, et al.: Blood pressure crisis following withdrawal of clonidine (catapres, catapresan), with special reference to arterial and urinary catecholamine levels, and suggestions for acute management. *Am Heart J* 85:605, 1973.
48. Hunyor SN, Hansson L, Harrison TS, Hoobler SW: Effects of clonidine withdrawal. Possible mechanisms and suggestions for management. *Br Med J* 2:209, 1973.
49. Stelzer FP, Sturenbord JS, Sreenevasan V, et al.: Late toxicity of clonidine withdrawal. *NEJM* 294:1182, 1976.
50. Whitsett TL, Chrysant SG, Dillard B, Czerwinski AW: Withdrawal of clonidine. *JAMA* 235:2717, 1976.
51. Koch-Wesser J: Hydralazine. *NEJM* 295:320, 1976.
52. Gifford RW: Drug combinations as rational antihypertensive therapy. *Arch Intern Med* 133:1053, 1974.

53. Gottlieb TB, Chidsey CA: The clinicians guide to pharmacology of antihypertensive agents. *Geriatrics* 99, 1976.
54. Mundy GR, Raisz LG: Applied pharmacology of anti-hypertensive drugs. *Conn Med* 40:169, 1976.
55. Ngai SH: Parkinsonism, levodopa, and anesthesia. *Anesthesiology* 37:344, 1972.
56. Ngai SH, Wiklund RA: Levodopa and surgical anesthesia. *Neurology* (suppl) 22:38, 1972.
57. Wiklund RA, Ngai SH: Rigidity and pulmonary edema after Innovar in a patient on levo-dopa therapy. Report of a case. *Anesthesiology* 35:545, 1971.
58. Bevan, DR, Monks PS, Calne DB: Cardiovascular reactions to anaesthesia during treatment with levodopa. *Anaesthesia* 28:29, 1973.
59. Byck R: Drugs and the treatment of psychiatric disorders. In: Goodman LS, Gilman A, *The Pharmacol Basis of Therapeutics*, Vol. 5, p. 152, N.Y.: MacMillan, 1975.
60. Ballin JC: Toxicity of tricyclic antidepressants. *JAMA* 231:1369, 1975.
61. Prys-Roberts C, Meloche R, Foex P: Studies of anaesthesia in relation to hypertension: I. Cardiovascular responses of treated and untreated patients. *Br J Anaesth* 43:122, 1971.
62. Prys-Roberts C, Greene LT, Meloche R, Foex P: Studies of anaesthesia in relation to hypertension. II: Haemodynamic consequences of induction and endotracheal intubation. *Brit J Anaesth* 43:531, 1971.
63. Foex P, Meloche R, Prys-Roberts C: Studies of anaesthesia in relation to hypertension III: Pulmonary gas exchange during spontaneous ventilation. *Brit J Anaesth* 43:644, 1971.
64. Prys-Roberts C, Foex P, Greene LT, Waterhouse TD: Studies of anaesthesia in relation to hypertension. IV: The effects of artificial ventilation on the circulation and pulmonary gas exchanges. *Brit J Anaesth* 44:335, 1972.
65. Prys-Roberts C, Foex P, Biro GP, Roberts JG: Studies of anaesthesia in relation to hypertension. V: Adrenergic beta-receptor blockade. *Brit J Anaesth* 45:671, 1973.
66. Foex P, Prys-Roberts C: Anesthesia and the hypertensive patient. *Brit J Anaesth* 46:575, 1974.
67. Goldman L, Caldera DL, Nussbaum SR, et al.: Multifactorial index of cardiac risk in non-cardiac surgical procedures. *N Engl J Med* 297:845, 1977.
68. Mauney FM, Jr, Ebert PA, Sabiston DC Jr: Postoperative myocardial infarction. *Ann Surg,* 172:497, 1970.
69. Breslin DJ, Swinton NW Jr: Elective surgery in hypertensive patients: Preoperative considerations. *Surg Clin N Am* 50:585, 1970.
70. Kimbrough HM, Crampton RS, Gillenwater JY: Cardiac rhythm in men during cystoscopy. *J of Urol* 113:846, 1975.

CHAPTER XVI

Congestive Heart Failure

Willard S. Harris, M.D.

Cardiological advances have recently improved the chances that a patient with left ventricular (LV) dysfunction will survive a major noncardiac operation. This chapter will define LV dysfunction, list its causes, discuss its preoperative bedside diagnosis, analyze the cardiac risks of noncardiac surgery as they apply to such a patient and, finally, describe the advances that have markedly bettered his preoperative management.

Left Ventricular Dysfunction

Definition

In the patient with dysfunction of the LV, this chamber performs suboptimally as a pump. Two kinds of dysfunction occur, often together. In one kind, LV stroke work is less than expected for a given end-diastolic volume.[1-3] The Starling curve (end-diastolic LV volume or myocardial stretch on the horizontal axis and stroke work on the vertical axis) is depressed. The stroke work, stroke volume, or cardiac output needed for tissue perfusion either is inadequate or requires an abnormally great increase in end-diastolic LV volume and pressure, which may disturb breathing through pulmonary venous congestion and its effects. In the second kind of dysfunction, stiffening of the LV, i.e., reduction in its diastolic compliance, impairs LV filling.[4] The end-diastolic LV compliance curve (end-diastolic LV volume on the horizontal axis and pressure on the vertical axis) is shifted upward and to the left

305

(Figure 1). In a normal adult, the average end-diastolic LV volume is 70 ml per m^2 body surface area,[5] which occurs at a pressure within the range of 4 to 12 mmHg.[6,7] Almost all disorders causing LV dysfunction—including LV hypertrophy, cardiomyopathy and coronary artery disease—may be accompanied by stiffening of the LV, distention of which even to a normal end-diastolic volume requires an abnormally great increment of end-diastolic pressure, sometimes to one exceeding 20 mmHg. The myocardial stretch needed for a full Starling effect occurs, therefore, only at the cost of an elevated end-diastolic LV pressure and of pulmonary venous congestion, which may, if severe enough and the patient is awake, cause shortness of breath.

Causes

The causes of LV dysfunction are, most commonly, coronary artery disease and, because of LV hypertrophy and increased vascular resistance, systemic arterial hypertension; then, the specific valvular disorders of aortic stenosis, mitral regurgitation, and aortic regurgitation and, finally, the cardiomyopathies,[8,9] which may be classified as congestive cardiomyopathy, restrictive cardiomyopathy, or hypertrophic subaortic stenosis. Restrictive cardiomyopathies, such as amyloidosis, are uncommon but do occur; they impede LV filling.

In coronary artery disease, there are currently identified seven causes for LV dysfunction, many of them combined in a given patient. These are a lack of synchronous movement of the LV wall during systole, called asynergy; acute myocardial infarct; loss of LV myocardium so that the chamber is a weaker pump; LV aneurysm, which puts the contracting remnant of the LV at a mechanical disadvantage; papillary muscle dysfunction, which results in mitral regurgitation; acute ischemia which, of course, may occur without pain in the anesthetized patient but produces very striking LV dysfunction; and, finally, fibrosis due to so-called microinfarcts.

Preoperative Diagnosis

The bedside diagnosis of LV dysfunction depends mostly on the symptoms of cardiac decompensation or failure. Most patients di-

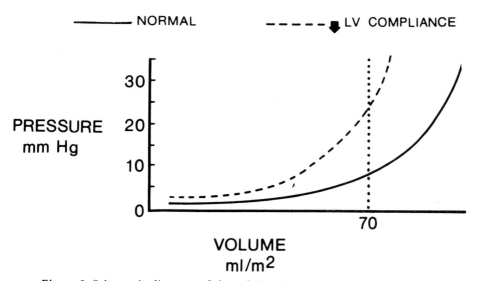

Figure 1. Schematic diagram of the relation between left ventricular (LV) volume and pressure at end-diastole. In normal adults (solid line) the average (± SD) LV end-diastolic volume is 70 (± 20) ml/m² body surface area,[5] indicated by the dotted vertical line, and the end-diastolic pressure is in the range from 4 to 12 mmHg .[6,7] In patients with a less compliant LV (dashed line) due, e.g., to LV hypertrophy, cardiomyopathy, or coronary artery disease, the same LV end-diastolic volume would require a much higher distending pressure, sometimes exceeding 20 mmHg, as shown here.

agnosed as having LV dysfunction have symptoms but no physical signs of decompensation. The clinical importance to perioperative management of LV dysfunction detected by laboratory findings but lacking symptoms or physical signs is unclear.

Cardiac decompensation due to LV dysfunction may give rise to any of the following symptoms: dyspnea, orthopnea, paroxysmal nocturnal dyspnea, cough, insomnia, nocturnal angina, fatigue, weakness, nocturia, edema, ascites, abdominal pain, or hemoptysis. Several of these symptoms occur particularly at night. Cough at night may be a single manifestation of LV failure. Insomnia is not an uncommon finding if you press the issue enough and may be caused, in part, by cough, paroxysmal nocturnal dyspnea, or Cheyne-Stokes respiration in which, during the hyperpneic phase, the patient is struggling and anxious. Insomnia may also be due to nocturia, frequently found in heart failure. Finally, nocturnal angina is often due to augmented venous return in the recumbent position, an effect that increases LV wall stress and the tendency of the ventricle with narrowed coronary arteries to become ischemic. Edema, ascites, and abdominal pain may occur when the right ventricle fails in response to LV failure.

Cardiac decompensation in LV dysfunction may be accompanied by any of the following physical signs; enlarged heart, S_3 gallop, murmur of mitral and/or tricuspid regurgitation, pulsus alternans, tachycardia, basilar rales, evidence of pleural effusion (usually right-sided or bilateral), tachypnea, Cheyne-Stokes respiration, elevated jugular venous pressure, peripheral edema, or hepatomegaly. Among these signs, elevated jugular venous pressure, which would be a manifestation of right ventricular failure secondary to LV failure, and the S_3 gallop are particularly important preoperative risk factors, discussed later. Pulsus alternans may be overlooked if the patient is lying in bed. It is increased by having the patient stand and by a rise in heart rate. It may begin after a premature contraction and then last for a few beats. Whenever present, pulsus alternans indicates LV dysfunction. Tachypnea, one of the most common signs of cardiac decompensation, is nonspecific but, often, in patients who then go on to develop frank pulmonary edema may be the first change the astute physician will note.

Cardiac Risks of Noncardiac Surgery

Risk of Cardiac Death

In 1977 and 1978, Goldman and associates[10,11] reported on 1,001 consecutive patients at Massachusetts General Hospital with major operations not on the heart. All patients were over the age of forty. While 866, or most, had general anesthesia, 116 had spinal or epidural anesthesia. The overall death rate was 5.9%, and the cardiac death rate was 1.9%. Thus, people over the age of forty who come to a teaching hospital and consecutively undergo major noncardiac surgery can be expected to have approximately a 2% cardiac mortality.

Univariate Analysis of Risk Factors

Table 1 lists in ascending order the approximate risk ratio, or increased chances, for a perioperative cardiac death as determined by Goldman and colleagues with univariate analysis, i.e., when each preoperative variable is considered by itself. Either rales or atrial fibrillation taken by itself, for example, increases the risk of a perioperative cardiac death five-fold. An S_3 gallop by itself increases it nine-fold. Either being seventy years or older or having a history of pulmonary edema any time in the past, even if the patient is now completely over it, increases it fourteen-fold. Of interest, any cardiac rhythm other than normal sinus or atrial fibrillation increases the risk by 20 to 1. Sinus arrhythmia, not discussed in the article by Goldman and associates, should probably be excluded. Preoperative jugular venous distention (elevation of jugular venous pressure)[10] is extremely important and ominous. By contrast, in patients who have noncardiac surgery, the risk of cardiac death

Table 1

Increased Risk of Cardiac Death from Noncardiac Surgery when Preoperative Variable Is Present*

Preoperative Variable	Approximate Risk Ratio†
Myocardial ischemia (history or ECG), ST-T abnormalities on ECG, cardiomegaly, atrial fibrillation, rales, mitral regurgitation murmur, or CHF despite treatment	5:1
S_3 gallop	9:1
Age more than 70 years, significant aortic stenosis, or history of pulmonary edema	14:1
Rhythm other than normal sinus or atrial fibrillation, or jugular venous distention	20:1

*Based on univariate analysis, with each preoperative variable considered by itself, by Goldman L., et al.: *Medicine* 57:357, 1978.

†Ratio between the cardiac mortality (percent dying a cardiac death) of those patients who had the preoperative variable and the cardiac mortality of those patients who did not have the preoperative variable. For each preoperative variable listed here differences in cardiac mortality between patients with and without that variable were significant (Chi square analysis with Yates correction) at $p < 0.05$.

Abbreviations: ECG = electrocardiogram; CHF = congestive heart failure.

is *not* increased by high blood pressure, past or present, an S_4 gallop, which is usually due to reduced LV compliance, a systolic ejection murmur if significant aortic stenosis is not present, diabetes, hyperlipidemia, or body build.

Multivariate Analysis of Risk Factors

The total risk for a patient is defined better when the risk factors are weighed not one by one, but all together through multivariate analysis. Goldman and co-workers found only nine preoperative or operative variables that had independent significance by multivariate analysis as risk factors for the patient postoperatively either dying from a cardiac complication or having such a serious one, e.g., pulmonary edema, that he comes close to death. These nine factors are listed in descending order of risk, as follows: S_3 gallop or elevated jugular venous pressure; myocardial infarct less than six months earlier; abnormal cardiac rhythm on the last preoperative electrocardiogram; more than five premature ventricular beats per minute on any preoperative electrocardiogram; age more than seventy years; emergency operation; intraperitoneal, intrathoracic, or aortic operation; important aortic stenosis; and general status.

Goldman and associates[10] have devised a cardiac risk index, which indicates prognosis and is computed by addition of the risk points (derived from the discriminant-function coefficients) listed in Table 2. By history, for example, age more than seventy years gives five points and myocardial infarct during the six months previously gives 10 points. On physical examination, either an S_3 gallop or increased jugular venous pressure gives 11 points. Intraperitoneal, intrathoracic, or aortic operation gives three points. The maximum possible risk points are 53.

Table 3 lists four classes defined by the total risk points found and gives the prognosis for a patient in a class. If the preoperative patient has 26 or more points in this multivariate analysis, for example, then the incidence of a life-threatening cardiac event—which is limited to three, viz., a perioperative myocardial infarct, pulmonary edema, or ventricular tachycardia—without cardiac death occurring is 22% and, in addition to that, the risk of dying a cardiac death is 56%. With 26 or more risk points determined

Table 2
Computation of Cardiac Risk Index*

	Criteria	Points
History	Age more than 70 years	5
	Myocardial infarct less than 6 months previously	10
Physical Examination	S₃ gallop or elevated jugular venous pressure	11
	Important valvular aortic stenosis	3
ECG	Last preoperative ECG: Rhythm other than sinus or PACs	7
	Any preoperative ECG: more than 5 PVCs/min	7
General Status	$PO_2 < 60$ mm Hg, $PCO_2 > 50$ mmHg, $K < 3$ meq/liter, $HCO_3 < 20$ meq/dl, BUN > 50 mg/dl, Cr > 3 mg/dl, SGOT abnormal, chronic liver disease or bedridden from noncardiac causes	3
Operation	Emergency	4
	Intraperitoneal, intrathoracic, or aortic	3
		53

*Adapted from Goldman L. et al.: *N Engl J Med* 297:845, 1977.

Abbreviations: ECG = electrocardiogram; PACs = premature atrial contractions; PVCs = premature ventricular contractions, PO_2 = partial pressure of oxygen; PCO_2 = partial pressure of carbon dioxide; K = potassium; HCO_3 = bicarbonate; BUN = blood urea nitrogen; Cr = creatinine; SGOT = serum glutamic oxaloacetic transaminase.

preoperatively, therefore, the chances during or shortly after operation of either dying from the heart or coming very close to it is 78%, or approximately three out of four.

As an example of the clinical use of the cardiac risk index, consider the following patient, whose risk points are in parentheses. A 72-year-old patient (5) with an S₃ gallop (11) and atrial fibrillation (7) having an intraperitoneal operation (3) would be in the worst class, Class IV, with 26 risk points. Perioperatively, according to the findings of Goldman and colleagues, he would have a 22% chance of a life-threatening, but nonfatal, cardiac complication and a 56% chance of cardiac death, for a total of three out of four

Table 3
Cardiac Risk Index*

Class	Points	Life-threatening Cardiac Event† %	Cardiac Death %	Total Cardiac Death or Near-death %
I (n = 537)	0–5	0.7	0.2	0.9
II (n = 316)	6–12	5	2	7
III (n = 130)	13–25	11	2	13
IV (n = 18)	≥ 26	22	56	78

*Adapted from Goldman L. et al.: *N Engl J Med* 297:845, 1977.
†Intraoperative or postoperative myocardial infarct, pulmonary edema, or ventricular tachycardia without cardiac death.
Abbreviation: n = number of patients in that Class in the study by Goldman and associates.

chances of either dying a cardiac death from that operation or coming very close to it.

Pulmonary Edema

Incidence and Prognosis

In the study by Goldman and co-workers[11] pulmonary edema occurred during or shortly after the operation twice as often, 3.6%, as myocardial infarct and was followed by cardiac death 40% of the time and death of any kind 57% of the time. In contrast, postoperative heart failure without pulmonary edema, which occurred 2.7% of the time, was followed by no cardiac deaths and by 15% total deaths. Thus, postoperative pulmonary edema (and not heart failure in the absence of pulmonary edema) is extremely serious, and anything that could prevent it should help a cardiac patient survive a noncardiac operation.

Risk Factors

Certain preoperative variables predict the risk of pulmonary edema that a patient in general, over the age of forty, faces from a noncardiac operation.[11] If congestive heart failure once occurred, but there is no evidence of it at the time of surgery, or if the patient is in Class III (is comfortable at rest, but has symptoms with less than ordinary activity) by the New York Heart Association criteria, the risk of postoperative pulmonary edema is 6%, a bad prognosis, but not horrendous. Preoperative variables associated with a peri-operative incidence (given in parentheses) of pulmonary edema 16% or greater, however, are any of the following five: persistence of heart failure despite treatment (16%), Class IV (symptoms at bed rest) by the New York Heart Association criteria (25%), jugular venous distention (30%), S_3 gallop (35%), and a history of pulmonary edema, even if the patient has none at all immediately preoperatively (23%).

The work of Goldman and associates as well as a canvass of the literature suggests that the risk of postoperative heart failure—with or without pulmonary edema—is increased by the preoperative risk factors of heart failure, either by past history or currently present, a history of pulmonary edema any time in the past, or valvular heart disease. In the category of operative risk factors, heart failure is more likely to occur if the operation is an emergency procedure, is intrathoracic or intra-abdominal, lasts more than five hours, or is done under general anesthesia rather than spinal or other kinds of anesthesia.

Characteristics of Postoperative Pulmonary Edema

In the forty patients with operative and postoperative pulmonary edema studied by Cooperman and Price,[12] the edema began in 22 (55%) during the first half-hour after the anesthetic was discontinued and in another six (15%) during the second half-hour. Thus, most instances (70%) of operative or postoperative pulmonary edema had their onset during the first hour after the anesthetic was stopped.

The early signs are tachypnea, decreased tidal volume, wheezes (due to bronchial edema and distention of bronchial veins), and tachycardia. These should be manifest to the anesthesiologist who is keeping careful records on the patient. Rales and jugular venous distention may be absent until later.[12]

The precipitating causes are thought to be the end of positive pressure breathing; the respiratory depression and obstruction that may occur at this time and produce hypoxemia, which impairs LV function, particularly if there is coronary artery disease; arterial hypertension, which is common in this period as the analgesic actions of the anesthetic and the effects of other drugs wear off and which diminishes the ability of the LV to empty itself; and residual myocardial depression by the general anesthetic.[12]

Fluid overinfusion has been found to contribute in at least 50% of cases.[12] Not giving excessive fluid during the operation, therefore, can reduce the likelihood of postoperative pulmonary edema in half or more of such patients, a point relevant to the discussion later in this chapter of hemodynamic monitoring.

Spinal anesthesia protects against postoperative pulmonary edema.[11,12] According to statistics, however, it does not protect against death or other cardiac complications.[11] Spinal anesthesia produces venodilation and reduces afterload, as evidenced by its tendency to cause hypotension. It does not cause myocardial depression, which all volatile anesthetics used in general anesthesia do. For these reasons, if one suspects strongly that pulmonary edema may occur in a patient, spinal anesthesia would be better than general anesthesia.

The study of Goldman and co-workers[11] gives further important information about postoperative pulmonary edema. Two separate sets of features identify preoperatively patients more likely than others to develop postoperative pulmonary edema. If the patient has heart failure before operation, his chances of getting pulmonary edema postoperatively are 16%. On the other hand, more than half of those who have postoperative pulmonary edema have *not* had previous heart failure, but they are usually over the age of sixty, have preoperative electrocardiograms that are abnormal in any kind of way, and have intra-abdominal or intrathoracic surgery.

In the study by Goldman and associates,[11] 15 (42%) of the 36 patients who developed postoperative pulmonary edema had neither previous heart failure nor perioperative myocardial infarct. Presumably, the causes of their postoperative pulmonary edema were myocardial depression due to either hypoxemia or the general anesthetic, increased afterload—i.e., increased resistance to LV emptying—excessive fluid infusion, or the increased metabolic rate due to such perioperative events as shivering after the end of anesthesia and surgical trauma.

Major Advances in Perioperative Management

Better Knowledge of Cardiovascular Effects of Anesthetics

All inhalational anesthetics that are now used depress myocardial contractility.[13–15] These myocardial depressant anesthetics do not include ether or cyclopropane, which are no longer employed, but do include halothane, methoxyflurane, enflurane and, at inspired concentrations of 40% or higher, nitrous oxide. The depression is dose-dependent. An attempt to overcome something like arterial hypertension by giving more anesthetic will further depress LV contractility, with the consequent danger of pulmonary edema. In the usual doses, halothane does not itself change vascular resistance or heart rate. If the anesthesiologist gives more halothane to lower arterial pressure, he does this lowering by a depression of myocardial contractility, which may increase pulmonary capillary wedge pressure. Not only does nitrous oxide at 40% and higher inspired concentrations depress myocardial function, but if narcotics have been given, which is likely today, then nitrous oxide also decreases cardiac output and raises systemic vascular resistance, i.e., increases the afterload of a LV that now has depressed contractility.[15,16] Nitrous oxide is not safe, therefore, for the avoidance of pulmonary edema.[14–16]

A second important point about anesthetics is that, to avoid their effects on the cardiovascular system, the common practice now is to use quite light anesthesia. Unlike the deep anesthesia of years ago, light anesthesia does not block the autonomic reflex responses to the noxious stimuli that are rampant during any surgical procedure.[14,15] In almost all patients, for example, direct laryngoscopy and endotracheal intubation reflexly raise heart rate and arterial pressure by marked amounts and elevate systemic vascular resistance, thereby increasing the myocardial oxygen demand and afterload of the LV.[17] Anesthesiologists are generally aware of the autonomic reflex responses that light anesthesia permits and should use nonanesthetic means to prevent them, especially in patients at increased risk for cardiac complications, e.g., giving intra-venous nitroprusside or nitroglycerin to lower afterload or preload or giving fluid to maintain preload and cardiac output.[15,17–19]

Hemodynamic Monitoring

In those patients with LV dysfunction who are considered to be at risk for developing perioperative pulmonary edema, myocardial damage, or other cardiovascular problems that will be discussed later in this chapter, perioperative hemodynamic monitoring with a flow-directed balloon-tipped (balloon flotation) catheter, such as the Swan-Ganz catheter, passed intravenously into the pulmonary artery is extremely useful.[20–24] The information such monitoring can provide includes pulmonary artery, pulmonary capillary wedge (LV filling), and right atrial pressures and cardiac output determined by thermodilution. These measurements permit cal-culation of stroke volume, systemic vascular resistance, and stroke work and even, if desired, the construction of Starling-type curves.

Certain patients with LV dysfunction need perioperative he-modynamic monitoring for three reasons. First, especially when symptoms or signs of cardiac decompensation are present, the pa-tient's LV is operating on the flat part of a depressed Starling curve and is highly sensitive to conditions of loading. Not only will an increase of afterload lower the cardiac output, but too great an increase of afterload or preload—i.e., too high a rise of systemic vascular resistance or too much fluid given—will elevate the pul-monary capillary wedge pressure and lead to pulmonary edema.[3]

Second, if a patient with coronary artery disease has hypotension or hypertension (both of which are common events throughout the induction of anesthesia and the operation itself), he is prone to develop myocardial ischemia, which may lead either to myocar-dial infarct resulting in obvious LV dysfunction or to LV failure and pulmonary edema without actual myocardial necrosis.[17,25–27]

Finally, hemodynamic monitoring provides the only way at any time during the operation to know whether arterial hypotension is due to low cardiac output or decreased systemic vascular resis-tance. The cardiac output might fall, for example, either because

LV dysfunction has been induced or worsened by halothane or myocardial ischemia or because not enough fluid has been given. The anesthesiologist needs some measure of preload, such as pulmonary capillary wedge pressure, to know if inadequacy of LV filling is the cause for the arterial hypotension and to take the right steps then and there to rectify it.

Current indications for perioperative Swan-Ganz catheterization during major noncardiac surgery in cardiac patients are the following six: significant heart disease if large shifts of volume are expected during the operative or postoperative period; severe coronary artery disease; the need for positive inotropic agents or vasodilators for the treatment of heart failure, such as characterizes patients entering the operation already in heart failure; aortic surgery with aortic cross-clamping, which always occurs during repair of an abdominal aortic aneurysm; significant mitral or aortic valvular disease; and significant cardiomyopathy or the presence of hypertrophic subaortic stenosis.[24,26,28]

Newer Therapies

Vasodilator therapy has become important in the perioperative management of the patient with heart failure. There are two kinds, or sites and effects, of vasodilation. One is the dilation of arterioles, which lowers aortic input impedance, resulting in a rise of cardiac output. The other is venous dilation, such as nitrates produce, which increases the volume capacity of the veins, causing a fall of LV filling pressure and pulmonary capillary wedge pressure and, consequently, reducing the tendency toward pulmonary edema.[29,30]

Vasodilators act on one or both vascular sites. Given intravenously, nitroprusside dilates both arterioles and veins; nitroglycerine dilates veins predominantly and, to a lesser extent, arterioles; and phentolamine dilates arterioles predominantly and, to a lesser extent, veins. Given by routes other than the intravenous, nitroglycerin (sublingual or in skin ointment) and isosorbide dinitrate (sublingual or oral) dilate only veins, hydralazine (oral) dilates only arterioles, and prazosin (oral) dilates both arteries and veins[29,30] (Table XVI-4).

Table 4
Vasodilator Drugs

	Venous	Arterial
Parenteral		
phentolamine	+	+ + +
trimethaphan (Arfonad)	+ + +	+ +
nitroprusside	+ + +	+ + +
Nonparenteral		
nitrates	+ + +	+
hydralazine (Apresoline)	0	+ + +
prazosin (Minipress)	+ +	+ +
captopril	+ + +	+ + +

In the patient endangered by the manifestations of LV dysfunction, the operative use, as needed, of intravenous nitroprusside or intravenous nitroglycerin is highly recommended for the lowering of LV afterload and preload, provided that Swan-Ganz catheterization is present. In heart failure, the elevated pulmonary capillary wedge pressure can be reduced by venodilators; in addition, the depressed Starling-type curve can be raised toward normal not only by the positive inotropic action such agents as digitalis, dopamine, or dobutamine provide, but also by the lowering of LV afterload arteriolar dilators induce.[31]

If an operation must be delayed for the treatment of chronic refractory heart failure, the administration by other than the intravenous route of vasodilators would be helpful. According to Massie and co-workers,[29] if the cardiac index (cardiac output expressed as liters/min/m^2 body surface area) is normal but LV filling pressure is markedly elevated (above 20 mmHg), venodilation with nitroglycerin, isosorbide dinitrate, or prazosin is recommended. When the cardiac index is low (below 2.5 liters/min/m^2), however, an arteriolar dilator such as oral hydralazine should be given. With a low cardiac index, if the LV filling pressure is adequate (12–20 mmHg), hydralazine would be given and if the LV filling pressure is markedly elevated (above 20 mmHg), either hydralazine and a nitrate or prazosin would be given.

When the patient with heart failure due to LV dysfunction does not respond adequately to the usual therapy with digitalis and diuretics before operation,[32] vasodilators are extremely helpful before or during the operation.[29–32] Especially if mitral regurgitation is present, lowering of afterload and preload is of benefit. If the increase in cardiac output or fall in pulmonary capillary wedge pressure induced by vasodilators is inadequate, potent positive inotropic agents (dopamine, dobutamine) can be given by intravenous infusion to improve contractility.[18,32] Finally, if heart failure persists despite maximal vasodilation and positive inotropic therapy and the patient needs the operation on an emergency basis, intra-aortic balloon counterpulsation can be added perioperatively. Counterpulsation has been used to pull such patients through noncardiac surgery even in the presence of heart failure.[33]

During operations, systemic arterial pressure rises commonly with direct laryngoscopy and endotracheal intubation, bronchoscopy or tracheal suction, surgical incision, mesenteric traction, aortic cross-clamping (during repair of an aortic aneurysm), and recovery from anesthesia.[17] Except for aortic cross-clamping, which affects hemodynamics directly, this hypertension is a reflex response. The ability moment-to-moment to keep arterial pressure from rising is made possible by the use of fast-acting, intravenously administered vasodilators combined with Swan-Ganz catheterization and intra-arterial cannulation in the patient who is at high risk.

Cautions in Specific Diseases

Preoperative Management of Systemic Arterial Hypertension

Look for complications of the disease or its treatment; e.g., cardiac, renal, cerebrovascular, or electrolyte abnormalities. If the patient is on antihypertensive therapy, continue it. If the hypertension is severe (arterial diastolic pressure greater than 110 mmHg), successful preoperative therapy diminishes dangerous increases and decreases of arterial pressure during the operation.[17,34]

Atrial Systole

A properly timed atrial systole is enormously important to LV function when LV filling is impeded by mitral stenosis[35-40] or a decrease in LV compliance, particularly when the LV is extremely thick due to aortic stenosis or cardiomyopathy (especially hypertrophic subaortic stenosis).[38-42] On average, atrial systole occurring just before end-diastole contributes to LV end-diastolic volume normally 20% (29 ml) but in severe aortic stenosis has been shown to contribute 29% (40 ml).[38] The loss of a properly timed atrial systole due to the onset of atrial fibrillation, which may occur during the operation, can be catastrophic in hypertrophic subaortic stenosis or severe aortic stenosis.[4,39-44]

In patients with LV dysfunction, the loss of atrial systole and its transport function when atrial fibrillation occurs raises mean left atrial and pulmonary capillary wedge pressures, lowers LV end-diastolic pressure and cardiac output, and causes a rise in peripheral resistance.[45] In these patients, the increase of ventricular rate with atrial fibrillation also may impede filling of the LV.[39,40,45] In someone with LV dysfunction, atrial fibrillation can be the "straw that breaks the camel's back" during the operation but, if its presence and effects are recognized, can be treated by electrical cardioversion or drugs.[46]

Operative Dangers of Mitral Stenosis

Pulmonary capillary wedge pressure and the pressure gradient from the left atrium to the LV are increased in mitral stenosis by either tachycardia or fluid overload.[40] Tachycardia, which impairs left atrial emptying by shortening the diastolic filling period of the LV, must be avoided. Excessive overload of fluid by either its administration or its redistribution into the thorax through the head-down position must be guarded against.[39] Procedures causing redistribution of fluid into the thorax can be done, but only if the pulmonary capillary wedge pressure is monitored. Mitral stenosis is critical if the mitral orifice is less than 1 cm^2/m^2 body surface area and the patient is in New York Heart Association functional Class III or IV, i.e., has symptoms with less than ordinary physical activity or at bed rest.[40,47,48] In the patient with *critical* mitral stenosis, elective noncardiac surgery should not be done until the valve has been repaired or replaced.[49] If the mitral orifice is close to 1 cm^2/m^2 body surface area and the patient is in functional Class II, i.e., is comfortable at rest but has symptoms with ordinary activity, the decision whether to have the valve operated on before elective noncardiac surgery is done must be made on an individual basis.[40]

Severe Aortic Stenosis

Properly timed atrial systole is critical. Atrial fibrillation, sinus tachycardia, or severe bradycardia (heart rate less than 45 beats per minute) is poorly tolerated by patients with severe aortic stenosis.[39,43,50,51] These patients should be monitored for myocardial ischemia with a lateral precordial electrocardiographic lead, e.g., V_5. Aortic stenosis is critical in the adult if the aortic orifice is 0.5 to 0.7 cm^2/m^2 body surface area or less[47] (but can be critical with a somewhat larger orifice if other heart disease, e.g., aortic or mitral regurgitation or coronary artery disease is also present)[43] and the patient either has symptoms (angina, syncope, or heart failure) due to aortic stenosis or has serious LV dysfunction and increasing cardiomegaly.[40] In the patient with *critical* aortic stenosis, the valve must be replaced before elective noncardiac surgery is done.[49]

Aortic Regurgitation

In patients with aortic regurgitation, either slowing of heart rate or increase of peripheral resistance, both of which may occur during the operation, tends to increase the regurgitation per beat and the LV end-diastolic volume and pressure.[52-57] In contrast to patients with aortic stenosis, patients with aortic regurgitation tolerate tachycardia well because it reduces the time during diastole for regurgitation to raise LV end-diastolic pressure[52] and for arterial diastolic pressure to fall.[39,50-52] Bradycardia is poorly tolerated, however, by patients with aortic regurgitation.[39,52] The anesthesiologist or person giving postoperative care has to keep this intolerance to bradycardia in mind. Vasodilators can be of help in aortic regurgitation[54-57] but must be given with special care because some of these patients can be excessively sensitive to them, probably owing to the reduction of coronary artery perfusion if arterial diastolic pressure falls too much.[39]

Hypertrophic Subaortic Stenosis

Swan-Ganz catheterization is important, particularly in symptomatic patients. Left ventricular preload cannot be permitted to fall because, if it did, the decreased LV size would worsen the LV outflow obstruction, preventing the ventricle from ejecting its required cardiac output.[58-60] Thus, a high mean airway pressure should be avoided and a properly timed atrial contraction maintained.[39] Atrial fibrillation or junctional rhythm, which loses the booster pump function of left atrial systole,[45] will markedly decrease cardiac output and arterial pressure.[44] In hypertrophic subaortic stenosis, in contrast to most other causes of LV dysfunction, vasodilators are harmful because they increase the LV outflow obstruction.[60] Propranolol[61,62] or, more recently, verapamil[63-65] therapy has been shown to benefit patients with hypertrophic subaortic stenosis.

Summary

Recently, the chances of a patient with LV dysfunction surviving noncardiac surgery have markedly improved, owing to a better understanding of LV function, preoperative risks, perioperative hemodynamics, and the effects of anesthetics; the introduction of important hemodynamic monitoring when required; the rational use of old and new therapy, particularly the newer diuretics, vasodilators, and positive inotropic agents; and the knowledge of when to repair the valve surgically before elective noncardiac surgery.

References

1. Starling EH: Linacre Lecture on the Law of the Heart (1915). London, Longmans, Green and Co., Ltd., 1918.
2. Braunwald E: The control of ventricular function in man. *Br Heart J* 27:1, 1965.
3. Braunwald E, Ross J Jr, Sonnenblick EH: *Mechanisms of Contraction of the Normal and Failing Heart*, 2nd ed. Boston: Little, Brown and Co., 1976.

4. Grossman W, McLaurin LP: Diastolic properties of the left ventricle. *Ann Intern Med* 84:316, 1976.
5. Kennedy JW, Baxley WA, Figley MM, et al.: Quantitative angiocardiography. I. The normal left ventricle in man. *Circulation* 34:272, 1966.
6. Braunwald E, Brockenbrough EC, Frahm CJ, Ross J Jr: Left atrial and left ventricular pressures in subjects without cardiovascular disease. Observations in eighteen patients studied by transseptal left heart catheterization. *Circulation* 24:267, 1961.
7. Parker JO, DiGiorgi S, West RO: A hemodynamic study of acute coronary insufficiency precipitated by exercise. With observations on the effect of nitroglycerin. *Am J Cardiol* 17:470, 1966.
8. Goodwin JF: Prospects and predictions for the cardiomyopathies. *Circulation* 50:210, 1974.
9. Goodwin JF, Braunwald E: Cardiomyopathy. In: *The Heart*, 4th ed, edited by Hurst JW. New York: McGraw-Hill, pp. 1556–1590, 1978.
10. Goldman L, Caldera DL, Nussbaum SR, et al.: Multifactorial index of cardiac risk in noncardiac surgical procedures. *N Engl J Med* 297:845, 1977.
11. Goldman L, Caldera DL, Southwick FS, et al.: Cardiac risk factors and complications in non-cardiac surgery. *Medicine* 57:357, 1978.
12. Cooperman LH, Price HL: Pulmonary edema in the operative and postoperative period: A review of 40 cases. *Ann Surg* 172:883, 1970.
13. Merin RG: Effect of anesthetic drugs on myocardial performance in man. *Annu Rev Med* 28:75, 1977.
14. Hug CC, Jr: Pharmacology—Anesthetic drugs. In: *Cardiac Anesthesia*, edited by Kaplan JA. New York: Grune and Stratton, pp. 3–37, 1979.
15. Ngai SH: Effects of anesthetics on various organs. *N Engl J Med* 302:564, 1980.
16. McDermott RW, Stanley TH: The cardiovascular effects of low concentrations of nitrous oxide during morphine anesthesia. *Anesthesiology* 41:89, 1974.
17. Prys-Roberts C: Medical problems of surgical patients: Hypertension and ischaemic heart disease. *Ann Roy Coll Surg Engl* 58:465, 1976.
18. Hug CC, Jr, Kaplan JA: Pharmacology—Cardiac drugs. In: *Cardiac Anesthesia*, edited by Kaplan JA, New York: Grune and Stratton, pp. 39–69, 1979.
19. Laver MB, Lowenstein E: Anesthesia and the patient with heart disease. In: *The Practice of Cardiology*, edited by Johnson RA, Haber E, Austen WG. Boston: Little, Brown and Co., pp. 1090–1109, 1980.
20. Swan HJC, Ganz W, Forrester JS, et al.: Catheterization of the heart in man with use of a flow-directed balloon-tipped catheter. *N Engl J Med* 283:447, 1970.
21. Ganz W, Donoso R, Marcus HS, et al.: A new technique for measurement of cardiac output by thermodilution in man. *Am J Cardiol* 27:392, 1971.
22. Ganz W, Swan HJC: Measurement of blood flow by thermodilution. *Am J Cardiol* 29:241, 1972.

23. Pace NL: A critique of flow-directed pulmonary arterial catheterization. *Anesthesiology* 47:455, 1977.
24. Kaplan JA: Hemodynamic monitoring. In: *Cardiac Anesthesia,* edited by Kaplan JA. New York: Grune and Stratton, pp. 71–115, 1979.
25. Gray RJ, Harris WS, Shah PK, et al.: Coronary sinus blood flow and sampling for detection of unrecognized myocardial ischemia and injury. *Circulation* 56, Suppl 2: II-58–61, 1977
26. Attia RR, Murphy JD, Snider M, et al.: Myocardial ischemia due to infrarenal aortic cross-clamping during aortic surgery in patients with severe coronary artery disease. *Circulation* 53:961, 1976.
27. Waller JL, Kaplan JA, Jones EL: Anesthesia for coronary revascularization. In: *Cardiac Anesthesia,* edited by Kaplan JA. New York: Grune and Stratton, pp. 241–280, 1979.
28. Carroll RM, Laravuso RB, Schauble JF: Left ventricular function during aortic surgery. Arch Surg 111:740, 1976.
29. Massie BM, Chatterjee K, Parmley WW: Vasodilator therapy for acute and chronic heart failure. In: *Progress in Cardiology,* vol 8, edited by Yu PN, Goodwin JF. Philadelphia: Lea and Febiger, pp. 197–234, 1979.
30. Chatterjee K, Parmley WW: Vasodilator therapy for chronic heart failure. *Ann Rev Pharmacol Toxicol* 20:475, 1980.
31. Cohn JN: Physiologic basis of vasodilator therapy for heart failure. *Am J Med* 71:135, 1981.
32. Gazes PC, Assey ME: The management of congestive heart failure. *Current Problems in Cardiol* 4:1, 1980.
33. Foster ED, Olsson CA, Rutenberg AM, Berger RL: Mechanical circulatory assistance with intra-aortic balloon counterpulsation for major abdominal surgery. *Ann Surg* 183:73, 1976.
34. Goldman L, Caldera DL: Risks of general anesthesia and elective operation in the hypertensive patient. *Anesthesiology* 50:285, 1979.
35. Heidenreich FP, Thompson ME, Shaver JA, Leonard JJ: Left atrial transport in mitral stenosis. *Circulation* 40:545, 1969.
36. Mitchell JH, Shapiro W: Atrial function and the hemodynamic consequences of atrial fibrillation in man. *Am J Cardiol* 23:556, 1969.
37. Thompson ME, Shaver JA, Leon DF: Effect of tachycardia on atrial transport in mitral stenosis. *Am Heart J* 94:297, 1977.
38. Stott DK, Marpole DGF, Bristow JD, et al.: The role of atrial transport in aortic and mitral stenosis. *Circulation* 41:1031, 1970.
39. Chambers DA: Anesthesia for the patient with acquired valvular heart disease. In: *Cardiac Anesthesia,* edited by Kaplan JA. New York: Grune and Stratton, pp. 197–240, 1979.
40. Braunwald E: Valvular heart disease. In: *Heart Disease,* edited by Braunwald E. Philadelphia: WB Saunders Co., pp. 1095–1165, 1980.
41. Frank S, Braunwald E: Idiopathic hypertrophic subaortic stenosis. Clinical analysis of 126 patients with emphasis on the natural history. *Circulation* 37:759, 1968.
42. Wigle ED, Felderhof CH, Silver MD, Adelman AG: Hypertrophic obstructive cardiomyopathy (muscular or hypertrophic subaortic ste-

nosis). In: *Myocardial Diseases,* edited by Fowler NO. New York: Grune and Stratton, pp. 297–318, 1973.

43. Schlant RC, Nutter DO: Heart failure in valvular heart disease. *Medicine* 50:421, 1971.

44. Braunwald E: Idiopathic hypertrophic subaortic stenosis (obstructive cardiomyopathy, asymmetric septal hypertrophy). In: *The Heart,* 4th ed, edited by Hurst JW. New York: McGraw-Hill, pp. 1560–1567, 1978.

45. Morris DC, Hurst JW: Atrial fibrillation. *Current Problems in Cardiol,* 5:1, 1980.

46. Bigger JT, Jr.: Management of arrhythmias. In: *Heart Disease,* edited by Braunwald E. Philadelphia: WB Saunders Co., pp. 691–743, 1980.

47. Schlant RC: Altered cardiovascular function of rheumatic heart disease and other acquired valvular disease. In: *The Heart,* 4th ed, edited by Hurst JW. New York: McGraw-Hill, pp. 965–981, 1978.

48. The Criteria Committee of the New York Heart Association: *Diseases of the Heart and Blood Vessels. Nomenclature and Criteria for Diagnosis,* 6th ed. Boston: Little, Brown and Co., pp. 110–114, 1964.

49. Perlroth MG, Hultgren HN: The cardiac patient and general surgery. JAMA 232:1279, 1975.

50. Trenouth RS, Phelps NC, Neill WA: Determinants of left ventricular hypertrophy and oxygen supply in chronic aortic valve disease. *Circulation* 53:644, 1976.

51. Vincent WR, Buckberg GD, Hoffman JIE: Left ventricular subendocardial ischemia in severe valvar and supravalvar aortic stenosis. A common mechanism. *Circulation* 49:326, 1974.

52. Judge TP, Kennedy JW, Bennett LJ, et al.: Quantitative hemodynamic effects of heart rate in aortic regurgitation. *Circulation* 44:355, 1971.

53. Bolen JL, Holloway EL, Zener JC, et al.: Evaluation of left ventricular function in patients with aortic regurgitation using afterload stress. *Circulation* 53:132, 1976.

54. Bolen JL, Alderman EL: Hemodynamic consequences of afterload reduction in patients with chronic aortic regurgitation. *Circulation* 53:879, 1976.

55. Miller RR, Vismara LA, DeMaria AN, et al.: Afterload reduction therapy with nitroprusside in severe aortic regurgitation: Improved cardiac performance and reduced regurgitant volume. *Am J Cardiol* 38:564, 1976.

56. Greenberg BH, DeMots H, Murphy E, Rahimtoola SH: Beneficial effects of hydralazine on rest and exercise hemodynamics in patients with chronic severe aortic insufficiency. *Circulation* 62:49, 1980.

57. Greenberg BH, DeMots H, Murphy E, Rahimtoola SH: Mechanism for improved cardiac performance with arteriolar dilators in aortic insufficiency. *Circulation* 63:263, 1981.

58. Pierce GE, Morrow AG, Braunwald E: Idiopathic hypertrophic subaortic stenosis. III. Intraoperative studies of the mechanism of ob-

struction and its hemodynamic consequences. *Circulation* 30, Suppl IV: IV–152, 1964.

59. Braunwald E, Lambrew CT, Rockoff SD, et al.: Idiopathic hypertrophic subaortic stenosis: I. A description of the disease based upon an analysis of 64 patients. *Circulation* 30, Suppl IV: IV–3, 1964.

60. Wigle ED, David PR, Labrosse CJ, McMeekan J: Muscular subaortic stenosis: The interrelation of wall tension, outflow tract "distending pressure" and orifice radius. *Am J Cardiol* 15:761, 1965.

61. Goodwin JF: Congestive and hypertrophic cardiomyopathies. A decade of study. *Lancet* 1:731, 1970.

62. Stenson RE, Flamm MD, Harrison DC, Hancock EW: Hypertrophic subaortic stenosis. Clinical and hemodynamic effects of long-term propranolol therapy. *Am J Cardiol* 31:763, 1973.

63. Kaltenbach M, Hopf R, Kober G, et al.: Treatment of hypertrophic obstructive cardiomyopathy with verapamil. *Brit Heart J* 42:35, 1979.

64. Rosing DR, Kent KM, Borer JS, et al.: Verapamil therapy: A new approach to the pharmacologic treatment of hypertrophic cardiomyopathy. I. Hemodynamic effects. *Circulation* 60:1201, 1979.

65. Rosing DR, Kent KM, Maron BJ, Epstein SE: Verapamil therapy: A new approach to the pharmacologic treatment of hypertrophic cardiomyopathy. II. Effects on exercise capacity and symptomatic status. *Circulation* 60:1208, 1979.

CHAPTER XVII

The Pregnant Cardiac Patient

Randy B. Hartman, M.D.

With the advent of modern obstetrical practices, antibiotics, and antihypertensive agents, the risk of pregnancy and childbirth has been greatly reduced. At the present time, maternal mortality occurs less than one time in 1,000 pregnancies.[1] Heart disease is present in approximately 0.5 to 2.0% of all pregnancies,[2,3] and now constitutes the principal nonobstetrical cause of maternal death.[1] In order to appreciate and manage the special problems involved with successful surgery or delivery in the pregnant woman with cardiac disease, a thorough knowledge of the hemodynamic changes of pregnancy and of the common cardiac disorders is necessary.

Cardiovascular Physiology of Pregnancy

Multiple physiologic changes occur in pregnancy in order to meet the metabolic needs of the developing fetus via the placenta. These changes place enormous stress on the maternal circulation (Table 1). Cardiac output begins to increase during the first trimester, and reaches a peak of 30–40% above the prepregnancy level by the twentieth to twenty-fourth week.[4] This high output is then sustained until delivery. It was once believed that the cardiac output decreased in late pregnancy, but recently this has been shown to be an artifact of supine measurement.[5,6] Late pregnancy vena cava arteriograms demonstrate complete occlusion of the vena cava by the gravid uterus, which may be partially relieved by assumption of lateral position.[7] Even though substantial collateral blood flow

327

Table 1
Circulatory Changes in Pregnancy[21]

Heart Rate	Increase	10 to 15 beats/min
Blood Volume	Increase	40 to 50%
Stroke Volume	Increase	
Cardiac Output	Increase	30 to 50%
Systemic Blood Pressure	Decrease	slightly until term
Systemic Vascular Resistance	Decrease	
Pulmonary Vascular Resistance	Decrease	

occurs through the azygous, lumbar, and paraspinal veins, this mechanical caval compression greatly increases the lower extremity venous pressure (producing pedal edema), decreases the blood return to the right atrium (decreasing right ventricular preload) and, thus, decreases the cardiac output. With this in mind, many authorities recommend delivery in the Sims (lateral) position for most cardiac patients in order to minimize these effects.

An occasional patient may suffer a vasovagal episode while supine, and the combination of bradycardia and decreased cardiac output secondary to caval obstruction may produce presyncope or syncope.[7,8] These symptoms may be dramatically relieved by turning the patient on her side to relieve caval obstruction. In addition, the enlarged uterus may partially compress the abdominal aorta[9] and further decrease blood flow to the fetus during uterine contractions.

Heart rate increases about ten to twenty beats per minute, especially during early pregnancy,[10] and remains relatively constant even in conditions of changing cardiac output, as detailed above. Stroke volume is increased to a greater degree than heart rate during the later phase of pregnancy.[10] This is tolerated quite well by the normal heart, but adds additional burden to an already compromised left ventricle.

Blood volume, especially plasma volume, begins to rise as early as the sixth week of pregnancy. It increases rapidly until the fifth month, then slowly increases until term, when it is forty to fifty percent greater than normal.[5,11] The total body water during pregnancy increases by about six to eight liters.[12] Total red cell volume increases steadily throughout pregnancy, but never increases to the degree of the plasma volume, resulting in the so-called "physiologic anemia of pregnancy."[13] Systolic blood pressure changes relatively little during pregnancy, but a measurable decline in the diastolic pressure occurs early in the mid-trimester. There may be small increases in right atrial pressure but, for the most part, intracardiac pressures are unchanged in the patient without cardiac disease.[14] It is obvious that with significant increases in cardiac output and little change in systemic and intracardiac pressures, both systemic and pulmonary vascular resistance are greatly decreased. It was once thought that this resulted from the placenta acting as a giant arteriovenous fistula, but recent evidence suggests that the effects of estrogen and progesterone may also be major factors.[15-17] Estrogen has been found to decrease peripheral vascular resistance, while progesterone promotes venous relaxation.[18] Other hemodynamic changes in pregnancy may be related to increasing levels of these hormones, as animal studies have shown that estrogen can increase heart rate, myocardial contractility, cardiac output, and blood flow to the breast and uterus.[15,17,19] Also, estrogen and progesterone in combination may stimulate an increase in aldosterone, serving to increase sodium and water retention.[20,21]

Circulatory changes during labor and delivery may further stress the cardiovascular system (Table 2). During uterine contraction, 300 to 500 ml of blood is expressed into the maternal circulation.[22] With each contraction, mean blood pressure rises approximately 10%, probably because of peripheral sympathetic stimulation. These combine to increase cardiac output 15 to 20% and increase left ventricular work.[23] Because epidural anesthesia seems to mitigate these changes, it is the preferred anesthesia for most patients with heart disease.[24,25]

Immediately following delivery (Table 3), blood volume increases secondary to autotransfusion from the contracting empty

Table 2
Circulatory Changes During Labor

Engagement of fetal head
—Decrease of vena cava obstruction
—Increase venous return to right atrium
Major uterine contractions
—300 ml to 500 ml blood expressed into maternal circulation
—Increased sympathetic stimulation
—Increased heart rate, blood pressure, cardiac output
Above combined to increase heart work

Table 3

Circulatory Changes During Early Puerperium

Blood volume increases secondary to:
    Autotransfusion from contracting empty uterus
    Relief of vena cava compression
    Absorption of extracellular fluid
Cardiac output increases 10 to 20% with relative bradycardia
Above combine to increase cardiac stroke volume

uterus, relief of vena cava compression, and absorption of extracellular fluid. These physiologic changes more than equal the usual blood loss of 500 ml during vaginal delivery[26,27] and in fact, the normal nongravid blood volume is not reached until four to six weeks after delivery.[6] Cardiac output increases about 10 to 20% following delivery, while the heart rhythm is characterized by relative bradycardia.[28] Thus, the puerperium is a critical and stressful time for a marginal maternal cardiovascular system. Close observation is mandatory during and after delivery, as many patients will suffer cardiac decompensation and will go into pulmonary edema during this period.

The Spectrum of Heart Disease

The types of heart disease encountered in pregnant women has undergone significant changes over the past few decades. Rheumatic heart disease was once predominant, being seen twenty times as often as congenital lesions.[29] Because of recent major advances made in cardiovascular surgery, partial or complete repair of congenital lesions is now seen more frequently, and a new category of lesions, the prosthetic heart valve, now requires management during pregnancy. However, rheumatic heart disease still comprises a large proportion of heart disease complicating pregnancy.

Mitral Stenosis

Up to 75% of pregnant patients with rheumatic heart disease will have pure or predominant mitral stenosis.[11] The great majority of these patients can be successfully managed through pregnancy; however, definite risk is present. About one-fourth of pregnant patients with rheumatic heart disease will suffer complications, including pulmonary venous congestion of varying degrees, atrial fibrillation, severe hemoptosis, systemic and pulmonary emboli, and infective endocarditis.

The basic hemodynamic defect is mechanical obstruction to left ventricular filling by the stenosed mitral valve. This obstruction is exacerbated during pregnancy by the increased cardiac output and heart rate. Generally, patients who are asymptomatic or only mildly symptomatic before pregnancy [New York Heart Association (NYHA) Class I or II)], have few problems, although an occasional asymptomatic patient may develop severe or even lethal pulmonary edema during pregnancy.[30] Pain-induced tachycardia or excessive intravenous fluids may also produce pulmonary edema. Patients with more severe disease (Class III or IV) may have major complications, and if pregnancy continues in this group, then close monitoring is essential. During labor and delivery, invasive monitoring of intracardiac pressures with prompt utilization of preload reducers is mandatory (see Invasive Monitoring).

In all patients, close observation is recommended with special attention to weight gain and heart rate. It is difficult to monitor for signs of increasing pulmonary congestion, as mild dyspnea and hyperventilation occur normally in pregnancy.[31] Also, third heart sounds, basilar rales, increased jugular venous pulses, and peripheral edema frequently occur in normal pregnancy.[32] Thus, one must be especially sensitive to changes in symptoms and to weight gain and tachycardia above physiologic limits. Management and, in some cases, prevention of pulmonary congestion may be accomplished by salt restriction, daily bed rest, and, if needed, diuretics. Mitral valve replacement should be offered those patients with severe pulmonary edema or hemoptosis which occur prior to a time of possible delivery and do not promptly respond to medical management.[21] The more optimum situation, of course, is to apply maximum medical and surgical therapy before a planned pregnancy occurs.

Some authorities recommend prophylactic digitalization throughout pregnancy in patients with moderate mitral valve obstruction in order to protect against a rapid ventricular rate should atrial fibrillation develop.[4] This would seem a judicious preoperative procedure in patients with mitral valve obstruction as the hemodynamic changes and catecholamine release perioperatively may also precipitate atrial fibrillation. If cardiac decompensation occurs with the onset of atrial fibrillation, prompt cardioversion is indicated,[29] but if atrial fibrillation is tolerated, digoxin and quinidine may successfully convert the rhythm to sinus.

The intrapartum period is one of special danger. Increased venous return and pain-induced tachycardia may cause the barely-compromised circulation to quickly decompensate. Here, pain relief is very important, and epidural analgesia (if the patient is not anticoagulated) may be quite helpful. Vaginal delivery is considered optimal unless there are obstetrical indications for Caesarean section.

As in any patient with rheumatic valvular disease, penicillin prophylaxis should be continued throughout pregnancy, and broad spectrum antibiotics used in the perioperative period to protect against bacterial endocarditis.

Aortic Stenosis

This is a lesion only infrequently found in pregnant patients, with fewer than twenty-five cases reported.[33] Thus, it is difficult to formulate risk profiles or treatment regimens. Patients with mild to moderate aortic stenosis tolerate pregnancy relatively well,[21] but if cerebral symptoms, severe dyspnea, or angina pectoris develop, consideration should be given to interruption of the pregnancy in the first trimester, or aortic valve replacement if encountered later in pregnancy. Unfortunately, both procedures are associated with considerable maternal and fetal morbidity.[33]

Regurgitant Valve Lesions

Chronic mitral regurgitation and aortic regurgitation are generally well tolerated during pregnancy, and the cardiovascular system of the majority of these patients can cope with the increase in cardiac output unless the heart is barely compensated prior to pregnancy.[21] General measures of weight control and attention to blood pressure should guarantee a reasonably uneventful pregnancy. On the other hand, acute mitral regurgitation secondary to ruptured chordae tendinae might well lead to cardiac decompensation and pulmonary congestion. Also, the major cause of ruptured chordae tendinae is endocarditis, which must be carefully sought and treated.[34]

Prosthetic Heart Valves

Since the first prosthetic heart valve was implanted in the descending aorta in 1952,[35] countless people have benefited from this procedure—including many women still in their reproductive years. The first report of a term pregnancy in a patient with a prosthetic valve was as recent as 1966,[36] but numerous successful pregnancies have been reported since that time. Some authorities suggest that less risk is involved in patients with aortic valves as opposed to those with mitral valves, but this may only reflect the greater number of patients with mitral valves taking anticoagulation therapy. Although patients with mitral valve prostheses tend to have a lower fixed cardiac output and a subnormal rise in cardiac output with exercise,[37] most tolerate the hemodynamic load of pregnancy easily and without excessive hazard.[38] Multiple prosthetic valves in the same patient increase the chance for major complications.[39] This is probably also related to the increasing incidence of anticoagulation therapy, plus the greater severity of organic heart disease.

Generally, the maternal mortality is low in patients with prosthetic heart valves and, as a rule, complications are related to thromboembolism. Patients in the NYHA functional Classes I and II are good candidates for safe and successful pregnancy, while patients in Classes III and IV have definite increased risks.

In past years, there was fear that hearts with prosthetic valves would be incapable of meeting the metabolic needs of the fetus[29]; this seldom, if ever, occurs. Rather, the major risks to the fetus are complications arising from the anticoagulation therapy instituted to protect the mother. In pregnancies not requiring anticoagulation, fetal survival is much improved.[40] (See discussion of anticoagulation below.) Tissue valves do not often necessitate anticoagulation when placed in the aortic position. Current recommendations for tissue mitral valve prostheses suggest anticoagulation only when complicated by atrial fibrillation, a significantly enlarged left atrium, or atrial thrombi.[41] Thus, in women who desire pregnancy, the choice of a tissue valve would seem optimal from the standpoint of fetal survival.

Pulmonary Hypertension

Severe pulmonary hypertension usually results from primary idiopathic pulmonary hypertension or the development of Eisenmenger's syndrome secondary to cardiac shunt lesions. Because these patients have fixed restrictions of their pulmonary blood flow and often have right-to-left intracardiac shunts, the physiologic changes of pregnancy (reduced systemic resistance and increased cardiac output) further stress an already compromised circulation. These patients have a very high mortality rate, greater than 50% in some series,[42] being at risk for sudden death throughout the gestational period, and particularly during the peripartum period. Morbidity can be roughly related to the severity of pulmonary hypertension.[43]

Surgery or Caesarean section may be particularly hazardous. For example, Caesarean section in the Eisenmenger's syndrome carries a mortality of 60% in the few reported cases,[44,45] although successful outcomes are reported.[46] Monitoring of systemic and pulmonary artery pressures in these patients is essential since major hemodynamic changes may occur with anesthesia or delivery. Epidural anesthesia is recommended because pain, valsalva, and venous dilatation are minimized with this form of anesthesia.[46,47] High concentration oxygen (high flow with rebreathing bag) may lessen so-called "fixed" pulmonary hypertension and decrease pulmonary shunt flow.[47] Oxygen should be offered preoperatively and postoperatively and as long as necessary for cardiovascular stability, as many patients may decompensate several days after delivery.[44] In fact, up to 40% of the mortality associated with Eisenmenger's syndrome occurs within one to seven days postpartum.[44,48]

Full-dose heparin anticoagulation before and after surgery or delivery has been widely recommended in patients with Eisenmenger's syndrome to protect against the high risk of pulmonary intravascular thrombosis.[29,44] However, some authorities feel that full-dose anticoagulation may actually contribute to maternal mortality.[49] Perhaps, a reasonable alternative would be to utilize mini-dose heparin until further data is available.

Systemic hypotension should be promptly reversed with vaso-pressors; otherwise, increased right-to-left shunting of blood may occur, which can lead to profound cyanosis.[50] If bradycardia occurs, insertion of a temporary pacemaker is indicated and may be life-saving.[50]

Tetralogy of Fallot

The most common cyanotic congenital lesion found in adults is tetralogy of Fallot. Seldom do women with tetralogy of Fallot have full-term pregnancies and, if they do, the offspring are usually small for gestational age.[51] The decline in systemic resistance during pregnancy increases the degree of maternal cyanosis by increasing the right-to-left shunting of blood through the ventricular septal defect. Maternal and fetal prognosis is proportional to the degree of maternal shunting, cyanosis, and the hemoglobin level.[29,52] If the maternal hematocrit is 65% or greater, over 75% of the pregnancies will terminate in spontaneous abortion or premature labor.[53,54]

The labile hemodynamic changes of the intrapartum period are especially hazardous, and most maternal deaths occur during this time.[29] Further decreases in peripheral vascular resistance result in even greater right-to-left shunting of venous blood. Decreased venous pressures may lead to decreased pulmonary blood flow, which also reduces total oxygenation. Thus, preload and afterload must be closely monitored. Elastic support stockings, delivery in the Sims position, volume replacement to maintain preload, and pressor agents to maintain systemic blood pressure have been utilized to optimize maternal and fetal survival.[29]

Coarctation of the Aorta

Coarctation of the aorta is reported to occur in between 1 in 1,000 and 1 in 3,000 women.[43,55] The incidence of associated problems in pregnancy has decreased because of earlier diagnosis and repair, and there does not appear to be a risk in pregnancy in patients who have had coarctation repair or who have uncomplicated coarctation of the aorta.[55-57] If, however, the patient has complicated coarctation, that is, coarctation with associated heart defects (bicuspid aortic valve, ventricular septal defect, or patent ductus arteriosis), then her risk of congestive heart failure, rupture of the aorta, dissecting aneurysm, or infective endocarditis is much greater.[57,58] Many feel that pregnancy is contraindicated in patients with "complicated" coarctation and recommend therapeutic abortion in those seen in the first trimester.[58] Successful surgical correction of coarctation of the aorta has been accomplished during pregnancy, but most authorities recommend medical management unless serious complications arise.[57] Coarctation of the aorta discovered during pregnancy should generally be repaired postpartum.

Although labor and delivery do not seem to be a time of as high a risk as was once believed,[29] adequate analgesia is important during labor to decrease the maternal bearing-down efforts. Epidural analgesia followed by vaginal forceps delivery in the second stage of labor is recommended.[56,59]

Peripartum Cardiomyopathy

A condition of unknown etiology, peripartum cardiomyopathy, presents a wide spectrum of clinical disease with a maternal mortality rate of 30 to 60%.[30] Those patients who survive seem to be at great risk for recurrence in subsequent pregnancies; therefore, further pregnancies should be strongly advised against.[60] The clinical manifestation of this disorder is essentially that of severe congestive heart failure, and management should be directed toward aggressive therapy of the heart failure.

Congestive Heart Failure

Congestive heart failure is a serious risk factor for problems during pregnancy, with maternal mortality varying directly with cardiac reserve. Thus, patients in NYHA functional Classes I and II have a mortality rate of less than 1%, while those in Classes III and IV have a mortality of between 5 and 10%.[29]

Patients with congestive heart failure and particularly patients with peripartum cardiomyopathy are prone to develop pulmonary emboli secondary to the hypercoagulabile state of pregnancy, venous stasis, and relative immobility.[61] Thus, subcutaneous minidose heparin is highly recommended.[61,62] Invasive monitoring of patients with severe congestive heart failure with a Swan-Ganz catheter during labor and delivery is requisite for optimal management. Only then may diuretics and afterload reduction agents be properly utilized to decrease the heart's hemodynamic burden by skillful manipulation of the peripheral vascular resistance and wedge pressure.

Contraindications to Pregnancy

Certain cardiovascular lesions place the pregnant patient and fetus at substantial risk for major morbidity and mortality (see Table 4). Severe pulmonary hypertension, cyanotic heart disease, prior episodes of peripartum cardiomyopathy, congestive heart failure, and coarctation of the aorta usually represent unacceptable

Table 4
Cardiovascular Disease and Pregnancy

Cardiovascular Lesion	Maternal Mortality	Risk
Septal defects	Nil	
Patent ductus	if corrected	Minimal
Simple coarctation	or	
Rheumatic disease	Class I or II	
Mitral Stenosis		
Class III or IV	5	
Atrial fibrillation	15	Moderate
Congestive Heart Failure		to
Class III or IV	5 to 10	Severe
Tetralogy of Fallot	10	
Complicated coarctation	20	
Eisenmenger's Syndrome	33	
Marfan's Syndrome	50	
Primary Pulmonary	50	Severe
Hypertension		
Peripartum cardiomyopathy	30 to 60	

risk. The decision to proceed with a pregnancy in the presence of these lesions is a difficult one, and serious consideration should be given to abortion as a preferred alternative in the first trimester of pregnancy. If the patient is past the first trimester, then abortion itself may be dangerous,[43,61] and probably meticulous medical, surgical, and obstetrical management gives the best hope of maternal and fetal survival.

Anticoagulation During Pregnancy

The risk of thromboembolism in pregnancy is increased because of a rise in the levels of coagulation factors II, VII, VIII, and X.[62] There is some evidence to suggest an increase in the number and adhesiveness of circulating platelets, and significant depression of the fibrinolytic system occurs.[62] All of these changes result in a hypercoagulable state during normal pregnancy.

In patients with chronic atrial fibrillation, there is an increase in maternal morbidity, and anticoagulation should be strongly considered.[29] Both prosthetic heart valves and thrombophlebitis can lead to serious complications in the thrombotic milieu of pregnancy, especially without concomitant anticoagulation therapy. In nonpregnant patients with prosthetic heart valves, the value of anticoagulation in preventing emboli is well established.[63,64] There are scant data regarding the incidence of embolism in non-anticoagulated pregnant patients with prosthetic heart valves[65]; however, Limet and Grondin[66] have reviewed the literature and found that six of twenty-four patients with mechanical valves, but without anticoagulation, had embolic complications. Numerous studies attest to a reduced embolic rate in anticoagulated pregnant patients with prosthetic heart valves.[65-67]

Venous thromboembolism remains one of the chief causes of maternal deaths.[62,68] Extensive data on the comparative risks of treated and untreated thrombophlebitis show that the death rate of untreated antepartum thromboembolism is at least 15%, whereas in patients with anticoagulants, the mortality is less than 1%.[68-70]

Anticoagulant therapy, on the other hand, leads to an array of iatrogenic problems. Coumarin derivatives readily cross the placenta and have long been recognized as leading to increased fetal morbidity and mortality by predisposing to stillbirth and fetal hemorrhage.

A specific teratogenic effect of coumarin derivative was recognized in 1973[67] and has been termed the Warfarin Embryopathy Snydrome or Fetal Warfarin Syndrome.[71] A constellation of malformations, including midface hypoplasia, nasal hypoplasia, stippling of the bony epiphyses of the axial skeleton, premature delivery, and respiratory distress secondary to small nasal airway or prematurity may occur when the fetus is exposed to coumarin derivatives during first trimester, especially between the sixth and ninth week of gestation.[71]

Serious central nervous system malformations thought to be related to the use of coumarin derivatives in the second and third trimester may occur.[71,72] These include optic atrophy resulting in blindness and faulty brain growth with attendant mental retardation, spasticity, seizure, deafness, and developmental retardation. Sequelae of these developmental failures are usually serious and have resulted in significant personal and societal burdens.

No precise figure for the risk of development of the Fetal Warfarin Syndrome is available, but the risk of malformations from first trimester oral anticoagulant exposure has been estimated to be as high as 15% to 20%.[73]

How coumarin derivatives interfere with fetal organogenesis is not known. Postulates have included focal microhemorrhages and deficiency of vitamin K-dependent protein production.[72]

Hall and associates[71] recently reviewed all published cases of pregnancy in which coumarin derivatives were administered. They found approximately one-sixth of pregnancies resulted in abortion or stillbirth, one-sixth ended in abnormal newborn infants with malformations related to either embryogenesis or organögenesis and, at most, two-thirds were normal (Table 5).

Heparin would appear to be the appropriate drug for anticoagulation during pregnancy since it does not pass the placental barrier and, thus, no teratogenic effects have been ascribed to it. However, several problems are associated with its use. A review of the small number of reports describing osteoporosis and bone fractures resulting from heparin use reveals that dosage and length of treatment are determinants of its development.[75–77] Osteoporosis has not been reported in patients receiving less than 10,000 units per day of heparin, regardless of the duration of therapy. If

Table 5
Outcome of Anticoagulant Use During Pregnancy[71]

	Coumarins	Heparin
Abortion or stillbirths	1/6	1/8
Abnormal or premature infants	1/6	1/5
Normal infants	2/3	2/3
Maternal complications	Minimal	Minimal

Greater number of normal newborns with heparin, but offset by increase in maternal complications

greater dosages are given, then spinal fractures have occurred with as little as four months' usage. Squires and Pinch[77] recently reported the occurrence of osteoporosis and a thoracic vertebrae compression fracture in a pregnant patient treated because of thrombophletitis with subcutaneous heparin for approximately 130 days.

Heparin-induced thrombocytopenia is seen mainly in patients on long-term parental heparin, but may be seen after less than one week of therapy.[78-81] The incidence and seriousness of this immunologic reaction awaits further study, but lethal hemorrhage has been reported.[81] Recent evidence suggests that porcine-derived heparin may induce only minimal thrombocytopenia.[82]

A review[71] of 135 published cases involving the use of heparin during pregnancy noted a maternal complication rate related to antepartum hemorrhage of approximately 10%. Many of these were serious in nature, and several resulted in maternal and fetal death. Fetal morbidity and mortality were particularly high, with one-eighth of the pregnancies ending in stillbirth, one-fifth premature, and approximately two-thirds having a normal outcome. Why heparin should jeopardize pregnancy is not known, but its chelating ability might indirectly affect the fetus.[71]

The experience with platelet-affecting drugs used for anticoagulation during pregnancy is minimal. Dipyridamole's successful but limited use has been reported in pregnancies in which the patient had mitral or aortic mechanical valves.[83,84] More extensive experience must be gained with these drugs before their use can be recommended in patients with prosthetic heart valves.[85] Antiplatelet drugs have not been helpful in therapy of venous thromboembolism in the nonpregnant patient and, thus, would not be expected to be of value in the pregnant patient with thrombophlebitis.

Thus, no ideal anticoagulant for use in pregnancy exists. Current recommendations attempt to skirt the major adverse effects of both drugs.[70,86] Utilizing heparin as the first trimester anticoagulant of choice eliminates the possibility of the Fetal Warfarin Syndrome, and maternal hemorrhage associated with heparin is low during the first trimester. Therefore, for pregnancies in patients with prosthetic heart valves or as initial treatment for thrombophletitis, heparin has wide support. No data exist on optimum dosages of heparin, but most studies report adequate anticoagulation with either 10,000 units subcutaneously bid or 5,000 subcutaneously tid.[86–88]

Coumarin derivatives may cause fetal abnormalities during the second and third trimesters; however, most authorities suggest that they be used for anticoagulation during this period and until near term. The minimum time necessary for fetal coagulation parameters to return to normal after discontinuing coumarin derivatives is unknown. Hirsh[70] showed that if coumarin were stopped three weeks before labor, neonatal coagulation was normal at delivery, and others have confirmed the clinical value of substituting heparin for coumarin in the late stage of pregnancy.[66,89] By this method, fetal and placental hemorrhage secondary to trauma during labor and delivery can be avoided.

Thus, present recommendations (Table 6) are to use subcutaneous heparin during the first trimester. Warfarin should then be given between the 13th and 37th weeks of pregnancy, after which heparin should be administered until labor begins. Heparin should

Table 6
Recommendations for Anticoagulation During Pregnancy

1st trimester—subcutaneous heparin, 10,000 μ bid or 5,000 μ tid
13th to 37th week—warfarin by mouth
37th week to labor—subcutaneous heparin
Postpartum—subcutaneous heparin 4 to 6 hours after delivery if uterus is empty, fully contracted, and not actively bleeding
    Restart warfarin by mouth and wean heparin

---

be reintroduced four to six hours after delivery if the uterus is empty, fully contracted, and not actively bleeding. Warfarin can be restarted any time after complete hemostasis occurs. Warfarin use by the mother who is breast-feeding is not contraindicated, as it is not known to be secreted into breast milk.[90]

The above regimen, though safer to the mother than elimination of all anticoagulants, and safer for the fetus than continuous coumarin use, still poses some risk and is logistically difficult to utilize. There are no large series reporting maternal and fetal morbidity and mortality using the method. Several small studies report excellent results,[69,70] but greater experience must be gained before this method can be pronounced as safe. Its major problem involves timing; plans for both conception and delivery must be thoroughly discussed and understood by the patient. Pregnancies in patients with artificial heart valves should be planned particularly well in advance so that heparin can be utilized during the first trimester. Patients on coumarin drugs are more apt to have premature deliveries and, thus, may not be weaned from oral anticoagulants when their labor begins. This, unfortunately, increases hemorrhagic complications in the fetus as noted above, but there does not seem to be an increase in blood loss during pregnancy or delivery in women receiving oral anticoagulants.[91]

Because of the manifold problems associated with this complicated dosage schedule, many practitioners are utilizing subcutaneous heparin alone throughout pregnancy. This has been successful in some small, poorly documented reports,[87,92,93] but, unfortunately, studies with large numbers of patients and carefully enumerated complications have yet to be published.

Scant data are available on pregnancies involving patients with tissue valves.[42] It would appear, however, that if anticoagulation is not required prior to pregnancy, little increased danger of embolism during pregnancy exists in these patients. Indeed, young women who require prosthetic heart valve insertion and who desire subsequent pregnancy should possibly be offered a tissue valve even though people in this younger age group have more frequent tissue valve dysfunction.[94]

At any rate, the maternal and fetal risks of anticoagulation during pregnancy should be thoroughly explained to any woman of child-bearing age who has or is about to undergo valve replacement or who develops thrombophlebitis during pregnancy.

Use of Drugs During Pregnancy

Drug use during pregnancy should be kept to the absolute minimum, but numerous drugs may be and should be used if there is a clear and specific indication.

Digitalis

Digitalis has a mild uterine stimulant action in vitro[95] and at one time was felt to decrease the length of labor[96]; however, further studies have cast doubt on any oxytocic activity in vivo.[23,95] Although considerable evidence for transplacental movement exists, there have been no reported teratogenic effects of the cardiac glycosides.[23,97]

Thiazide Diuretics

These have been and are the preferred drugs for treating essential hypertension during pregnancy, but they offer no benefit in the treatment of pregnancy-induced hypertension (PIH).[97] They can, in fact, be detrimental, as further reduction of an already reduced blood volume may occur. No specific fetal problems are known except for a possible association with neonatal thrombocytopenia.[97,98]

Furosemide (Lasix)

Very little data are available on the use of oral furosemide for long-term use in pregnancy. If a fast-acting, powerful, intravenous diuretic is needed for either preload reduction or diuresis, then furosemide is probably the drug of choice.[24]

Methyldopa (Aldomet)

This drug is effective in the control of hypertension during pregnancy and has become the drug of choice for treatment of essential hypertension.[99] Methyldopa seems to be well tolerated by the fetus, which accounts in part for its popularity.

Hydralazine (Apresoline)

Given by mouth, hydralazine is an effective agent for control of PIH. It decreases maternal blood pressure while preserving uterine blood flow.[97] Intravenous hydralazine is a powerful antihypertensive agent, but cannot be as easily titrated as other available agents.

Nitroprusside (Nipride)

This is an excellent drug for acute reduction of preload and afterload, and is the drug of choice in nonpregnant patients for these hemodynamic maneuvers. A recent report[100] documenting cyanide levels in the fetus after administration of nitroprusside gives cause for concern, and until further data are available, cautious use of this drug during pregnancy is in order.

Nitroglycerin

Intravenous nitroglycerin has recently become widely available and, generally, is an excellent drug for acute control of elevated preload or afterload. At the present time, this is probably the drug of choice for immediate control of severe hypertension during pregnancy.[101]

Sympathomimetic Drugs

Multiple sympathomimetic drugs which work predominantly by alpha agonist activity have been employed to increase the pressure in the arterial circuit. Extensive reviews are available,[97] but there seems to be little practical advantage to any one of these agents or for their specific indication in any clinical situation.

Dopamine (Intropin)

Having documented efficacy in the management of anesthesia-induced spinal/hypotension[102] dopamine has also been successfully used in the treatment of hypotension of diverse etiologies. It increases the maternal blood pressure and seems to maintain uterine blood flow,[103] but sparse data are available.

Propranolol (Inderal)

Propranolol increases uterine tone and has been used clinically to correct dysfunctional labor.[104] Prolonged use of the drug, however, has led to several adverse fetal effects. Prolonged increase in uterine tone has been thought responsible for intrauterine growth retardation, resulting in low birth-weight infants.[105] There is also evidence that propranolol interferes with the fetal response to hypoxia, which has resulted in cases of neonatal respiratory depression.[106,107] Sustained postdelivery bradycardia and hypoglycemia are additional vexing problems associated with maternal use of this drug.[106,107] Although there have been no teratogenic problems associated with its usage, propranolol should be prescribed judiciously.

In spite of these side-effects, propranolol should be used throughout pregnancy in patients with Marfan's syndrome to decrease the blood pressure and pulse pressure wave in hopes of improving the dismal maternal mortality statistics in this condition.[4] Propranolol is also quite properly used in thyroid storm to control the cardiovascular effects of excessive thyroxin.[108,109]

When propranolol is used chronically, one must be cognizant of its side effects and closely monitor the infant's respiratory status, heart rate, and blood glucose during the post-delivery phase. Recent evidence suggests that maternal ingestion after delivery should not contraindicate breast-feeding, as the breast milk drug concentration is quite small.[110]

Metoprolol (Lopressor)

The results of metoprolol use in PIH have been recently documented.[111] Although giving excellent control of PIH and seeming to cause fewer infant side. effects than propranolol, unreserved recommendations for its use will have to await more extensive study.

Quinidine

The antiarrhythmic drug of choice during pregnancy, no major fetal or neonatal problems from quinidine have been reported.[23,112]

Disopyramide (Norpace)

Disopyramide is pharmacologically similar to quinidine. Although the experience with this drug during pregnancy is limited, it should be used with caution at the present time because a recent report has documented its possible production of hypertonic uterine contractions.[113]

Procainamide (Pronestyl)

Although used successfully to control various cardiac arrhythmias during pregnancy, little actual data on the use of procainamide in this setting have been reported

Electrical Cardioversion During Pregnancy

Although cardioversion is now frequently utilized, little information concerning its application during pregnancy exists, and fewer than 15 cases have been reported.[114] None of the reported cases has resulted in major fetal problems, even though shocks of up to 300 joules have been delivered to the mother. However, fetal dysrhythmias have been reported following cardioversion, and monitoring of the fetal ECG is recommended.[114] Certainly, if the maternal safety is jeopardized, immediate cardioversion is indicated.

Invasive Monitoring

Insertion of a Swan-Ganz catheter is a relatively benign procedure in experienced hands and is indicated for optimal management in women with severe toxemia (who invariably have contracted intravascular volumes antepartum),[113–115] congestive heart failure of any etiology, septic shock, adult respiratory distress syndrome, or hypotension of any etiology.[115–117] Intraoperative hemodynamic monitoring is not indicated in a normal pregnancy, but in patients with potentially abnormal hemodynamics, intracardiac pressures may be or become abnormal, especially during the stress of surgery or the pain of delivery. Catecholamine release during surgical induction, together with the hemodynamic changes of supine position (as outlined above), may cause major changes in right ventricular or left ventricular end-diastolic pressure. In order to quickly and properly respond to these changes, pulmonary artery and wedge pressures must be closely monitored. Only then can one make proper choices concerning administration of diuretic therapy, volume expanders, afterload reduction agents, or pressor agents.

Bacterial Endocarditis Prophylaxis

The proper role of prophylactic antibiotics in the prevention of bacterial endocarditis is yet to be determined.[21] The well known recommendations of the American Heart Association have never been subjected to systematic evaluation in man.

There are few published studies of bacteremia during pregnancy.[118–120] The best study reveals a bacteremia frequency of approximately 5%,[120] a rather small percentage, considering that other reports document a frequency of transient bacteremia as high as 25% after brushing one's teeth![121,122] The American Heart Association does not recommend prophylaxis for uncomplicated vaginal deliveries. Nevertheless, the force of custom dictates that patients with rheumatic or congenital heart disease (except, perhaps, the secundum type ASD[123]) and, more so, those with prosthetic heart valves be given bacterial endocarditis prophylaxis. Current recommendations for surgery (except dental and upper

Table 7
Recommended Bacterial Endocarditis Prophylaxis[124]

Aqueous Penicillin G 2 Million U IM Or IV
Or
Ampicillin 1.0 GM IM Or IV
Plus
Gentamicin 1.5 MG/KG IM Or IV
Or
Streptomycin 1.0 GM IM

Give prior to delivery or preoperatively, then two additional doses every 8 to 12 hours

respiratory procedures) are found in Table 7.[124] The initial dosage should be given at the beginning of labor. Controversy exists on the optimal length of prophylaxis, but recent recommendations rarely favor greater than twenty-four hours of antibiotic coverage.[24]

Prevention of Conception for the Woman with Heart Disease

Effective birth control is a major problem for women with cardiac disorders who wish or need to avoid pregnancy. The rhythm method, spermicidal foams, condoms, or diaphragms all have a high failure rate. The only two contraceptive methods with high protection rates are the oral steroids (birth control pill) and the intrauterine device (IUD).

There are several deleterious effects of the estrogen component of the oral steroid contraceptive, including an increased thromboembolic rate, frequent hypertensive responses, fluid and water retention, and various degrees of increased hyperlipidemia.[125–127] Oral contraceptives containing 50 μg or less of estrogen are associated with fewer complications and are probably reasonable for use in those patients with mild cardiac disease.[125,127] The progesterone component of the birth control pills does not seem to have any adverse cardiovascular effects, [126,127] and if contraceptives consisting solely of progestins are available in the future, these may be suitable for cardiac patients.[128]

The IUD is associated with two major problems in the cardiac patient. There is a small risk of a vagal reaction occurring during the insertion of the device, with resultant transient hypotension which may be dangerous, depending on the type of cardiac disorder.[129–131] This occurs much less frequently with small IUDs (less than 1% with a CU-7).[132]

Another potential problem is a transient bacteremia occurring during the insertion of the IUD, which could lead to bacterial endocarditis. Studies, however, have showed bacteremia to rarely, if ever, occur during insertion or removal of an IUD,[133] and Mishell et al.[134] have documented that the endometrium is sterile in 80% of patients within forty-eight hours of insertion of an IUD. These findings plus the additional insurance of IV antibiotics for bacterial endocarditis prophylaxis prior to IUD insertion suggest a very small risk for development of bacterial endocarditis. The IUD is, therefore, an excellent method of contraception in the young female with cardiac disease who does not desire surgical sterilization .

References

1. Hibbard LT: Maternal mortality due to cardiac disease. *Clin Obstet Gynecol* 18:27, 1975.
2. Ehrenfeld EN, Brezizinski A, Braon K, et al.: Heart disease in pregnancy. *Obstet Gynecol* 23:363, 1964.
3. Metcalfe J: Rheumatic heart disease in pregnancy. *Clin Obstet Gynecol* 11:1010, 1968.
4. Metcalfe J, Ueland K: The heart and pregnancy. In: Hurst JW (Ed.): *The Heart.* New York: McGraw-Hill, 1980.
5. Chesley LC, Duffus GM: Posture and apparent plasma volume in late pregnancy. *J Obstet Gynaecol Brit Commonw* 78:406, 1971.
6. Talwar KK, Waki PL: Pregnancy with heart disease. *Jr Assoc Phys Ind* 27:995, 1979.
7. Kerr MG: The mechanical effects of the gravid uterus in late pregnancy. *J Obstet Gynaecol Brit Commonw* 72:543, 1965.
8. Courtney L: Supine hypotension syndrome during Caesarean section. *Brit Med J* 1:797, 1970.
9. Bieniarz J, Crottegini JJ, Curuchet E, et al.: Aortocaval compression by the uterus in late human pregnancy. *Am J Obstet Gynecol* 100:203, 1968.
10. Laird-Meeter K, Van De Ley G, Bom TH, et al.: Cardiocirculatory adjustments during pregnancy—An echocardiographic study. *Clin Cardiol* 2:328, 1979.
11. Burwell CS, Metcalfe J: *Heart Disease and Pregnancy: Physiology and Management.* Boston: Little, Brown, and Churchill, 1958.

12. Hytten FE, Thomson AM: Water and electrolytes in pregnancy. *Brit Med Bull* 24:15, 1968.
13. Chesley LC: Plasma and red cell volumes during pregnancy. *Am J Obstet Gynecol* 112:440, 1972.
14. Bader RA, Bader ME, Rose OJ, Braunwald E: Haemodynamics at rest and during exercise in normal pregnancy as studied by cardiac catheterization. *J Clin Investigation* 34:1524, 1953.
15. Ueland K, Parer JT: Effects of estrogen on the cardiovascular system of the ewe. *Am J Obstet Gynecol* 96:400, 1966.
16. Bryant EE, Douglas BH, Asburn AD: Circulatory changes following prolactin administration. *Am J Obstet Gynecol* 115:53, 1973.
17. King TM, Whitehorn WV, Reeves, B: Effects of estrogen on composition and function of cardiac muscle. *Am J Physiol* 196:1282, 1959.
18. Wood JE: Cardiovascular effects of oral contraceptives. *Mod Concepts Cardiovasc Dis* 41:37, 1972.
19. Csapo A: Actomyocin formation by estrogen action. *Am J Physiol* 162:406, 1950.
20. Hytten FE, Thompson AM: Water and electrolytes in pregnancy. *Brit Med Bull* 24:15, 1958.
21. Perloff JK: Pregnancy and cardiovascular disease. In: Braunwald E (Ed.): *Heart Disease—A Textbook of Cardiovascular Medicine.* Philadelphia: WB Saunders Co., 1980.
22. Ueland K, Hansen JM: Maternal cardiovascular dynamics. II. Posture and uterine contractions. *Am J Obstet Gynecol* 103:1, 1969.
23. Metcalfe J, Ueland K: Maternal cardiovascular adjustment to pregnancy. *Prog Cardiovasc Dis* 16:363, 1974.
24. Ueland K: Intrapartum management of the cardiac patient. *Clin Perinat* 8:155, 1981.
25. Ostheimer GW, Alper MH: Intrapartum anesthetic management of the pregnant patient with heart disease. *Clin Obstet Gynecol* 18:81, 1975.
26. Pritchard JA: Changes in the blood volume during pregnancy and delivery. *Anesthesiology* 26:393, 1965.
27. Ueland K: Maternal cardiovascular dynamics. VII. Intrapartum blood volume changes. *Am J Obstet Gynecol* 126:671, 1976.
28. Ueland K, Hansen JM: Maternal cardiovascular dynamics. III. Labor and delivery under local and caudal analgesia. *Am J Obstet Gynecol* 103:8, 1969.
29. Ueland K: Cardiovascular diseases complicating pregnancy. *Clin Obstet Gynecol* 21:430, 1978.
30. Szekely P, Snaith L: *Heart Disease and Pregnancy.* Edinburgh & London: Churchill Livingstone, 1974.
31. Milne JA, Howie AD, Pack AI: Dyspnoea during normal pregnancy. *Brit J Obstet Gynaecol* 85:260, 1978.
32. Cutforth R, MacDonald CB: Heart sounds and murmurs in pregnancy. *Am Heart J* 71:740, l966.
33. Arias F, Pineda J: Aortic stenosis and pregnancy. *J Reprod Med* 20:229, 1978.

34. Reichak N, Shelburne JD, Perloff JK: Clinical aspects of rheumatic valvular disease. *Prog Cardiovasc Dis* 15:491, 1973.
35. Hufnagel CA, Harvey WP: The surgical correction of aortic regurgitation: Preliminary report. *Bull Georgetown Univ Med Center* 6:60, 1953.
36. DiSaia PJ: Pregnancy and delivery of a patient with a Starr-Edwards mitral valve prosthesis: Report of a case. *Obstet Gynecol* 28:469, 1966.
37. McHenry MM, Smaloff EA, Davey TB, et al.: Hemodynamic results with full-flow orifice prosthetic valves. *Circulation* 35 (suppl):24, 1967.
38. Hultgren H, Hubis H, Shumway N: Cardiac function following mitral valve replacement. *Am Heart J* 75:302, 1968.
39. Lutz DJ, Noller KL, Spittell JA Jr, et al.: Pregnancy and its complications following cardiac valve prostheses. *Am J Obstet Gynecol* 131:460, 1978.
40. Harrison EC, Roschke EJ: Pregnancy in patients with cardiac valve prostheses. *Clin Obstet Gynecol* 18:107, 1975.
41. Beadle EM Jr, Luepker RV, Williams PP: Pregnancy in a patient with porcine valve xenografts. *Am Heart J* 98:510, 1979.
42. McCaffrey RM, Dunn LJ: Primary pulmonary hypertension in pregnancy. *Obstet Gynecol Surv* 19:567, 1964.
43. Ueland K, Metcalfe J: Heart disease in pregnancy. *Clin Perinat* 1:349, 1974.
44. Gleicher N, Midwall J, Hochberger D, Joffin H: Eisenmenger's syndrome and pregnancy. *Obstet Gynecol Surv* 34:721, 1979.
45. Lumley J, Whitman JG, Morgan M: General anesthesia in the presence of Eisenmenger's syndrome. *Anesth Analg* 56:543, 1977.
46. Spinnato JA, Kraynack BJ, Cooper MW: Eisenmenger's syndrome in pregnancy: Epidural anesthesia for elective Cesarean section. *N Engl J Med* 304:1215, 1981.
47. Midwall J, Jaffin H, Herman MV, Kupersmith J: Shunt flow and pulmonary hemodynamics during labor and delivery in the Eisenmenger syndrome. *Am J Cardiol* 42:299, 1978.
48. Sinnenberg RJ Jr: Pulmonary hypertension in pregnancy. *Southern Med J* 73:1529, 1980.
49. Pitts JA, Crosby WM, Basta LL: Eisenmenger's syndrome in pregnancy. *Am Heart J* 93:321, 1977.
50. Arias F: Maternal death in a patient with Eisenmenger's syndrome. *Obstet Gynecol* 50:76, 1977.
51. Batson GA: Cyanotic congenital heart disease and pregnancy. *J Obstet Gynaecol Brit Commonw* 81:549, 1974.
52. Meyer EC, Tulsky AS, Sigmann P, Silber EN: Pregnancy in the presence of Tetralogy of Fallot. *Am J Cardiol* 14:874, 1964.
53. Neill CA, Swanson S: Outcome of pregnancy in congenital heart disease. (Abstr) *Circulation* 24:1003, 1973.
54. Cannell DE, Vernon CP: Congenital heart disease and pregnancy. *Am J Obstet Gynecol* 85:744, 1963.
55. Pritchard JA: Co-arctation of the aorta and pregnancy. *Obstet Gynecol Surv* 8:775, 1953.

56. Goodwin JF: Pregnancy and coarctation of the aorta. *Clin Obstet Gynecol* 4:645, 1961.
57. Deal K, Wooley CF: Coarctation of the aorta and pregnancy. *Ann Intern Med* 78:706, 1973.
58. Ueland K: Pregnancy and cardiovascular disease. *Med Clin of N A* 61:17, 1977.
59. Benny PS, Prasad J, Macvicar J: Pregnancy and coarctation of the aorta—Case report. *Brit J Obstet Gynaecol* 87:1159, 1980.
60. Demakis JG, Rahimtoola SH: Peripartum cardiomyopathy. *Circulation* 44:964, 1971.
61. Goodwin JF: Peripartal heart disease. *Clin Obstet Gynecol* 18:125, 1975.
62. Howie PW: Thromboembolism. *Clin Obstet Gynaecol* 4:397, 1977.
63. Gadboys HL, Litwak RS, Niemetz J, Wisch N: Role of anticoagulants in preventing embolization from prosthetic heart valves. *JAMA* 202:134, 1967.
64. Limet R, Lepage G, Grondin CM: Thromboembolic complications with the cloth-covered Starr-Edwards aortic prosthesis in patients not receiving anticoagulants. *Ann Thorac Surg* 23:529, 1977.
65. Buxbaum A, Aygen MM, Shahin W, et al.: Pregnancy in patients with prosthetic heart valves. *Chest* 59:639, 1971.
66. Limet R, Grondin CM: Cardiac valve prostheses, anticoagulation, and pregnancy. *Ann Thorac Surg* 23:337, 1977.
67. Tejani N: Anticoagulant therapy with cardiac valve prosthesis during pregnancy. *Obstet Gynecol* 42:785, 1973.
68. Hirsh J, Cade JF, Gallus AS: Anticoagulants in pregnancy: A review of indications and complications. *Am Heart J* 83:301, 1972.
69. Finnerty JJ, MacKay BR: Antepartum thrombophlebitis and pulmonary embolism. Report of a case and review of the literature. *Obstet Gynecol* 19:405, 1962.
70. Hirsh J, Cade JF, O'Sullivan EF: Clinical experience with anticoagulant therapy during pregnancy. *Brit Med J* 1:270, 1970.
71. Hall JG, Pauli RM, Wilson KM: Maternal and fetal sequelae of anticoagulation during pregnancy. *Am J Med* 63:122, 1980.
72. Stevenson RE, Burton OM, Ferlauto GJ, Taylor HA: Hazards of oral anticoagulants during pregnancy. *JAMA* 243:1549, 1980.
73. Fillmore SJ, McDevitt E: Effects of coumarin compounds on the fetus. *Ann Intern Med* 73:731, 1970.
74. Griffith GC, Nichols G Jr, Asher JD, Flanagan B: Heparin osteoporosis. *JAMA* 193:91, 1965.
75. Miller WH, DeWolfe VG: Osteoporosis resulting from heparin therapy. *Cleveland Clinic Quarterly* 33:31, 1966.
76. Sackler JP, Lin L: Heparin-induced osteoporosis. *Brit J Radiol* 46:548, 1973.
77. Squires JW, Pinch LW: Heparin-induced spinal fractures. *JAMA* 241:2417, 1979.
78. Gollub S, Ulin AW: Heparin-induced thrombocytopenia, *Man J Lab Clin Med* 59:430, 1962.

79. Bell W, Tomasulo P, Alving B, et al.: Thrombocytopenia occuring during the administration of heparin. *Ann Intern Med* 85:155, 1976.

80. Nelson J, Lerner R, Goldstein R, et al.: Heparin-induced thrombocytopenia. *Arch Intern Med* 138:548, 1978.

81. Kapsch DN, Adelstein EH, Rhodes GR, Silver D: Heparin-induced thrombocytopenia, thrombosis, and hemorrhage. *Surgery* 86:148, 1979.

82. Powers PJ, Cuthbert D, Hirsh J: Thrombocytopenia found uncommonly during heparin therapy. *JAMA* 241:2396, 1979.

83. Ahmad R, Rajah SM, Mearns AJ, Deverall PB: Dipyridamole in successful management of pregnant woman with prosthetic heart valve. (Letter) *Lancet* Dec 25, 1976.

84. Biale Y, Cantor A, Lewenthal H, Gueron M: The course of pregnancy in patients with artificial heart valves treated with dipyridamole. *Int J Gynaecol Obstet* 18:128, 1980.

85. Taguchi K: Pregnancy in patients with a prosthetic heart valve. *Surg Gynecol Obstet* 145:206, 1977.

86. Anticoagulants and heart valve replacement in pregnancy. Editorial. *Brit Med J* 1:1047, 1977.

87. Spearing G, Fraser I, Turner G, Dixon G: Long-term self-administered subcutaneous heparin in pregnancy. *Brit Med J* 1:1457, 1978.

88. Venous thromboembolism and anticoagulants in pregnancy. Editorial. *Brit Med J* 4:421, 1975.

89. Ramsay DM: Thromboembolism in pregnancy. *Obstet Gynecol* 45:129, 1975.

90. Orme ML'E, Lewis PJ, DeSwiet M, et al.: May mothers given warfarin breast-feed their infants? *Brit Med J* 1:1564, 1977.

91. Lutz DJ, Noller KL, Spittell JA Jr, et al.: Pregnancy and its complications following cardiac valve prosthesis. *Am J Obstet Gynecol* 131:460, 1978.

92. Bonnar J: Venous Thrombo-embolism and pregnancy. In: *Recent Advances in Obstetrics and Gynecology.* Boston: Little, Brown & Churchill, 1979.

93. Flessa HC, Glueck HI, Dritschilo A: Thromboembolic disorders in pregnancy: Pathophysiology, diagnosis and treatment with emphasis on heparin. *Clin Obstet Gynecol* 17(4):195, 1974.

94. Geha AS, Laks MS, Stansel HD Jr, et al.: Late failure of porcine valve heterografts in children. *J Thorac Cardiovasc Surg* 78:351, 1979.

95. Norris PR: The action of cardiac glycosides on the human uterus. *J Obstet Gynaecol Brit Commonw* 68:916, 1961.

96. Weaver JB, Pearson JF: Influence of digitalis on time of onset and duration of labour in women with cardiac disease. *Brit Med J* 3:519, 1973.

97. Brinkman CR III, Woods JR Jr: Effects of cardiovascular drugs during pregnancy. *Cardiovasc Med* 1:231, 1976.

98. Rodriguez SV: Neonatal thrombocytopenia associated with antepartum administration of thiazide drugs. *N Engl J Med* 270:881, 1964.

99. Treatment of moderate hypertension in pregnancy. Editoral. *Brit Med J* 280:1483, 1980.
100. Lewis PE, Cefalo RC, Naulty JS, et al.: Placental transfer and fetal toxicity of sodium nitroprusside. *Gynecol Invest* 8:46, 1977.
101. Snyder SW, Wheeler AS, James FM: The use of nitroglycerin to control severe hypertension of pregnancy during Cesarean section. *Anesthesiology* 51:563, 1979.
102. Cabalum T, Zugaib M, Lieb S, et al.: Effect of dopamine on hypotension induced by spinal anesthesia. *Am J Obstet Gynecol* 133:630, 1979.
103. Blanchard K, Dandavino A, Nuwayhid B, et al.: Systemic and uterine hemodynamic responses to dopamine in pregnant and non-pregnant sheep. *Am J Obstet Gynecol* 130:669, 1978.
104. Mitrani A, Oettinger M, Abinader EG, et al.: Use of propranolol in dysfunctional labor. *Brit J Obstet Gynaecol* 82:651, 1975.
105. Datta S, Kitzmiller JL, Ostheimer GW, et al.: Propranolol and parturition. *Obstet Gynecol* 51:577, 1978.
106. Gladstone GR, Hardof A, Gersony WM: Propranolol administration during pregnancy: Effects on the fetus. *J Pediatr* 86:962, 1975.
107. Habib A, McCarthy JS: Effects on the neonate of propranolol administered during pregnancy. *J Pediatr* 91:808, 1977.
108. Langer A, Hung CT, McA'Nulty JA, et al.: Adrenergic blockade: A new approach to hyperthyroidism during pregnancy. *Obstet Gynecol* 44:181, 1974.
109. Bullock JL, Harris RE, Young R: Treatment of thyrotoxicosis during pregnancy with propranolol. *Am J Obstet Gynecol* 121:242, 1975.
110. Bauer JH, Pope B, Zajicek J, Groshong T: Propranolol in human plasma and breast milk. *Am J Cardiol* 43:860, 1979.
111. Sandstrom B: Antihypertensive treatment with the adrenergic beta-receptor blocker metoprolol during pregnancy. *Gynecol Obstet Invest* 9:195, 1978.
112. Hill LM, Malkasian GD Jr: The use of quinidine sulfate throughout pregnancy. *Obstet Gynecol* 54:366, 1979.
113. Leonard RF, Braun TE, Levy AM: Initiation of uterine contractions by disopyramide during pregnancy. *N Engl J Med* 299:84, 1978.
114. Finlay AY, Edmunds V: D.C. cardioversion in pregnancy. *Brit J Clin Pract* 33:88, 1979.
115. Soffronoff EC, Kaufmann BM, Connaughton JR: Intravascular volume determinations and fetal outcome in hypertensive disease of pregnancy. *Am J Obstet Gynecol* 127:4, 1977.
116. Berkowitz RL, Rafferty TD: Pulmonary artery flow-directed catheter use in the obstetric patient. *Obstet Gynecol* 55:507, 1980.
117. Strauss RG, Keefer JR, Burke T, Civetta RM: Hemodynamic monitoring of cardiogenic pulmonary edema complicating toxemia of pregnancy. *Obstet Gynecol* 55:170, 1980.
118. Redleaf PD, Fadell EJ: Bacteremia during parturition. *JAMA* 169:1284, 1959.

119. Baker TH, Hubbell R: Reappraisal of a symptomatic puerperal bacteremia. *Am J Obstet Gynecol* 97:575, 1967.
120. McCormack WM, Rosner B, Lee YH, et al.: Isolation of genital mycoplasmas from blood obtained shortly after vaginal delivery. *Lancet* 1:596, 1975.
121. Rise E, Smith JF, Bell J: Reduction of bacteremia after oral manipulations. *Arch Otolaryngol* 90:106, 1969.
122. Cobe HM: Transitory bacteremia. *Oral Surg* 7:609, 1954.
123. Everett ED, Hirschmann JV: Transient bacteremia and endocarditis prophylaxis. A review. *Medicine* 56:61, 1977.
124. AHA Committee Report: Prevention of bacterial endocarditis. *Circulation* 56:139A, 1977.
125. Brenner PF, Mishell DR: Contraception for the woman with significant cardiac disease. *Clin Obstet Gynecol* 18:155, 1975.
126. Oparil S: Hypertension and oral contraceptives. *J Cardiovasc Med* 6:381, 1981.
127. Dalen JE, Hickler RB: Oral contraceptives and cardiovascular disease. *Am Heart J* 101:626, 1981.
128. Shah SH, Deshmukh MA, Sharma RK, Purandare VN: Contraception in cardiac cases. *J Postgrad Med* 21:180, 1975.
129. Acker D, Boehm FH, Askew DE, Rothman H: Electrocardiogram changes with intrauterine contraceptive device insertion. *Am J Obstet Gynecol* 115:458, 1973.
130. Conrad CC, Ghazi M, Kitay DZ: Acute neurovascular sequelae of intrauterine device insertion or removal. *J Reprod Med* 11:211, 1973.
131. Johnson FL, Doerffer FR, Tyson JEA: Clinical experience with the Marquiles intrauterine contraceptive device. *Can Med Assoc J* 95:14, 1966.
132. Newton J, Elias J, McEwan J: Intrauterine contraception using the copper-seven device. *Lancet* 2:951, 1972.
133. Everett ED, Reller LB, Droegemueller W, Greer BE: Absence of bacteremia after insertion or removal of intrauterine devices. *Obstet Gynecol* 47:207, 1976.
134. Mishell DR Jr, Bell JH, Good RG, Moyer DL: The intrauterine device: A bacteriologic study of the endometrial cavity. *Am J Obstet Gynecol* 96:119, 1966.

CHAPTER XVIII

The Cardiac Patient with Dental Disease

Stephen P. Glasser, M.D.

There has long been a close professional association between the internist and the dentist but, although the medical and dental professions have much in common, their knowledge about each other is disparate. Unfortunately, medical schools usually do not teach students much about dental disease, despite the fact that the problems of dental care for the cardiac patient are significant and both are common. The maintenance of oral health in the cardiac patient, if ignored, can create sequela of major consequence.

For purposes of orientation, a partial classification of dental disease is presented in Table 1. Most physicians are aware that the most common problem faced by the dentist is exodontia, or removal of teeth. The trauma of extraction with its forceful manipulation is one of the most important factors in producing bacteremia. Laceration of the venules and capillaries creates a portal through which bacteria can enter the blood stream. The number of teeth extracted at one session is often related to the degree of trauma.[1] Another procedure that exposes patients to manipulative trauma is endodontia, or root canal therapy. Of all dental manipulative procedures, this is least likely to result in the complications of hemorrhage and bacteremia, because the area of manipulation is small and limited. Periodontic procedures are performed to curtail and eliminate gingival inflammation and to prevent reabsorption of alveolar bone.

By far, the conditions of greatest concern to the physician are those which involve infection of the oral tissues, primarily dental caries and disease involving the supportive periodontal structures.[2]

Table 1
Partial Classification of Dental Disease

Abnormalities of Dentition
Developmental Defects
Functional Changes (Erosion, Abrasion)
Trauma
Caries
Infection
       Pulp infection
       Suppurative periodontitis
       Subperiosteal abscess
       Gingival abscess
Periodontal Disease (Atrophy, Gingivitis, Trauma, etc.)

Tooth decay begins when the outer enamel and, then, the underlying dentin break down. The dentin is then invaded by bacteria, which results in further destruction. Eventually, if the decay is not arrested, it leads to inflammation and necrosis of the dental pulp. A dental alveolar abscess may form and can result in systemic illness as well as lead the patient with heart disease to the dentist's office.

Periodontal disease is not as easily recognized compared to other dental diseases. There is chronic inflammation of the gingival tissues and underlying alveolar bone. The early stages are asymptomatic, although the gums tend to bleed. If the inflammation is not properly controlled, it progresses to a breakdown of the gingival tissues and bone with resultant infection. Underlying systemic disease, particularly diabetes mellitus, may markedly accelerate the degenerative process.

With this in mind, the dental aspects of particular cardiac problems can be considered and these are listed in Table 2.[3]

Arteriosclerotic Heart Disease

Because of its frequency, the patient with coronary artery disease is perhaps the most important patient to consider for concomitant dental disease. Dental care in such patients presents special problems since these patients tend to be in the older age groups and

Table 2
Potential Danger from Dental Problems in Patients with
Cardiovascular Disease[3]

Condition	Potential Danger
Arteriosclerotic Heart Disease	Apprehension Hypotension Angina, Arrhythmias Myocardial Infarction Heart Failure
Valvular Heart Disease	Endocarditis Arrhythmias Heart Failure
Hypertensive Heart Disease	Lability of Blood Pressure Hypertensive Crisis Orthostatic Hypotension
Congenital Heart Disease	Endocarditis Septic Emboli

[3]Adapted from Klatell J, et al: Dental care for the cardiac patient. *Primary Cardiology* Nov:56, 1978.

may require extensive dental therapy. The pain, anxiety, and fear associated with dental procedures and its resultant increase in endogenous catecholamine release may be deleterious to patients with coronary lesions. They are also patients who may be taking a number of cardiovascular drugs which need to be considered in the setting of contemplated dental therapy (e.g., anticoagulant, digitalis, antihypertensives, antiarrhythmia agents, etc.). Thus, the concept of preventive dentistry and the importance of early and complete dental care should be carefully explained to the coronary patient. The risks of dental surgery in this group of patients are similar to the risks of other types of surgery. The values and limitations of local versus general anesthesia must be similarly evaluated.[4] If an acute or recent (within the preceding three to six months) myocardial infarction has occurred, elective dental surgery should be delayed. Symptoms of new onset or unstable angina and worsening heart failure should be sought. When present, these should be stabilized before anything less than acute emergency procedure is being considered.

Valvular Heart Disease

The reader is referred to Chapter 14, discussing this subject in detail, but some general remarks as it pertains to the patient with dental disease are warranted. The causal relationship between dental extraction and bacterial endocarditis is probably related to a dental infection or previous extractions. It has, therefore, become generally acceptable to give patients with congenital or rheumatic valvular heart disease antibiotics (preferably penicillin) prophylactically before dental extraction.[5]

In general, patients with a structural lesion of the heart that can serve as a nidus for bacterial endocarditis should receive subacute bacterial endocarditis prophylaxis. This includes almost all patients with cardiac murmurs (except those that are clearly functional) and those with congenital heart disease. Patients with repaired congenital heart disease do not need prophylaxis unless there is a residual defect. Even if the repair included the use of artificial material, bacterial endocarditis prophylaxis is still not warranted. One major exception is after the repair of coarctation of the aorta. Since 25% to 75% of these patients have associated bicuspid aortic valves that may not be clinically manifest, subacute bacterial endocarditis prophylaxis is justified. Since bacterial endocarditis is relatively common, even with mild valvular lesions,[4] the hemodynamic severity of the valvular lesion plays no part in the decision for prophylactic therapy.

Patients who have had rheumatic fever without cardiac involvement do not require prophylaxis. Important here is the knowledge that the doctor must specifically seek out information on the need for prophylaxis. He cannot depend on patient knowledge. Harvey and Capone[6] demonstrated that in patients with rheumatic heart disease, only 24.3% (of 181 patients) knew that they should have antibiotic coverage for dental extractions, and only 8.3% knew that they should be protected during extractions and amalgam restorations. Patients with congenital heart disease had even less knowledge of their needs (Table 3).

The amount of trauma induced by a procedure has a great bearing on the amount of bacteremia that develops. Bender et al.[7] demonstrated an 85% incidence of bacteremia immediately after multiple extractions and gingivectomy. With deep scaling, the incidence was 53% and with light scaling, 30% (Table 4). They con-

Table 3
Knowledge of Cardiac Patients Concerning Need for Antibiotic
Prophylaxis for Extractions vs. Cleaning and Filling of Teeth[6]

Type of Heart Disease	No. of Patients	Knowledge of Patient Concerning Prophylaxis for:			
		Extractions		Cleaning and Filling	
Rheumatic	181	44	24.3%	15	8.3%
Congenital	55	9	16.4%	4	7.3%
Functional vs. Organic	22	3	13.6%	1	4.5%
Total	258	56	21.7%	20	7.7%

[6]Harvey WP, Capone MA: The American Journal of Cardiology, June, 1961, p 795. Reproduced with permission of *The American Journal of Cardiology,* publisher, and W. Proctor Harvey, M.D., author.

Table 4
Incidence of Bacteremia Following Dental Manipulation[7]

Procedure	Positive Cultures	
	Immediately After Manipulation Per Cent	Ten Minutes After Manipulation Per Cent
Endodontic		
Within Root Canal	0	0
Beyond Root Canal	31	0
Exodontic		
Multiple Extraction	85	44
Single Extraction	52	24
Periodontic		
Gingivectomy	83	25
Deep Scaling	53	13
Light Scaling	30	5

(The incidence of positive cultures is also related to the state of oral hygiene.)
[7]Adapted from Klatell J, et al: Dental care for the cardiac patient. *Primary Cardiology,* Nov:56, 1978.

cluded that procedures such as fabrication of crowns, orthodontic manipulation, impression-taking, and amalgam restorations, should cause no concern since they are not associated with hemorrhage or bacteremia. Harvey and Capone,[6] however, reported two patients with subacute bacterial endocarditis preceded by only an amalgam restoration two and three months prior. In recent years, the illicit use of intravenous drugs (primarily heroin) has become an important associated factor. Mostaghim and Millard's study[8] revealed that 10% of their patients with bacterial endocarditis were "mainliners."

There is some controversy as to who should receive bacterial endocarditis prophylaxis, but there is almost no question on what constitutes prophylaxis. Penicillin is the drug of choice, and there is no disagreement on the advisability of using penicillin immediately before and after dental treatment.[9] There is some argument on how long antibiotics should be given before the procedure, but it is generally agreed to be one to two days.[9] A longer period is not likely to cause sterilized root abscesses or infected tonsils, but may cause sensitive bacteria to be replaced by penicillin-resistant strains. The American Heart Association[9] suggests 500 mg of penicillin V or phenethicillin one hour before the procedure and then 250 mg every six hours for at least two days after the procedure; 600,000 units of procaine penicillin G mixed with 200,000 units of crystalline penicillin G given by intramuscular injection one hour before the procedure and then once daily for at least two days.

For patients allergic to penicillin, erythromycin can be used with an initial dose of 500 mg one to one and one-half hours before the procedure and then 250 mg four times daily. For small children, 10 mg/kg should be given every six hours. In the past, this drug has not been given intramuscularly because of its proclivity to sterile abscess but since, erythromycin preparations for parenteral use have become available.

The antibiotic coverage should be broadened for patients who require emergency dental procedures during active subacute bacterial endocarditis. In some patients with prosthetic heart valves, staphylococcal infection can become a problem. Cohn et al.[10] described three patients with bacterial endocarditis involving an aortic valve prosthesis. This occurred after dental extractions, despite the use of penicillin prophylaxis. Because of this, they suggested a more comprehensive antibiotic regimen consisting of broad spectrum antibiotic troches for two days before the procedure, 600,000 units of procaine penicillin every six hours, 500 mg of streptomycin every 12 hours on the day before and on the day of the procedure, and three to five days after it. Methicillin sodium (5g) should be given intravenously on the day of surgery, and sodium oxacillin (4g) should be given orally for three to five days after the procedure.

Congenital Heart Disease

Without question, the risk of SBE after dental surgery is greater in patients with congenital heart disease than it is in patients with normal hearts, not only because of the cardiac defect itself but also, in some cases, because of changes in periodontal tissues which predispose to poor oral hygiene and chronic periodontal infection.[13] The most characteristic changes in the periodontal tissues consist of dilatation of the gingival capillaries, which results in edema of the gums and decreased resistance to infection. The dilatation of the gingival capillaries is thought to be a result of increased salivary kallikrein.[2] Frequent infections of the upper respiratory tract, loss of lip seal, and mouth breathing expose the periodontal tissues to bacterial attack. In the presence of lowered resistance of the periodontal tissue, even normal oral flora may establish infection.

Other problems in patients with certain types of congenital heart disease also occur. In patients with coarctation of the aorta, the mandibular arteries, as well as the arteries leading to the individual teeth, may be enlarged. Tooth extraction in such patients may result in excessive bleeding. The problems of anesthesia in cyanotic patients is also a consideration.

Anesthetics

When complete and total, anesthesia effectively minimizes apprehension and reduces the amount of endogenous epinephrine excretion. Adequate premedication is equally important and must be individualized. This also reduces apprehension and minimizes blood pressure elevation during the waiting room period. Pentobarbital (30–60 mg) or secobarbital (50–100 mg) are satisfactory for most patients. The importance of aspiration technique when administering anesthetics cannot be overemphasized. Harris[14] demonstrated that up to 3.2% of taps are "bloody" and cannot be detected unless the plunger of the syringe is slightly, but definitely, withdrawn. By this maneuver, he was able to reduce the frequency of undesirable side effects from 8.8% to 3.8%. Intra-arterial injections cause distant anesthesia and blanching of the immediate region. The most common cause of reactions to local anesthesia in dentistry is intravenous injection. This may cause central nervous system stimulation or depression, hypertensive crisis, or dangerous degrees of myocardial ischemia. Recent evidence claims it is safe and beneficial to use vasoconstrictors with local anesthesia. In 1955, the New York Heart Association recommended a dose of no more than 10 cc of a 1:50,000 dilution of epinephrine be administered in one session.[15] It has been found that since procaine itself has a slight vasodilating effect, this dose of epinephrine is necessary. When lidocaine is used, even smaller amounts of epinephrine (1:100,000, for instance) can be used. As long as the aspiration technique is utilized, the benefit engendered by the use of vasoconstriction with local anesthesia far outweighs the minimal risk.

Drugs to Consider

Antihypertensives

These are probably the most important group of agents to consider. In many instances, their most prominent side effect is orthostatic hypotension, resulting at times in syncope when the patient suddenly assumes the upright position. Guanethedine sulfate (Ismelin) and the ganglionic blocking drugs are the most important agents in this regard. Somewhat less commonly, methyldopa (Aldomet) may be the cause. The indiscriminate use of diuretic agents may result in hypovolemia and/or hypopotassemia, which can produce similar symptoms; and the latter may also exacerbate digitalis toxicity.

These agents, in addition to Rauwolfia preparations, also increase responsiveness to vasoconstrictors, so extra care should be used to prevent intravascular injection.

Nitroglycerin

If a patient develops angina pectoris during a dental procedure, nitroglycerin can be given for relief. A fresh supply should be available (the drug deteriorates and should not be more than six months to one year old for full effectiveness). Its side effects are primarily secondary to vasodilatation with resultant flushing and headache. Blood pressure generally falls after nitroglycerin is administered.

Saliva-inhibiting Drugs

Atropine and its prototypes are used in dentistry for obvious reasons. However, it is important to realize that because of their vagolytic effect, a tachycardia may result. In the cardiac-prone patient, this may result in breathlessness and angina pectoris.

Digitalis

This is a drug that many cardiac patients will be taking, but unless digitalis toxicity is present, it will usually cause little problem. This important drug is discussed in greater detail in Chapter 3.

Propranolol

Many patients with angina pectoris will be receiving this medication, which acts primarily by slowing the resting pulse and blunting the pulse rate response to exercise, anxiety, etc. Also important is the danger of sudden discontinuation of this medication. If dental treatment will result in the patient's inability to swallow oral medications, this must be considered (see Chapter 3).

Anticoagulants

Anticoagulants are now an accepted form of therapy for many patients with various forms of cardiovascular diseases, such as those that follow myocardial infarction, embolization in rheumatic and arteriosclerotic heart disease, certain types of strokes, venous disease, and pulmonary embolization. They are administered both as specific treatment for thromboembolic manifestations and as a prophylactic measure to prevent recurrence. In the latter instance, they are often continued for long periods of time, sometimes for the rest of the patient's life.

The aim of anticoagulant treatment is to retard or prevent intravascular coagulation. In the United States, the prothrombin time is used as an indicator of the effect of the drugs. One compares the normal prothrombin time to the therapeutic range, which is usually considered to be two to two and one-half times the control level.

Some of the earlier reports of oral surgical procedures performed purposely or inadvertently on patients receiving anticoagulant drugs revealed the occurrence of prolonged postoperative hemorrhage. Recommendations were made that no surgery be performed on patients during anticoagulant therapy so that if surgery was necessary, anticoagulant therapy was discontinued until the prothrombin time returned to an acceptable level. At the same time, however, there were reports in the literature on the danger of discontinuance of anticoagulant therapy because of an increased incidence of blood clots with embolization. This prompted a number of studies and, although there is still some controversy surrounding the question, many minor and major surgical procedures have been safely performed on patients taking anticoagulant drugs.[16] Although some reports have suggested that oral bleeding in anticoagulated patients after dental extractions is a significant problem, recent studies have not substantiated this.[17] It is now generally agreed that single or multiple extractions can be performed in these patients if proper attention is given to careful hemostatis procedures. In fact, Chamberlain[18] stated that the danger of clotting when anticoagulant drugs are discontinued is greater than the danger of bleeding when the drugs are continued, providing that the proper safeguards are used. The blood prothrombin time should be held in low optimal range ($1\frac{1}{2}$ times the control level).

Additional safeguards include advising hospitalization, applying constant pressure to the involved tissues during surgery, placing a foamed gelatin in each socket, placing multiple sutures under tension, having the patient apply heavy biting pressure for 30 minutes maintained by biting on gauze pressure packs, applying ice packs externally 30 minutes on and 30 minutes off for 48 hours, withholding mouth rinses and hot liquids for 48 hours, and maintaining a soft diet for 48 to 72 hours. If bleeding persists despite these measures, discontinuation of the drug is the first consideration (provided the situation is not emergent, since there will be a lag of 24 to 48 hours before the prothrombin time begins returning to normal). If the problem requires more immediate therapy, however, the administration of Aquamephyton Injection parenterally or orally, depending on the rapidity of correction necessary, is of value.

References

1. Bender IB, Seltzer S: Dental procedures of interest to the physician in the management of patients with cardiovascular disease. *Am Heart J* 66:697, 1963.
2. Burch GE, DePasquale NP: Relationship of dentistry to cardiology. *Am Heart J* 67:99, 1964.
3. Klatell J, Rubin M, Evans BE: Dental care for the cardiac patient. *Primary Cardiology* Nov/Dec:56, 1978.
4. Anderson TO, Harris SC, Duncan AH, et al.: Management of dental problems in patients with cardiovascular disease. *JAMA* 187:848, 1964.
5. ADA and American Heart Association (Report of a working conference jointly sponsored by them): Management of dental problems in patients with cardiovascular disease. *JADA* 68:333, 1964.
6. Harvey WP, Capone MA: Bacterial endocarditis related to cleaning and filling of teeth (with particular reference to the inadequacy of present day knowledge and practice of antibiotic prophylaxis for all dental procedures). *Am J Cardiol* 7:793, 1961.
7. Bender IB, Seltzer S, Tashman S, et al.: Dental procedures in patients with rheumatic heart disease. *Oral Surg* 16:466, 1963.
8. Mostaghim D, Millard HD: Bacterial endocarditis: A retrospective study. *Oral Surg* 40:219, 1975.
9. American Heart Association: Prevention of bacterial endocarditis. *Am Heart Assoc Bulletin* 7–72–200M, 1972.
10. Cohn LH, Roberts WC, Rockoff SD, et al.: Bacterial endocarditis following aortic valve replacement. Clinical and pathological correlations. *Circulation* 33:209, 1966.
11. Robinson L, Kraus FW, Lazansky JP, et al.: Bacteremia of dental origin. *Oral Surg, Oral Med, Oral Path* 3:519, 1950.

12. Peterson LJ, Peacock R: The incidence of bacteremia in pediatric patients following tooth extraction. *Circulation* 53:676, 1976.
13. Gould MSE, Picton DCA: The gingival condition of congenitally cyanotic individuals. *Brit Dent J* 109:96, 1960.
14. Harris SC: Action of local anesthetic agents. *Dent Clin North Am* July:231, 1961.
15. Report of the special committee of the New York Heart Association, Inc. on the use of epinephrine in connection with procaine in dental procedures. *Am Heart J* 50:108, 1955.
16. Behrman SJ, Wright IS: Dental surgery during continuous anticoagulant therapy. *JAMA* 175:483, 1961.
17. Shira RB, Hall RJ, Guernsey LH: Minor oral surgery during prolonged anticoagulant therapy. *J Oral Surg* 20:93, 1962.
18. Chamberlain FL: Management of medical-dental problems in patients with cardiovascular diseases. *Mod Concepts Cardiovasc Dis* 30:697, 1961.

CHAPTER XIX

The Cardiac Patient with Pulmonary Disease

Keith W. Chandler, M.D.
and David A. Solomon, M.D.

The Management of Postoperative Pulmonary Complications

There is no sound evidence that indicates that patients with cardiac disease are more prone to postoperative pulmonary complications. Morbidity and mortality after general surgery in all types of patients, including those with heart disease, are primarily caused by pulmonary complications (Table 1). Therefore, the management of these problems assumes importance whenever any patient has general surgery.

Intraoperative Factors

The development of such postoperative pulmonary complications as atelectasis, pneumonia, pleurisy, and pleural effusion correlates with the presence of preoperative lung disease. Nonetheless, consideration of other variables is warranted since even those patients with severe respiratory compromise prior to surgery may pursue an uncomplicated postoperative course, while those patients with no prior apparent lung disease can, on occasion, fall prey to postoperative respiratory complications.

369

Table 1
Postoperative Pulmonary Complications

Intraoperative Factors
General anesthesia
muscle weakness
diaphragm displacement
Endotracheal intubation
mucociliory transport
bacterial contamination
Surgical incision site
Pulmonary Aspiration of Gastric Contents
Arterial Hypoxemia
Atelectasis
Bronchitis
Pneumonia
Pleural Effusion
Respiratory Failure

General Anesthesia and Respiratory Muscles

The effects wrought on the lung by general anesthesia are manifold.[1] Induction of anesthesia, particularly when coupled with neuromuscular paralysis, dramatically alters ventilation-perfusion matching of the lung. General anesthesia, even with maintenance of spontaneous breathing, leads to a cephalad displacement of the diaphragm in the supine patient. With this displacement of the diaphragm, the amount of air remaining within the lung at the end of a normal breath (the functional residual capacity) is diminished. Concomitant neuromuscular paralysis with the requirement for positive pressure breathing produces changes in diaphragmatic displacement as well.

Endotracheal Intubation

In addition to the physical and physiological effects of general anesthesia and respiratory muscle paralysis, tracheal intubation and mechanical ventilation may interfere with pulmonary defense mechanisms. Endotracheal intubation with a cuffed tube compromises tracheal mucociliary transport. Contamination of the tracheobronchial tree with potentially pathogenic bacteria is a hazard frequently associated with endotracheal intubation.[2] If an endotracheal tube is required for a prolonged period of time (greater than six hours) as many as 45% of surgical patients demonstrate the presence of gram negative organisms in aspirates obtained from the trachea. The incidence of contamination rises with the preoperative use of antibiotics.[3]

Surgical Incision Site

The greatest operative determinant of postoperative pulmonary complications is the site of the surgical incision (Table 2). While superficial incisions and extrathoracic, extra-abdominal operations result in some modification of pulmonary function, the impairment produced is generally clinically insignificant and respiratory complications are infrequent and unpredictable. Although evidence is sketchy, simultaneous bilateral thoracotomy incisions appear to result in the greatest decline in immediate postoperative pulmonary function.[4] Thoracoabdominal incisions, because of injury to the diaphragm and entry into the pleural and peritoneal cavities, also induce a great deal of postoperative pulmonary functional impairment.[5] Following unilateral thoracotomy, the vital capacity on the first postoperative day may be but 25% of its preoperative value. Upper abdominal paramedian and midline incisions and long abdominal incisions are accompanied by a post-

Table 2
Incision Site and Vital Capacity (VC) Change

Superficial Incision
    Insignificant change in VC
Extrathoracic, Extra-abdominal Incision
    Insignificant change in VC
Thoracic Incision
    75% decline in VC
Abdominal Incision
    Upper abdominal
        65% decline in VC
    Subcostal and posterior flank
        50% decline in VC
    Lower abdominal
        40% decline in VC

operative vital capacity 33% to 38% of the preoperative level.[6] Subcostal or posterior (flank) incisions[7] are responsible for a 50% fall in the postoperative vital capacity. Lower abdominal incisions may be associated with a postoperative vital capacity 62% of the preoperative value,[6] while inguinal and femoral herniorrhaphy incisions produce much less vital capacity impairment.[5] The falls in vital capacity are paralleled by falls in the one-second forced expiratory volume (FEV_1),[6,7,8] and although gradual improvement is the rule, the vital capacity is still diminished on the seventh postoperative day and may not return to its preoperative level before four weeks have elapsed.[5] Knowledge of a patient's preoperative pulmonary function permits an educated prediction of postoperative ventilatory adequacy and an assessment of the risk of postoperative respiratory insufficiency.

Although the incidence of pulmonary complications following surgical procedures varies depending upon the definition of what constitutes a pulmonary complication, a tabulation of studies in which complications were subdivided on the basis of operative site[8] reinforces the paramount importance of this variable. Nonabdominal, nonthoracic surgery is attended by a 0.1% to 2.3% incidence of pulmonary complications, while the incidence of such complications following thoracic surgery is 60%. The complication rate following upper abdominal surgery is 7.5% to 56%, while with lower abdominal surgery, it is 0.7% to 33%. Monotonously shallow breathing and the inability to sigh, cough, or breathe deeply, when superimposed on perturbations initiated pre- and intraoperatively are reasons enough for the increase in respiratory morbidity following thoracic or upper abdominal surgery.

Pulmonary Aspiration of Gastric Contents

The incidence of pulmonary aspiration of gastric contents during the perioperative period is unclear because short of the use of bronchoscopy to verify the diagnosis, the direct observation of aspiration is required to establish the occurrence of this complication.[9] Patients who aspirate during general anesthesia often are those undergoing obstetric or emergency procedures that allow for little preoperative preparation.[10] An additional feature which favors pulmonary aspiration includes post-intubation laryngeal incompetence, a condition that may persist hours into the post-anesthesia period when full recovery from anesthesia has apparently occurred.[11]

Since pulmonary injury occurs almost instantaneously following the aspiration of gastric contents, lavage of the lung is not recommended.[12] The use of corticosteroids in aspiration pneumonitis is controversial and is not widely endorsed because of the lack of clinical evidence to support a beneficial effect on outcome.[10,12] The major thrust of treatment is symptomatic and includes correction of hypoxemia by providing supplemental oxygen. One-quarter of appropriately treated patients with aspiration pneumonia will initially demonstrate clinical improvement but, subsequently, will develop superimposed bacterial infection.[10] Since prophylactic use of antimicrobial drugs seemingly does not alter the incidence of subsequent bacterial infection, antibiotic treatment is characteristically not initiated until clinical evidence suggests the presence of infection.[12,13] Treatment then is based on results of well-collected expectorated sputum or tracheobronchial aspirate smear and culture specimens[12] and oftentimes includes the use of an aminoglycoside combined with oxacillin, clindamycin, or a cephalosporin[13] because gram negative and gram positive pathogens are frequently recovered from hospitalized patients following aspiration of gastric contents.[10] One possible exception to this approach of withholding antibiotics until the indications for their use develop would be their early implementation in patients who aspirate material grossly contaminated with large numbers of micro-organisms.[14]

Postoperative Arterial Hypoxemia

That general anesthesia with controlled ventilation leads to a decline in one's arterial oxygen tension (PaO_2) was established in 1959.[15] Since then, hundreds of investigations into the pathophysiology and clinical relevance of perioperative hypoxemia have been published. Many of these investigations were summarized and reviewed by Marshall and Wyche in 1972.[16] It is apparent that hypoxemia is undesirable, irrespective of the patient's underlying clinical status. But, in the patient with cardiac disease, arterial hypoxemia has even greater importance.

Collapse of peripheral, dependent alveoli during mechanical

ventilation is a phenomenon which has been documented anatomically in experimental animals.[17] Such atelectasis is manifested by falls in arterial oxygen tension and is often referred to as "microatelectasis" or "miliary atelectasis" (Figure 1) to distinguish it from radiographically apparent collapse ("macroatelectasis"). Intraoperatively, frequent, or sustained passive hyperinflation will restore arterial oxygen tension to control values presumably by reexpanding collapsed alveoli.[18] If surgery has been nonabdominal/nonthoracic, arterial oxygen tension gradually returns to its preoperative value during the initial one to three hours following general anesthesia.[19] The effects of general anesthesia in promoting alveolar collapse are largely dissipated within a short period following removal of the anesthetic agents. During this period, those who would tolerate hypoxemia poorly, particularly the elderly or those with cardiopulmonary disease, should receive supplemental oxygen therapy.

Following abdominal surgery, however, hypoxemia is more persistent. If patients undergo general anesthesia for abdominal operations, the arterial hypoxemia begins intraoperatively or immediately postoperatively and the arterial oxygen tension reaches its nadir between the first and third postoperative day. If patients undergo epidural anesthesia for abdominal operations, the arterial oxygen tension, normal in the immediate postoperative period, begins to decline by three hours reaching its nadir between the first and third postoperative day.[20]

While general anesthesia produces arterial hypoxemia via a variety of mechanisms, persistence of arterial hypoxemia well into the postoperative period is generally a result of disturbances related to the surgical procedure performed. The end result of these disturbances may well be similar to that produced by general anesthesia in terms of ventilation/perfusion mismatch with or without alveolar collapse.[21] Not uncommonly, the arterial blood oxygen tension falls to below 60 torr[22,23] and moderate hypoxemia may persist for days following upper abdominal surgery. The elderly and those with the greatest degree of arterial hypoxemia may show the least improvement in oxygen tension during supplemental oxygen therapy.[23,24] In such patients, higher concentrations of inspired oxygen may be required to reverse hypoxemia. Patients undergoing open heart surgery demonstrate comparable degrees of postoperative hypoxemia with a mean maximal decline of ar-

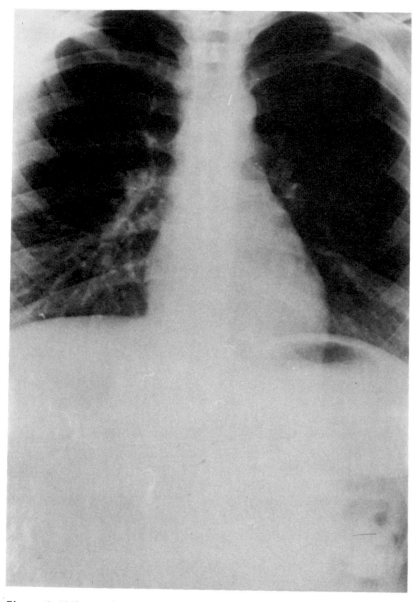

Figure 1. "Microatelectasis" in a 36-year-old woman one day postoperatively. Arterial hypoxemia is evident, but the chest roentgenogram appears to be normal.

terial oxygen tension of 17 torr being reached between the first and third postoperative days. Moderate hypoxemia may persist beyond ten days, however.

To summarize, then, arterial hypoxemia is a virtually universal concomitant to the administration of general anesthesia. In the absence of thoracic or abdominal incisions, this hypoxemia resolves within hours. When thoracic or abdominal operations have been performed, hypoxemia may persist for days. Arterial hypoxemia is most commonly a result of maldistribution of ventilation in combination with intrapulmonary shunting of blood through areas of alveolar collapse. The magnitude of the decline in arterial oxygenation is determined by multiple variables including age, body habitus, site of the surgical incision, presence of pre-existent cardiac or pulmonary disease, and administration of sympathomimetic agents. Oxygen therapy should be provided when a patient's condition would be expected to be adversely influenced by hypoxemia. When supplemental oxygen is used to correct arterial hypoxemia, arterial blood gas analysis is necessary to verify the adequacy of the prescribed flow rate. Oxygen therapy may be required for days following surgery, even in the absence of clinically overt pulmonary complications.

The inability to cough and breathe deeply following thoracic or abdominal surgery impedes the generation of sufficient transpulmonary pressures to maintain alveolar expansion. Further, the inability to expectorate retained tracheobronchial secretions promotes resorption of air trapped behind the more proximal obstructions. Central bronchial obstruction may then be critical in the development of atelectasis on occasion, but in a great many patients no identifiable obstructing material can be identified. The incidence of atelectasis varies in proportion to the presence of certain preoperative risk factors and with the site of the surgical incision. Following upper abdominal surgery, the incidence of atelectasis based on radiographic findings approaches forty percent.[8]

Characteristically, atelectasis is described as "plate-like" subsegmental, or segmental and is predominantly basal in location (Figure 2). Mid-lung field and apical involvement and lobar collapse, although occasional occurrences, are much less commonly encountered. Clearing of collapse generally occurs over the initial three to four postoperative days.[25]

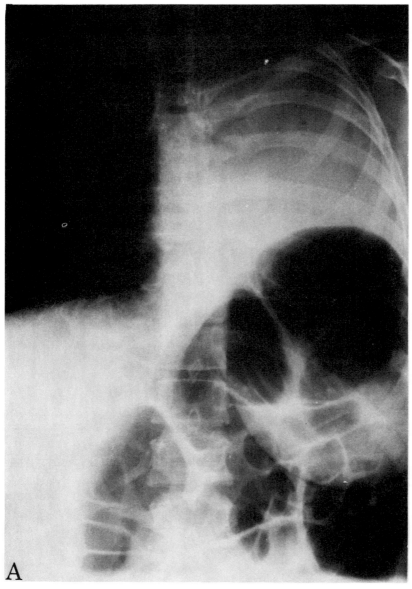

A

Figure 2. A 24-year-old woman three days after abdominal surgery.

A. 3–10–82. Complete atelectasis of the left lung.

Figure and legend continued on pp. 378–379

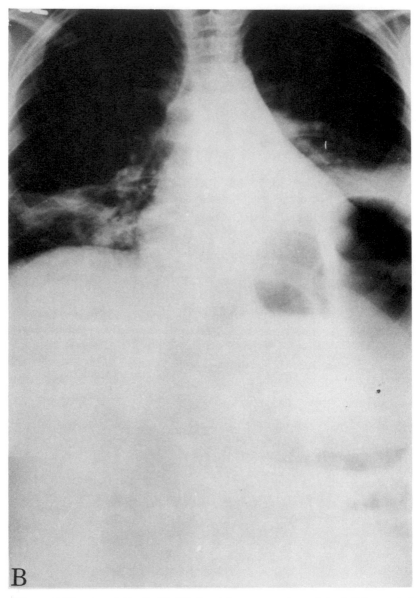

Figure 2 *(Continued)* B. 3–12–82. Partial re-expansion of the left lung and "plate-like" atelectasis on the right side.

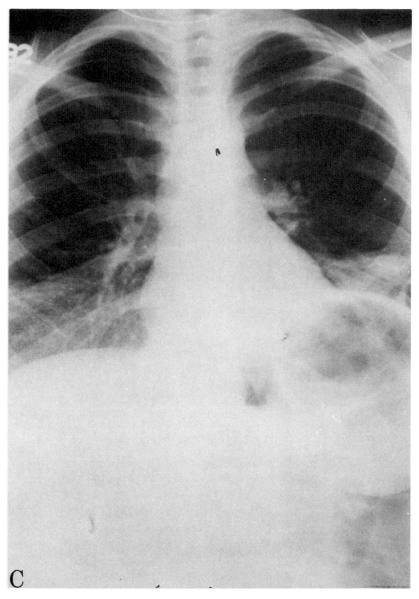

Figure 2 *(Continued)* C. 3–15–82. Continued improvement, but residual plate-like atelectasis bilaterally.

Prevention

Encouragement of deep breathing and coughing during the postoperative period should be routinely employed. Preoperative instruction should facilitate subsequent postoperative cooperation, even though obtundation and pain may blunt patient incentive. Respiratory maneuvers should begin in the recovery room during the "stir-up" period of arousal from anesthesia following surgery, and should continue until the patient is fully ambulatory.

Control of incisional pain may permit the effective performance of deep breathing maneuvers and coughing. Preoperative counseling and education may diminish the reactive component of pain, and splinting the incision with a pillow braced against the wound is a time-honored way of diminishing pain provoked by coughing. Opiate analgesics should not be withheld when indicated, but if used they should be used with the understanding that patients must be constantly encouraged to deep breathe. Intercostal nerve block following thoracic or upper abdominal surgery generally requires multiple injections unless an indwelling catheter is placed intraoperatively adjacent to the appropriate intercostal nerves.[26] Improvement over narcotic analgesia in regard to pulmonary function is probably minimal and the risk of pneumothorax attends the technique.[27]

Treatment

There are a variety of techniques available to treat atelectasis (Table 3). The institution of expiratory maneuvers as a means of reducing pulmonary complications following surgery has been traced to Harken, who in the early 1900s encouraged his postoperative patients to blow wind instruments to prevent respiratory complications.[28] The ability of expiratory maneuvers to prevent the development of atelectasis or to aid in the re-expansion of collapsed alveoli presumably depends on taking an initial large and sustained deep breath prior to exhalation. When blow bottles are used three to five times every three hours, they compare favorably with intermittent positive pressure breathing (IPPB) and with incentive spirometers (IS) in the prevention of postoperative atelectasis.[29] Since a high mouth pressure is necessary during expira-

Table 3
Treatment of Atelectasis

Blow Bottles
Intermittent Positive Pressure Breathing (IPPB)
Incentive Spirometer
Chest Physiotherapy
Voluntary Deep Breathing
Promotion of Tracheobronchial Clearance
   Ultrasonic nebulizer
   Tracheal suctioning
   Flexible fiberoptic bronchoscopy

---

tion with the technique and since forced expiration may enlist abdominal muscle contraction, some patients with incisional pain may find the use of blow bottles more disagreeable than maneuvers which emphasize sustained maximal inhalation.[29]

In order to augment inspiration, generate maximal transpulmonary pressure, and attain alveolar inflation, voluntary deep breathing devices known as incentive spirometers were designed.[28] An array of such devices exist, but clinically important differences in the incidence of postoperative complications were not demonstrated when different types of incentive spirometers were used in random fashion by patients following upper abdominal surgery.[30] After abdominal surgery, prescribed use of the incentive spirometer halves the incidence and reduces the severity of atelectasis in comparison with "routine" deep breathing,[31] chest physiotherapy performed twice daily,[32] or IPPB performed four times daily with volume adjusted "maximally" by the therapist.[33] Should atelectasis develop, use of the incentive spirometer may hasten the resolution of collapse.[32]

If the incentive spirometer is to be used, patients should be instructed in its use preoperatively. Ideally, the device should be used five to ten times per waking hour. Since less than one-third of patients will use the incentive spirometer as recommended, they should be encouraged to perform over one-hundred attempts per twenty-four-hour period and to achieve steadily larger inspired volumes or higher inspiratory flow rates with the passage of time.[32]

Intermittent positive pressure breathing (IPPB) by means of a pressure-limited respirator delivering humidified gas to a spontaneously breathing patient for brief periods is a controversial means of preventing or treating postoperative atelectasis. While IPPB is unquestionably overused,[34] the publicized failure of IPPB to prevent postoperative complications may lie in the method of its delivery.[28] Studies purporting to establish the ineffectiveness of IPPB treatments fail to specify the peak pressure generated or, more importantly, to record the inflating volumes achieved. Since inflating volume is the major consideration, the patient's maximal voluntary inspired volume should be compared with that achieved with IPPB.[35] When pressures of twenty-five to forty centimeters of water are employed and inflating volumes monitored, IPPB often allows significantly larger volumes to be achieved postoperatively than does coaching of a voluntary deep breath or inspiring through an incentive spirometer.[36,37]

Voluntary deep breathing with or without the incentive spirometer is, theoretically, preferable to IPPB when the latter is not required to deliver large inflating volumes. Concern about impaired venous return with diminished cardiac output,[34] nausea and gastric distension,[29] nosocomial infection, or hyperinflation and pneumothorax may limit the application of IPPB.[35] Because IPPB, when delivered with room air, results in brief periods of hypoxemia, the precaution of supplying supplemental oxygen to patients with borderline arterial oxygenation is prudent.[38] Finally, to minimize complications ensuing from the use of IPPB, the inspiratory flow rate should be as low as possible so that a high inflating volume is achieved over a long inspiratory time.[39] When aerosolized bronchodilators are delivered via IPPB, low flow rates may improve delivery to the lung.[37] When IPPB is prescribed for patients who are unable to voluntarily achieve large inspired volumes, and when measured inflating volumes are delivered at low flow rates with precautions taken to avoid hypoxemia and hyperventilation, its use may be advantageous.[28,31]

Chest physiotherapy as a means of preventing or treating postoperative atelectasis is perhaps as controversial a subject as is IPPB. Nonetheless, chest physiotherapy has frequently served as an integral component in regimens designed to diminish postoperative pulmonary complications. Perhaps more importantly, chest physiotherapy may hasten the resolution of atelectasis, once developed.[40,41]

Promotion of Tracheobronchial Clearance

Inhalation of ultrasonically nebulized water, preceded by inhalation of bronchodilators to diminish bronchospasm, may provoke coughing in patients who otherwise are unwilling or unable to cough following surgery. Cough pressures generated by spontaneous coughing following thoracotomy are but 29 percent of those achieved preoperatively and are ineffective in promoting the clearance of secretions. Cough pressures generated in response to delivery of ultrasonic mist approach 44 percent of the preoperative control values and are effective in promoting expectoration of mucous plugs.[42]

Tracheal suctioning may help clear tracheobronchial mucous obstructions. Because severe hypoxemia may occur during tracheal suctioning, preoxygenation with delivery of supplemental oxygen by nasal prongs, mask, or endotracheal tube, plus limitation of any suctioning period to fifteen seconds are advisable.[43,44] While blind nasotracheal suctioning is frequently performed, the risk of laryngospasm should limit this practice.[45] Insertion of an indwelling transtracheal catheter through the cricothyroid membrane so that coughing is provoked by periodic instillations of saline was once proposed as a means of reducing postoperative pulmonary complications.[46] Since this technique is attended by an unacceptable risk of complications, some of them fatal, it should not be used.

Flexible fiberoptic bronchoscopy is infrequently required to facilitate the removal of obstructing bronchial secretions. The absence of an air bronchogram predicts that proximal or large airway obstruction is the cause of atelectasis. When respiratory therapy cannot be performed or is ineffective in clearing the inspissated mucous secretions, fiberoptic bronchoscopy may be beneficial.[41] If an air bronchogram is present on the chest roentgenogram, proximal obstruction is unlikely and fiberoptic bronchoscopy generally will be of little benefit in resolving atelectasis.

With such an array of procedures to prevent and treat atelectasis following surgery, which approaches ought one take prophylactically and therapeutically? Patients at risk for the development of atelectasis should receive instruction prior to surgery in coughing, in deep breathing, and in the use of a device to encourage sustained maximal inspiration. Incentive spirometers offer an inex-

pensive means of encouraging sustained maximal inspiratory maneuvers. The frequent use of spirometers postoperatively is
effective in preventing and treating atelectasis. If atelectasis nonetheless occurs, re-expansion may be hastened by chest physiotherapy, tracheal suctioning, ultrasonic nebulization of water, or
maximal volume IPPB treatments. Patients weakening from prolonged reliance upon mechanical ventilation, neurologic, or mus-
culoskeletal disease who are unable voluntarily to perform a sustained maximal inspiration also may benefit from the use of IPPB.
If all these maneuvers fail, then flexible fiberoptic bronchoscopy
with suctioning may help re-expand the collapsed lung.

Postoperative Bronchitis and Pneumonia

Postoperative chest infections occur much less frequently than
does atelectasis. Patients with chronic bronchitis may continue to
expectorate purulent sputum in the postoperative period.[47] If
acute bronchitis is defined by the presence of a productive cough
with fever in the absence of chest roentgenographic evidence of
pneumonia, then 2 percent to 17 percent of patients undergoing
abdominal surgery will be diagnosed as developing acute bronchitis.[32,33]

Nosocomial pneumonia will follow abdominal or thoracic surgery in less than 5 percent of patients, but the results can be dev-
astating.[25,48] Pneumonia is the most frequent nosocomial infection
related to death[49] and in one investigation reporting the experience of nosocomial pneumonia in a respiratory-surgical intensive
care unit, the complication of pneumonia was associated with a
patient mortality more than ten-fold higher than that of the
nonpneumonia population.[50]

While pneumonia may originate via hematogenous spread from
a distant septic focus or from contaminated respiratory therapy
equipment, most patients are felt to acquire infections by aspirating
oropharyngeal secretions.[48] Although anaerobic and gram positive
aerobic bacteria may be involved in hospital-acquired pneumonia,
gram negative aerobes are the most clinically important pathogens
recovered.[50–52] Aspiration of contaminated oropharyngeal secretions into the tracheobronchial tree is facilitated by the presence
of a depressed sensorium,[53] and cuffed endotracheal[54] or trache-

otomy tubes[55] offer no guarantee against aspiration of secretions with subsequent tracheobronchial colonization or infection.[2,3]

The diagnosis of postoperative pneumonia is fraught with difficulty. Features suggestive of pneumonia include new or progressively worsening infiltrates on chest roentgenograms, fever, leukocytosis, and the recovery of potentially pathogenic bacteria from the tracheobronchial tree.[10] As has been emphasized, atelectasis is a frequent sequel to abdominal or thoracic surgery and may be radiographically indistinguishable from pneumonia.[41] Fever is considered by some investigators to be a concomitant of atelectasis alone without requiring superimposed bacterial infection.[8] Experimentally, however, fever only develops when atelectasis is associated with the presence of pathogenic bacteria within the atelectatic lung.[56,57] Presumably, then, when bacteria gain access to collapsed lung, fever may ensue and unless expectoration of purulent secretions is accomplished, pneumonia may follow without clear-cut distinctive signs and symptoms.[58]

Pneumonia is probably misdiagnosed with regularity.[59] Although nosocomial pneumonias develop in no more than five percent of patients following surgery, as many as ten percent receive treatment with antibiotics because of the initial clinical impression that pneumonia has supervened.[31] Frequent assessment of the situation and initiation of appropriate antibiotic treatment is the obvious proper course to pursue. Because nosocomial pneumonia may be caused by gram positive or negative aerobic or anaerobic organisms, appropriate initial antibiotic therapy should consist of an aminoglycoside combined with oxacillin, clindamycin, or a cephalosporin.[13,60] The most useful procedure to guide antibiotic therapy is often the least utilized. Clinically useful information will be obtained frequently by gram stain of expectorated secretions.[61,62] With the information imparted by gram stain of tracheobronchial secretions, appropriate antibiotic therapy for patients with suspected nosocomial pneumonias can be initiated, and subsequent cultural data can be interpreted knowledgeably.

Postoperative Pleural Effusions

Following abdominal surgery, pleural effusions, if searched for, occur in just fewer than fifty percent of patients.[63] Such effusions are characteristically small, presenting radiographically as obliteration of the posterior costophrenic sulcus. If the diagnosis of pleural effusion is in question and the postoperative patient is too unstable to tolerate transportation to the radiology suite, pleural effusions can be demonstrated by obtaining a bedside lateral decubitus radiograph with the patient lying on a "cardiac arrest board."[64] Postoperative effusions are commonly related to atelectasis, to the presence of free peritoneal fluid, and to upper abdominal surgery. They may be treated expectantly unless empyema is a strong consideration in the differential diagnosis. If the possibility of thoracic empyema is a concern, diagnostic thoracentesis should be performed. Accepted guidelines for the urgent drainage of a thoracic empyema via tube thoracostomy include the presence of gross pus, bacteria seen on gram stain or recovered from culture, a pleural fluid pH less than 7.00, or a pleural fluid glucose less than 40 mg%. The decision for tube thoracostomy is individualized if the pleural fluid pH is above 7.00 but below 7.20.[65] This therapeutic approach is advocated so that loculation and organization of the empyema will be avoided.

Postoperative Respiratory Failure

Postoperative respiratory failure is simply defined as a $PaO_2 <$ 50 torr and/or a $PaCO_2 > 50$ torr and results from a multiplicity of causes. Uncommon causes which merit consideration in postoperative patients include prolonged neuromuscular paralysis and upper airway obstruction.

Prolonged apnea following surgery should lead to investigation of possible untoward reactions to neuromuscular blocking agents. Incomplete neuromuscular block reversal is suggested by the inability of supine postoperative patients to perform movements against gravity and by their inability to maintain airway patency.[66] When supine postoperative patients are capable of sustaining a headlift for at least five seconds, neuromuscular recovery is at least 90 percent.[67]

Obstruction of the upper airway following surgery is often unrecognized and any associated respiratory distress may be incorrectly attributed to underlying lung disease. An endotracheal tube may obstruct if it becomes kinked, if its lumen is compromised by secretions or blood, or if the cuff herniates and occludes the tip. Following extubation, if neuromuscular blockade is not adequately reversed, the lax tongue may occlude the airway of the supine patient. If severe acute airway obstruction at the laryngeal level follows removal of an endotracheal tube, reintubation of the trachea is required. Acute postoperative laryngeal obstruction results from supraglottic, subglottic, or laryngeal edema and from laryngospasm.[68,69] Because of the difficulty accompanying reintubation of such patients, one skilled in endotracheal intubation always should be in attendance at the time of extubation.[70] If obstruction is not of such severity to require immediate re-establishment of an artificial airway, attempts may be directed toward providing an adequate inspired oxygen tension, inhaled nebulized racemic epinephrine and, if warranted by the severity of upper airway obstruction, intravenous infusion of glucocorticoids.

Once postoperative respiratory failure is apparent, steps should be taken to identify the specific causes contributing to ventilatory inadequacy. When these causes are identified, therapy should be directed to their reversal. Regardless of the root causes of acute respiratory failure, the fractional concentration of inspired oxygen should be high enough to maintain an arterial oxygen tension of 50 to 60 torr. Patients in acute respiratory failure with carbon dioxide retention require careful oxygen administration and if hypoxemia remains severe, progressive increments of inspired oxygen should be delivered until adequate oxygen saturation of arterial blood is verified. Progressive hypercapnia and acidosis leading to the inability of a patient to cooperate with his therapy is an indication for endotracheal intubation and mechanical ventilation.[71]

In the absence of respiratory acidosis, the concern in the management of acute respiratory failure is for the achievement of adequate tissue oxygenation. The adequacy of supplemental oxygen therapy in restoring arterial oxygen saturation must be verified and not assumed. While transcutaneous oxygen monitors and ear oximeters allow one to noninvasively assess the adequacy of supplemental oxygen in correcting hypoxemia when worsening carbon dioxide retention is not a concern, arterial blood gas analysis is the most readily available means for monitoring the response to oxygen therapy. The magnitude of the rise in arterial oxygen tension in response to oxygen therapy is determined by complex interactions among such variables as the nature of the underlying cause of respiratory failure, the means whereby supplemental oxygen is delivered, and the pattern of breathing exhibited by the patient.

If clinical improvement is not forthcoming when controlled oxygen is administered to a postoperative patient in acute respiratory failure and a readily reversible source of respiratory compromise is not evident, endotracheal intubation and mechanical ventilation are usually the next available recourses, especially when confronted by a patient with progressive hypercapnia, respiratory acidosis, and obtundation.[71] Guidelines for the implementation of ventilatory support in adults with acute respiratory failure include tachypnea with a respiratory rate greater than 35 per minute, a vital capacity less than 15 milliliters per kilogram of body weight, an inspiratory force less than 25 centimeters of water, persistent arterial hypoxemia in spite of an inspired oxygen concentration of 60 percent, and hypercapnia with the arterial carbon dioxide tension greater than 55 torr.[72] Those who have popularized these guidelines emphasize that "the trend of values is of utmost importance . . . (they) should obviously not be adopted to the exclusion of clinical judgement."[72] Once the decision to mechanically ventilate a patient is reached, endotracheal intubation must be accomplished. Recommendations for approaches which facilitate what otherwise would be difficult intubations have been published.[73] The ready availability of fiberoptic endoscopes permits tracheal intubation under direct vision when use of the laryngoscope blade is not practical. Use of the fiberoptic bronchoscope also allows the ready performance of endotracheal tube change in critically ill patients.[74]

Appropriate tube placement in terms of position above the carina is verifiable radiographically following intubation or endoscopically at the time of intubation. Because an endotracheal tube moves significantly in relationship to the main carina, the tip of the tube should be positioned so that it lies three to seven centimeters above the carina when the head is in a neutral position.[75]

Translaryngeal intubation is accomplished by either the nasal or the oral route. Nasotracheal intubation is reportedly less uncomfortable than orotracheal intubation. Because the size of the nasal passage constrains tube size and disposes to kinking of the tube, endotracheal suctioning may be made more difficult.[72] Nasotracheal intubation is attended by the risk of pressure necrosis of the external nares and of maxillary sinusitis.[76] When, with mechanical ventilation, the nasotracheal tube cuff is allowed to leak a minimal amount of air with each breath, massive gastric distension may rapidly develop.[77] Oral endotracheal tubes are more difficult to secure in place and, perhaps, because of the larger size tube employed, are more liable to traumatize the vocal cords.[78] However, oral endotracheal tubes with their generally larger diameter allow greater ease in suctioning of the bronchial tree. Both oral and nasal endotracheal tubes predispose patients to acute otitis.[79] For an adult, an endotracheal tube of 8.0 to 8.5 mm internal diameter is appropriate for nasal or oral endotracheal intubation under most circumstances. A tube of this size is small enough to minimize laryngeal damage, yet large enough to provide minimal airway resistance at all but the highest of flow rates.[80] Either size tube allows for the performance of flexible fiberoptic bronchoscopy during mechanical ventilation, should the need arise. At present, to limit laryngeal and tracheal damage, a low pressure, high compliance cuffed tube should be used, and excessive movement of the head and tube should be avoided during the period of intubation. Naturally, the insertion of the endotracheal tube should be accomplished as atraumatically as is possible.

Conclusion

The foregoing discussion omits reference to certain specialized or infrequently occurring postoperative pulmonary complications. Complications of pulmonary resection, pneumothorax, bronchospasm, pulmonary embolism, and a more extensive approach to the diagnosis of precipitants of respiratory failure were omitted for sake of conciseness. Those items selected for discussion were addressed because of their frequency of occurrence. While many patients will pursue courses uncomplicated by pulmonary impairment, the opportunity for mischance is ever present. Vigilance and intelligence are essential in the attempt to prevent those untoward events that are preventable and to minimize the consequences of those that, nonetheless, arise.

References

1. Rehderk K, Sessler AD, Marsh HM: General anesthesia and the lung. *Am Rev Respir Dis* 112:541, 1975.
2. DeVillota ED, Avello F, Granados MA, Arccas M, Mates B: Early postsurgical bacterial contamination of the airways: A study on twenty-eight open heart patients. *Acta Anaesth Scand* 22:227, 1978.
3. Redman LR, Lockey E: Colonization of the upper respiratory tract with gram negative bacilli after operation, endotracheal intubation, and prophylactic antibiotic therapy. *Anaesthesia* 22:220, 1967.
4. Pecora DV: Progressive changes in ventilation following bilateral pulmonary resection. *Surg Gynecol Obstet* 109:89, 1959.
5. Pecora DV: Predictability of effects of abdominal and thoracic surgery upon pulmonary function. *Ann Surg* 170:101, 1969.
6. Johnson WC: Postoperative ventilatory performance: Dependence upon surgical incision. *Am Surg* 41:615, 1975.
7. Ali J, Weisel RD, Layug AB, et al.: Consequences of postoperative alterations in respiratory mechanics. *Am J Surg* 128:376, 1974.
8. Latimer RG, Dickman M, Day WC, et al.: Ventilatory patterns and pulmonary complications after upper abdominal surgery determined by preoperative and postoperative computerized spirometry and blood gas analysis. *Am J Surg* 122:622, 1971.
9. Wolfe JE, Bone RC, Ruth WE: Diagnosis of gastric aspiration by fiberoptic bronchoscopy. *Chest* 70:458, 1970.
10. Bynum LJ, Pierce AK: Pulmonary aspiration of gastric contents. *Am Rev Respir Dis* 114:1129, 1976.
11. Tomlin PJ, Howarth FH, Robinson JS: Postoperative atelectasis and laryngeal incompetence. *Lancet* 1:1402, 1968.
12. Wynne JW, Modell JH: Respiratory aspiration of gastric contents. *Ann Intern Med* 87:466, 1977.
13. Bartlett JG: Aspiration pneumonia. *Clin Notes Respir Dis* 18:3, 1980.
14. Vilinskas J, Schweizer RT, Foster JH: Experimental studies on aspiration of contents of obstructed intestine. *Surg Gynecol Obstet* 135:568, 1972.
15. Frumin MJ, Bergman NA, Holaday DA, et al.: Alveolar-arterial O_2 differences during artificial respiration in man. *J Appl Physiol* 14:694, 1959.
16. Marshall BE, Wyche MQ Jr.: Hypoxemia during and after anesthesia. *Anesthesiology* 37:178, 1972.
17. Mead J, Collier C: Relation of volume history of lungs to respiratory mechanics in anesthetized dogs. *J Appl Physiol* 14:669, 1959.
18. Bendixen HH, Hedley-Whyte J, Laver MB: Impaired oxygenation in surgical patients during general anesthesia with controlled ventilation. *N Engl J Med* 269:991, 1963.
19. Marshall BE, Millar RA: Some factors influencing postoperative hypoxemia. *Anaesthesia* 20:408, 1965.

20. Boutros AR, Weisel M: Comparison of effects of three anesthetic techniques on patients with severe pulmonary obstructive disease. *Can Anaesth Soc J* 18:286, 1971.

21. Alexander JL, Spence AA, Parikh RK, Stuart B: The role of airway closure in postoperative hypoxemia. *Brit J Anaesth* 45:34, 1973.

22. Vaughan RW, Bauer S, Wise L: Effect of position (semirecumbent versus supine) or postoperative oxygenation in markedly obese subjects. *Anesth Analg* (Cleve) 55:37, 1976.

23. Drummond GB: Postoperative hypoxemia and oxygen therapy. *Brit J Anaesth* 47:491, 1975.

24. Davis AG, Spence AA: Postoperative hypoxemic and age. *Anesthesiology* 37:663, 1972.

25. Templeton AW, Almond CH, Seaber A, et al.: Postoperative pulmonary patients following cardiopulmonary bypass. *Am J Roentgenol Rad Therapy Nuclear Med* 96:1001, 1966.

26. Bryant LR, Trinkle JK, Wood RE: A technique for intercostal nerve block after thoracotomy. *Ann Thorac Surg* 11:388, 1971.

27. Utting JE, Smith JM: Postoperative analgesia. *Anaesthesia* 34:320, 1979.

28. Bartlett RH, Gazzaniga AB, Geraghty TR: Respiratory maneuvers to prevent postoperative pulmonary complications. A critical review. *JAMA* 224:1017, 1973.

29. Iverson LIG, Ecker RR, Fox HE, May IA: A comparative study of IPPB, the incentive spirometer, and blow bottles: The prevention of atelectasis following cardiac surgery. *Ann Thorac Surg* 25:197, 1978.

30. Lederer DH, Van de Water JM, Indech RB: Which deep breathing device should the postoperative patient use? *Chest* 77:610, 1980.

31. Bartlett RH, Brennan ML, Guzzaniga AB, Hanson EL: Studies on the pathogenesis and prevention of postoperative pulmonary complications. *Surg Gynecol Obstet* 137:925, 1973.

32. Craven JL, Evans GA, Davenport PJ, Williams RHP: The evaluation of the incentive spirometer in the management of postoperative pulmonary complications. *Br J Surg* 61:793, 1974.

33. Dohi S, Gold ML: Comparison of two methods of postoperative respiratory care. *Chest* 73:592, 1978.

34. McConnell DH, Maloney JV Jr, Buckberg GD: Postoperative intermittent positive-pressure breathing treatments: Physiological considerations. *J Thorac Cardiovasc Surg* 68:944, 1974.

35. Respiratory Care Committee of the American Thoracic Society. Intermittent positive pressure breathing (IPPB). *Clin Notes Respir Dis* 18:3, 1979.

36. Jones FL Jr: Increasing postoperative ventilation: A comparison of five methods. *Anesthesiology* 29:1212, 1968.

37. Bynum LJ, Wilson JE III, Pierce AK: Comparison of spontaneous and positive-pressure breathing in supine normal subjects. *J Appl Physiol* 41:341, 1976.

38. Wright FG Jr, Foley MF, Downs JB, Hodges MR: Hypoxemia and hypocarbia following intermittent positive pressure breathing. *Anesth Analg* (Cleve) 55:555, 1976.
39. Pfenninger J, Roth F: Intermittent positive pressure breathing (IPPB) versus incentive spirometer (IS) therapy in the postoperative period. *Intensive Care Med* 3:279, 1977.
40. Mackenzie CF, Shin B, McAslan TC: Chest physiotherapy: The effect on arterial oxygenation. *Anesth Analg* (Cleve) 57:28, 1978.
41. Marini JJ, Pierson DJ, Hudson LD: Acute lobar atelectasis: A prospective comparison of fiberoptic bronchoscopy and respiratory therapy. *Am Rev Respir Dis* 119:971, 1979.
42. Byrd RB, Burns JR: Cough dynamics in the post-thoracotomy state. *Chest* 67:654, 1975.
43. Harken AH: A routine for safe effective endotracheal suctioning. *Am Surg* 41:398, 1975.
44. Petersen GM, Pierson DJ, Hunter PM: Arterial oxygen saturation during nasotracheal suctioning. *Chest* 76:283, 1979.
45. Sykes MK, McNicol MW, Campbell EJM: Respiratory Failure. Oxford: Blackwell Scientific Publications, 1976.
46. Sizer JS, Frederick PL, Osborne MP: The prevention of postoperative pulmonary complications by percutaneous endotracheal catheterization. *Surg Gynecol Obstet* 123:336, 1966.
47. Laszlo G, Archer GG, Darrell JH, et al.: The diagnosis and prophylaxis of pulmonary complications of surgical operation. *Br J Surg* 60:129, 1973.
48. Eickhoff TC: Pulmonary infections in surgical patients. *Surg Clin N Amer* 60:175, 1980.
49. Gross PA, Neu HC, Aswapokee P, Van Antwerpen C, Aswapokee N: Deaths from nosocomial infections: Experience in a university hospital and a community hospital. *Am J Med* 68:219, 1980.
50. Stevens RM, Teres D, Skillman JJ, Feingold DS: Pneumonia in an intensive care unit. A 30-month experience. *Arch Intern Med* 134:106, 1974.
51. Bartlett JG, Gorbach SL, Finegold SM: The bacteriology of aspiration pneumonia. *Am J Med* 56:202, 1974.
52. Lorber B, Swenson RM: Bacteriology of aspiration pneumonia. A prospective study of community and hospital acquired cases. *Ann Intern Med* 81:329, 1974.
53. Huxley EJ, Viroslav J, Gray WR, Pierce AK: Pharyngeal aspiration in normal adults and patients with depressed consciousness. *Am J Med* 64:564, 1978.
54. Spray SB, Zuidema GD, Cameron JL: Aspiration pneumonia; incidence of aspiration with endotracheal tubes. *Am J Surg* 131:701, 1976.
55. Cameron JL, Reynolds J, Zuidema GD: Aspiration in patients with tracheostomies. *Surg Gynecol Obstet* 136:68, 1973.
56. Lansing AM, Jamieson WG: Mechanisms of fever in pulmonary atelectasis. *Arch Surg* 87:168, 1963.

57. Shields RT, Jr.: Pathogenesis of postoperative atelectasis. An experimental study. *Arch Surg* 58:489, 1949.
58. Coryllos PN: Postoperative pulmonary complications and bronchial obstruction. Postoperative bronchitis, atelectasis (apneumatosis) and pneumonitis considered as phases of the same syndrome. *Surg Gynecol Obstet* 50:795, 1930.
59. Bryant LR, Mobin-Uddin K, Dillon ML, Griffen WO: Misdiagnosis of pneumonia in patients needing mechanical respiration. *Arch Surg* 106:286, 1973.
60. Murray HW: Antimicrobial therapy in pulmonary aspiration. *Am J Med* 66:188, 1979.
61. Murray PR, Washington JA III; Microscopic and bacteriologic analysis of expectorated sputum. *Mayo Clin Proc* 50:339, 1975.
62. Heineman ITS, Chawla JK, Lofton WM: Misinformation from sputum cultures without microscopic examination. *J Clin Microbiol* 6:518, 1977.
63. Light RW, George RB: Incidence and significance of pleural effusion after abdominal surgery. *Chest* 69:621, 1976.
64. Goodman LR: Postoperative chest radiograph: Alterations after abdominal surgery. *Am J Roentgen* 134:533, 1980.
65. Light RW, Girard WM, Jenkinson SG, George RB: Parapneumonic effusions. *Am J Med* 69:507, 1980.
66. Brechner VL: Clinical syndrome of incomplete neuromuscular block reversal: Doctor look at your patient. *Anesth Analg* (Cleve) 50:876, 1971.
67. Ali HH, Savarese JJ: Monitoring of neuromuscular function. *Anesthesiology* 45:216, 1976.
68. Stoelting RK, Proctor J: Acute laryngeal obstruction after endotracheal anesthesia. *JAMA* 206:1558, 1968.
69. Rex MAE: A review of the structural and functional basis of laryngospasm and a discussion of the nerve pathways involved in the reflex and its clinical significance in man and animals. *Br J Anaesth* 42:891, 1970.
70. Johnstone RE, Brooks SM: Upper airway obstruction after extubation. *JAMA* 218:92, 1971.
71. Bone RC, Pierce AK, Johnson RL Jr: Controlled oxygen administration in acute respiratory failure in chronic obstructive pulmonary disease. A re-appraisal. *Am J Med* 65:896, 1978.
72. Pontoppidan H, Geffin B, Lowenstein E: Acute respiratory failure in the adult. *N Engl J Med* 287:690, 743, 799, 1972.
73. Salem MR, Mathrubhutham M, Bennett EJ: Difficult intubation. *N Engl J Med* 295:879, 1976.
74. Watson CB, Prough DS, Balestrieri FJ: Bronchoscopic tube change in critically ill patients (Abstract). *Crit Care Med* 8:246, 1980.
75. Conrardy PA, Goodman LR, Lainge F, Singer MM: Alteration of endotracheal tube position. Flexion and extension of the neck. *Crit Care Med* 4:8, 1976.

76. Arens JF, LeJeune FE Jr, Webre DR: Maxillary sinusitis, a complication of nasotracheal intubation. *Anesthesiology* 40:415, 1974.
77. Cooper JD, Malt RA: Meteorism produced by nasotracheal intubation and ventilatory assistance. *N Engl J Med* 287:652, 1972.
78. Dubrick MN, Wright BD: Comparison of laryngeal pathology following long-term oral and nasal endotracheal intubations. *Anesth Analg* (Cleve) 57:663, 1978.
79. Stauffer JL, Olson DE, Petty TL: Complications and consequences of endotracheal intubation and tracheotomy. *Am J Med* 70:65, 1981.
80. Nunn JF: *Applied Respiratory Physiology*. London: Butterworths & Co. Ltd. p. 109, 1977.

Index

395